ANNUAL REVIEW OF GERONTOLOGY AND GERIATRICS

Volume 23, 2003

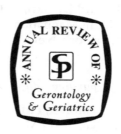

ANNUAL REVIEW of
Gerontology and Geriatrics

Volume 23, 2003

Focus On
Aging in Context: Socio-Physical Environments

Hans-Werner Wahl, PhD
Rick J. Scheidt, PhD
Paul G. Windley, PhD
Volume Editors

K. Warner Schaie, PhD
Series Editor

SPRINGER PUBLISHING COMPANY

Springer Publishing Company, Inc.
536 Broadway
New York, NY 10012-3955

Acquisitions Editor: Helvi Gold
Production Editor: Matt S. Fenton
Cover design by Joanne Honigman

04 05 06 07 08 / 5 4 3 2 1

ISBN 0-8261-1734-1
ISSN 0-198-8794

Printed in the United States by Maple Vail.

Contents

Preface

The focus of volume 23 of the *Annual Review of Gerontology and Geriatrics* is on "Aging in Context: Socio-Physical Environments." Although there were environment-related entries here and there in earlier volumes, such as the ones provided by Howell (1980), Lawton (1985), Carp (1994), and Gitlin (1998), this is the first comprehensive treatment of this scholarly area in this series. Besides its research impetus, we also believe that addressing the environment has much to do with the "good" life of aging persons (Lawton, 1983). Interestingly enough, the virulent gerontology issue of successful aging, which has found much conceptual and empirical research attention in recent time, is seldom also considered a strong *person-environment* (P-E) issue. This is particularly true when it comes to the physical-spatial environment traditionally emphasized in environmental gerontology work.

Historically, the emergence and growth of social and behavioral gerontology since the 1930s opened new gates to look at the role of environments in aging research (Wahl, 2001; Wahl & Weisman, in press). The term "context," frequently used interchangeably with the concept of environment, has meanwhile become a classic in aging research. It seems at first glance that gerontological scholars know quite well what they mean with such terms. Also, the critical role of P-E relations for the course and outcome of aging is normally taken for granted. The real struggle begins when the P-E perspective becomes subject to rigorous conceptual and empirical analysis. No one understood this better than M. Powell Lawton as reflected in his early writings on environmental issues (Lawton & Nahemow, 1973; Lawton & Simon, 1968). It was again Powell Lawton, together with Pat Parmelee, who raised concerns, in their contribution to the third edition of the *Handbook of the Psychology of Aging*, about the developmental dynamic and potential of environmental gerontology at the end of the 1980s. Parmelee and Lawton (1990) strongly advised us that there is a need "to move the field beyond its current languishing state" (p. 483). What is the current state-of-the-art in the field?

Tragic events sometimes come with hopeful new developments. Seen from this perspective, it is good to realize that the death of Powell Lawton in January 2001 has stimulated a series of activities, articles, and books aimed to further essential environmental gerontology issues in their broadest understanding. Illustratively, we would like to mention a recently published special issue of the *Journal of Housing for the Elderly* entitled "Physical Environments and Aging: Critical Contributions of M. Powell Lawton to Theory and Practice," which has been guest-edited by Rick Scheidt and Paul Windley (2003). There is also a recently published book, entitled *Aging Independently: Living Arrangements and Mobility* (Schaie, Wahl, Mollenkopf, & Oswald, 2003), containing many referrals to Powell Lawton's work (specifically in a chapter written by Laura Gitlin), as well as a forthcoming issue of *The Gerontologist* dealing with environmental issues, specifically with Powell Lawton's contributions to the field (with papers from Wahl & Weisman, Gitlin, Golant, and Kendig). The present volume of the *Annual Review of Gerontology and Geriatrics* acknowledges further the legacy of Powell Lawton. At the same time, the volume looks ahead to the serious challenges posed for theory, empirical research, and practice in gerontology.

We propose within this volume that current and future progress in environment-aging relations requires bridge building on two levels. First, there still is a need to build new bridges between different scholarly areas dealing with contextual aging within environmental gerontology. The classic issue that a major part of environmental research tends to focus on objective physical environments, whereas other studies predominantly address subjective P-E components, is illustrative in this regard. Second, and in our view equally important, is the search for new bridges between environmental gerontology and other areas of aging research dealing with environments. A good example for this is work addressing social environments without acknowledging at the same time that social relations are always framed within physical-spatial arrangements.

Thus, the major goal with this compilation of chapters is to provide and stimulate such multidirectional bridge building based on a purposefully selected set of authors from both within and outside of environmental gerontology. Such a task only naturally deserves intensive and explicit consideration of what Powell Lawton has contributed to the field. Hence, it is good to see that many of the authors take advantage of Powell Lawton's theoretical and empirical work in environmental gerontology. Also, it is quite clear that the consideration of environmental issues should focus on micro to macro levels as well as acknowledge "old" (such as traditional housing) and "new" (such as technology) environments. Taken as a whole, it is our hope that synergies between the different approaches, contents, and levels of analysis addressed in this volume will move the field beyond its languishing tendencies as requested by Parmelee and Lawton (1990).

The contributions to the volume proceed as follows: In Chapter 1, Wahl and Lang argue that there still is a widely unmet need to link the physical and social research world in aging much more strongly. A new concept entitled *Physical and Social Places Over Time* (SPOT) is suggested with the goal to connect available theories in environmental gerontology and social relations research in an adult lifespan developmental model. Scheidt and Norris-Baker provide, in Chapter 2, an in-depth analysis of the General Ecological Model proposed by Lawton and Nahemow (1973) 30 years ago. After reviewing and interpreting major transitions of the model since its introduction, suggestions in terms of enriching the model with a time dimension and making use of recent work in other fields of aging research such as the selective optimization with compensation approach are considered. Rubinstein and de Medeiros also rely heavily, in Chapter 3, on the Press-Competence model of Powell Lawton. In particular, searching for the self in environmental theorizing is disappointing according to these authors, but clearly needed to better understand meaning structure in P-E dynamics as people age.

In a complementary contrast to this, in Chapter 4, Iwarsson explores fit or misfit between aging persons and their environments based on an as objective as-possible assessment of both person competencies as well as home environments. The empirical pathway taken in this work adds substantially to a common complaint in the field, namely that environmental methods are diverse and mostly questionable with respect to validity and reliability.

Longino contributes, in Chapter 5, to environmental analysis by focusing on another major facet of the dynamics of P-E dynamics in the later years, namely migration. Descriptions of migration patterns within the U.S. are framed within a conceptual analysis of migration motives on the one hand and the consideration of different levels of impact on the other. A cohort perspective adds to a discussion of expectable migration changes of forthcoming older adults. A fruitful area of recent gerontology research normally not considered as a classic environmental gerontology theme is everyday competence. Diehl and Willis show, nevertheless, in Chapter 6, quite clearly that attention must be given to the person as well as his or her social and physical environment in order to understand the maintenance and loss of everyday competence across the adult lifespan.

Rowles, Oswald, and Hunter invite us, in Chapter 7, to consider the full scope of the experience of residential "inside" environments and "being in place" in old age. The argument that quality of life in the later years is, to a large degree, echoed in "negotiations" between the aging person, his or her maintained and lost capabilities, and interior environments is developed by touching upon houses, apartments, mobile homes, long-term care facilities, and other permanent living quarters.

Pinquart and Burmedi provide, in Chapter 8, the first meta-analysis (to our knowledge) of available findings targeting residential satisfaction in the adult life span as well as its correlates. Among their major results is a substantial positive association of age with housing and neighborhood satisfaction. The research of neighborhoods, in more general terms, is reviewed by Krause, in Chapter 9. The chapter detects a number of pitfalls in defining and measuring neighborhoods, which have major impact on interpreting potential empirical links between neighborhoods and aging persons' health and well-being.

Mollenkopf and Fozard address, in Chapter 10, a new gerontology field that has traditionally been subsumed under headings such as human factors research and which now is frequently labeled as gerontechnology. This analysis supports the view that "new" environments echoed in information and communication technology are a substantially growing research area, where the findings reveal many positive as well as negative implications of technology for older persons' quality of life. Golant envisages, in Chapter 11, still another level of environmental analysis by investigating the urban-rural distinction in light of a large body of work published since 1990 concerned with this classic environmental gerontology theme. Similar to the neighborhood concept, Golant raises conceptual and methodology concerns in this area still rarely considered when respective findings are reported in the literature. Fry, in Chapter 12, widens the scope of reflections on P-E dynamics in old age with her analysis of kinship and supportive environments of aging seen from a cross-cultural and anthropological point of view. Such a view underscores the relativity inherent in much social and physical environmental research in gerontology typically referring to Western cultures.

In Chapter 13, Windley and Weisman address classic challenges involved in the application of environmental gerontology research findings. Their analysis shows that major gaps between research and practice still exist; paths to shorten these gaps are discussed based on a revised action research paradigm.

Some readers may be disappointed that the issue of dementia has not found explicit consideration in this volume. We agree that P-E analyses of Alzheimer's disease and related cognitive disorders are important in terms of research and application. However, this topic has already received broad attention in excellent books, book chapters, review articles, and special issues (e.g., Day, Carreon, & Stump, 2000; Lawton, 2001; Weisman, 1997; Zarit & Pearlin, 2001; Zeisel, 1999). We therefore decided not to replicate what already has been said in quite a body of recent work.

Although the legacy of Powell Lawton has been acknowledged in an earlier volume of the *Annual Review of Gerontology and Geriatrics* (see Volume 21, 2001), we felt that addressing environmental issues in this series, for which he served as chief editor since 1989, comes simply with the duty to dedicate this volume to this giant in gerontology.

Finally, we would like to thank the editor-in-chief of the *Annual Review of Gerontology and Geriatrics*, K. Warner Schaie, PhD, for providing us with this opportunity to treat environmental gerontology issues in this series in such a comprehensive manner. In addition, we thank the authors of this volume for their outstanding contributions. We would also like to acknowledge the invaluable support of Ursula König in editorial assistance and the processing of papers, and we very much appreciate Springer Publishing Company and its excellent staff for supporting the publication of this volume in a most efficient way.

Hans-Werner Wahl, PhD
Rick J. Scheidt, PhD
Paul G. Windley, PhD

REFERENCES

Carp, F. M. (1994). Assessing the environment. In M. P. Lawton & J. A. Teresi (Eds.), *Annual review of gerontology and geriatrics* (Vol. 14, pp. 302-323). New York: Springer.

Day, K., Carreon, D., & Stump, C. (2000). The therapeutic design of environments for people with dementia: A review of the empirical research. *The Gerontologist, 40,* 397-416.

Gitlin, L. N. (1998). Testing home modification interventions: Issues of theory, measurement, design, and implementation. In R. Schulz, G. Maddox, & M. P. Lawton (Eds.), *Annual review of gerontology and geriatrics,* (Vol. 18, pp. 190-246). New York: Springer.

Howell, S. C. (1980). Environment and aging. In C. Eisdorfer (Ed.), *Annual review of gerontology and geriatrics* (Vol. 1, pp. 237-260). New York: Springer.

Lawton, M. P. (1983). Environment and other determinants of well-being in older people. *The Gerontologist, 23,* 349-357.

Lawton, M. P. (1985). Activities and leisure. In C. Eisdorfer, M. P. Lawton, & G. L. Maddox (Hrsg.), *Annual review of gerontology and geriatrics* (Vol. 5, pp. 127-165). New York: Springer.

Lawton, M. P. (2001). The physical environment of the person with Alzheimer's disease. *Aging & Mental Health, 5* (Suppl. 1), S56-S64.

Lawton, M. P., & Nahemow, L. (1973). Ecology and the aging process. In C. Eisdorfer & M. P. Lawton (Eds.), *The psychology of adult development and aging* (pp. 619-674). Washington, DC: American Psychological Association.

Lawton, M. P., & Simon, B. B. (1968). The ecology of social relationships in housing for the elderly. *The Gerontologist, 8,* 108-115.

Parmelee, P. A., & Lawton, M. P. (1990). The design of special environment for the aged. In J. E. Birren & K. W. Schaie (Eds.), *Handbook of the psychology of aging* (3rd ed., pp. 465-489). New York: Academic Press.

Schaie, K. W., Wahl, H.-W., Mollenkopf, H., & Oswald, F. (Eds.). (2003). *Aging independently: Living arrangements and mobility*. New York: Springer.

Scheidt, R. J., & Windley, P. G. (2003). Physical environments and aging: Critical contributions of M. Powell Lawton to theory and practice. *Journal of Housing for the Elderly, 17* (1/2).

Wahl, H. W. (2001). Environmental influences on aging and behavior. In J. E. Birren & K. W. Schaie (Eds.), *Handbook of the psychology of aging* (5th ed., pp. 215-237). San Diego: Academic Press.

Wahl, H. W., & Weisman, J. (in press). Environmental gerontology at the beginning of the new millennium: Reflections on its historical, empirical, and theoretical development. *The Gerontologist*.

Weisman, G. D. (1997). Environments for older persons with cognitive impairments. In G. Moore & R. Marans (Eds.), *Environment, behavior and design* (Vol. 4, pp. 315-346). New York: Plenum Press.

Zarit, S. H., & Pearlin, L. I. (2001). The contextual world of the person with Alzheimer's disease: Social and behavioral perspectives. *Aging & Mental Health, 5* (Suppl. 1).

Contributors

David Burmedi, PhD
German Center for Research on
   Aging at the University of
   Heidelberg
Heidelberg, Germany

Manfred Diehl, PhD
Institute on Aging
University of Florida
Gainesville, Florida

James L. Fozard, PhD
Florida Gerontological Research
   and Training Services
Palm Harbor, Florida

Christine L. Fry, PhD
Department of Sociology/
   Anthropology
Loyola University of Chicago
Chicago, Illinois

Stephen M. Golant, PhD
Department of Geography
University of Florida
Gainesville, Florida

Elizabeth G. Hunter, MS, OTR/L
Gheens Fellow
PhD Program in Gerontology
University of Kentucky
Lexington, Kentucky

Susanne Iwarsson, PhD, OTR
Division of Occupational Therapy
Lund University
Lund, Sweden

Neal Krause, PhD
School of Public Health II
University of Michigan
Ann Arbor, Michigan

Frieder R. Lang, PhD
Martin-Luther University
Halle-Wittenberg, Germany

Charles F. Longino, PhD
Department of Sociology
Wake Forest University
Winston-Salem, North Carolina

Kate de Medeiros, MA
Doctoral Program in Gerontology
UMBC: University of Maryland
   Baltimore County
Baltimore, Maryland

Heidrun Mollenkopf, PhD
German Center for Research on
   Aging at the University of
   Heidelberg
Heidelberg, Germany

Carolyn Norris-Baker, PhD
School of Family Studies and
    Human Services
Kansas State University
Manhattan, Kansas

Frank Oswald, PhD
German Center for Research on
    Aging at the University of
    Heidelberg
Heidelberg, Germany

Martin Pinquart, Dr. habil
Department of Developmental
    Psychology
Friedrich Schiller University
Jena, Germany

Graham D. Rowles, PhD
Professor of Geography,
    Behavioral Science and
    Nursing
Director, PhD Program in
    Gerontology
Associate Director Sanders-
    Brown Center on Aging
University of Kentucky
Lexington, Kentucky

Robert L. Rubenstein, PhD
Department of Sociology and
    Anthropology
University of Maryland
Baltimore, Maryland

Rick Scheidt, PhD
School of Family Studies and
    Human Services
Kansas State University
Manhattan, Kansas

Hans-Werner Wahl, PhD
German Center for Research on
    Aging at the University of
    Heidelberg
Heidelberg, Germany

Gerald R. Weisman, PhD
School of Architecture and
    Urban Planning
University of Wisconsin
Milwaukee, Wisconsin

Sherry L. Willis, PhD
The Pennsylvania State University

Paul Windley, PhD
College of Art and Architecture
University of Idaho
Moscow, Idaho

Forthcoming

ANNUAL REVIEW OF GERIATRICS AND GERONTOLOGY

Volume 24: The Life Course of Intergenerational Relations in Families as They Age

Editors: Merril Silverstein, Roseann Giarrusso, and Vern L. Bengtson

Contents

Section II. Intergenerational Relations Across Place

Intergenerational Relations in African-American Families:
Inner City vs. Rural Contexts
LINDA BURTON

Transmigration From India to the U.K. and the Maintenance of
Intergenerational Relationships
VANESSA BURHOLT AND G. CLARE WENGER

The Role of Social Context in Shaping Intergenerational Relations
in Indonesia and Bangladesh
ELIZABETH FRANKENBURG AND RANDALL KUHN

Intergenerational Norms and Support Across Five
European Nations
ARIELA LOWENSTEIN, RUTH KATZ, AND SVEIN OLAV DAATLAND

Intergenerational Exchange in the U.S. and Japan
TONI ANTONUCCI AND HIROKO AKIYAMA

Intergenerational Family Cohesion in the U.S. and China
JOHN LOGAN

Previous volumes include:

Volume 22: Focus on Economic Outcomes in Later Life
Editors: Stephen Crystal, PhD, and Dennis Shea, PhD

Volume 21: Focus on Modern Topics in the Biology of Aging
Editors: Vincent J. Cristofalo, PhD, and Richard Adelman, PhD

Volume 20: Focus on the End of Life: Scientific and Social Issues
Editor: M. Powell Lawton, PhD

Volume 19: Focus on Psychopharmacologic Interventions in Late Life
Editors: Ira Katz, MD, PhD, and David Oslin, MD

Volume 18: Focus on Interventions Research With Older Adults
Editors: Richard Schulz, PhD, George Maddox, PhD, and
M. Powell Lawton, PhD

Volume 17: Focus on Emotion and Adult Development
Editors: K. Warner Schaie, PhD, and M. Powell Lawton, PhD

CHAPTER 1

Aging in Context Across the Adult Life Course: Integrating Physical and Social Environmental Research Perspectives

HANS-WERNER WAHL
GERMAN CENTER FOR RESEARCH ON AGING AT THE UNIVERSITY OF HEIDELBERG

FRIEDER R. LANG
MARTIN-LUTHER UNIVERSITY HALLE-WITTENBERG, GERMANY

A ging occurs in context. Addressing the role of context for the course and direction of aging processes has become an essential element of lifecourse or lifespan perspectives in social and behavioral gerontology over the past five decades of research (e.g., P. B. Baltes, 1987; Carp, 1967; Dannefer, 1992; Kleemeier, 1959; Lawton, 1976, 1985; Rebok & Hoyer, 1977). When the process and outcome of aging is the target of analysis, such reference to resources (or constraints) in the person and her or his environment has even reached the status of a research paradigm in social and behavioral gerontology. However, it often remains unspoken what constitutes the context. One might even call it a "writing habit" to imply both social and physical environmental characteristics when addressing the context of aging. Furthermore, the "language game" (to use Wittgenstein's term) of referring to both the social and the physical context in order to describe and explain aging is very common in gerontology and lifespan literature. Normally, what is meant when scholars use such a language game is taken for granted. However, writing habits and the playing out of language games tend, over time, to pretend the existence of a proven knowledge, which no longer appears to deserve exact spelling out.

This chapter starts with the assumption that the rationale behind referring simultaneously to the social and physical environment still is in need of such spelling out. Perhaps there were even good reasons why this was

not so explicitly attempted before. Over the past decades, the aging literature has gone through a phase of flourishing of theoretical perspectives in
the realms of physical environments and of social environments (e.g.,
Lang, 2001, 2003; Wahl, 2001a, 2001b). Specific phenomenon in both areas
were explored and investigated by different researchers resulting in new
theoretical and empirical insights on the aging process. It appears that the
bodies of knowledge related to the physical context and to the social context of aging have grown apart and independent of each other.

The main purpose of the present work, combining the work of a physical environment and ecological researcher (HWW) with the work of a
social environment and social relations researcher (FRL), is to provide a
line of arguments in order to support the notion that this separation is
unjustified from a principal epistemology as well as an empirical aging
perspective. In fact, when ignoring either the physical or the social components in the context of aging, a wrong understanding of the fundamental processes of aging may be the consequence. Knowing about the
geographical, technical, and physical features together with their social-
relational implications, as well as knowing about the social contexts within
the opportunities and constraints of the physical world, are both needed
to develop an understanding of how aging is associated with contextual
processes. Also, we argue that the spelling out of links between the social
and physical environment in terms of theory and empirical work stimulates new and promising research avenues that have mostly been neglected
in recent time due to the schism of the physical and the social exerted in
the day-to-day research practice.

To be clear, we are not the first arguing in this direction in gerontology
or in lifespan developmental science. For example, one of the most outstanding protagonists of environmental gerontology, M. Powell Lawton,
has emphasized in his conceptual writings from the beginning the need to
address both the physical and the social environment (1982, 1999). In similar ways, Margret M. Baltes, in pointing to the critical role that the social
environment of elders can play as a dependency-provoking agency,
strongly emphasized the socio-physical setting (e.g., nursing homes versus private households), in which such person-to-environment interactions take place and exert impact on social interaction patterns (M. Baltes,
1996). Also, Leopold Rosenmayr, one of the pioneers of social gerontology
in German-speaking countries, advanced the concept of "intimacy at a distance" during the 1960s (Intimität auf Abstand). This acknowledges one
critical aspect of bonding between aged parents and their children, namely
that physical and spatial separation is an important prerequisite for the
preservation of emotional closeness (Rosenmayr & Köckeis, 1965; Tartler,
1961). Not much effort has been invested, however, in providing conceptual tools to better integrate the social and physical context of aging in
these writings and the other major works of gerontology to be discussed.

Thus, our major goal in this chapter is to prepare the ground for new pathways to better integrate the social and the physical environment.

NEED FOR LINKING THE PHYSICAL WITH THE SOCIAL ENVIRONMENT IN AGING: SUBSTANTIAL ARGUMENTS BUT LACK OF RESEARCH ATTENTION

Why is better integration of the social environment and the physical environment research world critical for gerontology and for life-span developmental perspectives? In order to answer this question, our use of the concepts of social and physical environment deserves clarification. Dannefer (1992) suggested to define the term context as composed of the social environment and of the physical environment. Following Dannefer, the social environment "refers to the totality of the diverse range of phenomena, events, and forces that exist outside the developing individual" (Dannefer, 1992, p. 84) and is directly linked to other persons. This includes research issues such as social networks, social support, or the regulation of social relationships in later adulthood (e.g., Antonucci, 2001; Lang, 2001). The physical environment "refers to the totality of the diverse range of phenomena, events, and forces that exist outside the developing individual" (Dannefer, p. 84) and are directly linked to the material and spatial sphere. This covers research issues such as the impact of the physical-spatial home environment on aging, the role of neighborhoods, institutional settings, or residential decisions (e.g., Lawton, 1985; Wahl, 2001a, 2001b). Although we will concentrate our discussion of the concepts of the social and physical environment at the micro- and meso-levels of analysis, the broader sociocultural or societal context and the interaction of social and physical elements therein, reflected in concepts such as cohort differences and the historical embeddedness of development and aging, always provide a major background for these lower levels of contextual analysis (P. B. Baltes, Reese, & Lipsitt, 1980; P. B. Baltes, 1987; Hagestad & Dannefer, 2001).

It is tempting, at first glance, to accept and acknowledge the separateness of the social and physical surroundings and their different roles in aging. On a surface level, one might view the social environment as one that is apparently alive and actively shaping the aging individual, whereas the physical environment appears to be dead and a "no response context." However, as we will argue, this is wrong. The social, like the physical, world is dynamic, malleable, and responsive in the context of aging individuals. In fact, the structural similarities between the social and the physical environments, as seen from an older person's point of view, are striking. On the one hand, both the social and physical environments are major resources or constraints for the individual's action potentials and quality of life. On the other hand, individuals appear to actively regulate the quality, structure, and function of their social and physical environments and thereby enhance their social and physical resources. This includes, for example, the choices individuals make with respect to social partners, their living arrangements, and the physical adaptation of their home environments. Furthermore, and most important for social and behavioral gerontology perspectives, is that the social and physical environments contribute in a closely interwoven manner to what has been coined "person-environment fit processes" (Carp, 1987; Kahana, 1982). To support this line of thought, it has first to be acknowledged that social relations are always framed within physical-spatial conditions (e.g., social contacts within institutions are shaped by physical-spatial dimensions; see already Lawton & Simon, 1968, and their well-known Docility Hypothesis). Inversely, physical environments are not lifeless entities; they symbolize, for example, most influential social experiences of one's biography. For example, objects in the home environment may serve as powerful memories of a lost loved one (Oswald & Wahl, in press; Rubinstein, 1989). Second, the social and physical environments interact in a complex and dynamic manner with respect to the proactive striving of aging individuals toward maintaining adaptation. For example, losing one's care-providing spouse in a remote area can produce a severe person-environment misfit. The decision to relocate to an assisted living facility located in a town far away from the former place of living as a consequence of this critical event might lead to a barrier-free physical environment and new developmental opportunities in terms of social interchange with other residents. However, the compensation and optimization associated with this relocation decision may not come without losses such as interruptions of former important social and physical ties (i.e., neighbors and landscapes).

By and large, we feel that such transactional processes related to person-environment fit or misfit, which always involve the person and his or her social and physical environment, are still not well understood in the aging literature (Lang, 2001; Wahl, 2001a; Wahl & Weisman, in press). This is critical because of the fact that the fragility of the person-environment system due to health decline and loss experiences is a fundamental dynamic of the aging experience. Although anthropological, empirical, and assessment-related arguments addressing the inter-relations between the social and the physical environment are nearby, they have not been applied yet in a sustainable manner or have led only to rare research exceptions.

From a basic anthropological perspective, substantial links are already being built between the physical and social environments, and thus both entities can only quite artificially be separated. Both are strongly culturally bound concepts; we see and experience the "objective" physical world based on cultural norms, habits, and perceptual styles. The physical part of the environment is always and unavoidably "loaded" with social and cultural elements that also reflect a basic position of phenomenology

(Kruse & Graumann, 1998). Similarly, we often rely on metaphors from the physical world to describe the quality (e.g., closeness) or quantity (e.g., network) of our social relationships. "Closeness" or "distance" are terms that are both equally fundamental in the material external world and its relation to the individual. Already in 1981, Canter and Craik suggested the term "socio-physical" instead of "physical" environment when person-environment constellations are the target of analysis. Moreover, social relations as well as physical environments both have been linked with the same classes of outcomes, such as subjective well-being, preservation of the self, and a positive future perspective. Probably, many would agree that this argumentation is persuasive enough to be used to drive theoretical approaches and empirical research, but this did not frequently happen in aging research, until today.

Empirically, we can rely on a wide scope of findings supporting the view that social life and social relations are closely related across the human lifespan to physical environmental contextual conditions. For example, it is a robust and well-known finding that in later adulthood an individual's life is centered very much around the immediate home environment, in which most everyday activities take place (e.g., M. Baltes, Wahl, & Schmid-Furstoss, 1990; Moss & Lawton, 1982). This is particularly true for the oldest old, who do not spend as much time outside their homes (M. Baltes, Maas, Wilms, Borchelt, & Little, 1999). Furthermore, most social interactions appear to take place in the near surroundings of the older individual's home (e.g., Rowles, 1983) and most older people report to have at least 1 child in a 10- to 15-minutes walking distance of their home (e.g., Kohli & Künemund, 2000). Social psychological research has also shown important links between environmental features and social behavior. For example, when individual space in a group of people (e.g., the individual's household) is scarce and limited, individuals typically experience distress (e.g. Altman, 1975; Baum & Paulus, 1987). Notably, such crowding effects are moderated both through social supportive behaviors (e.g., Evans & Lepore, 1993), personality characteristics (e.g., Fleming, Baum, & Weiss, 1987) as well as through architectural interventions (e.g., Evans, Lepore, & Schroeder, 1996). It is, however, at least with respect to the aging-related findings, the case that empirically supported coincidences have not found much theoretical reflection in this research.

In terms of assessment, a first issue is that physical and social elements of the environment are typically interwoven and are inseparable phenomena on the measurement level. For example, the quality of social relationships is known to depend on geographical proximity between social partners (e.g., the classic study of Festinger, Schachter, & Back, 1950) and vice versa. Geographical distance also constitutes a challenge as well as a constraint to many social ties (e.g., Adams & Stevenson, 2003). Not many instruments are around that take this explicitly into consideration. A second and related assessment issue results from narrow foci in research on either physical or social environments in which instruments are developed that tend to ignore either the physical material or the social-emotional aspects of the environment. One consequence of such narrow assessment procedures is that environments are often artificially separated in subsets. For example, housing problems are typically investigated without addressing the extent to which strong social bonds in the neighborhood exist. Additionally, social relationships are typically measured without assessing aspects of the place where social contact actually occurs, physical structures (e.g., room structure in nursing homes), or distances impacting on social relations. With few notable exceptions (e.g., the *Multiphasic Environmental Assessment Procedure* [MEAP], suggested for use in institutional settings by Moos & Lemke, 1996), most instruments are typically biased toward an emphasis on either the social or the physical environment.

CONCLUSIONS I

It seems that anthropological links between the social and physical environment are strongly demanded, but this has seldom stimulated more specified theories and theory-driven empirical research on aging. Inversely, the basic insights of the empirical literature support that both the social and physical environment form the "context" of aging, but the relations and interfaces between these are mostly ignored as a conceptual challenge. On the operational and assessment levels, there also are more or less tacit links between the physical and the social environment, but again, not reflected much in terms of theories. That said, we proceed with an exploration of how major theories, which have explicitly addressed the social as well as the physical environment, have dealt with the need to link the social with the physical context of aging. Due to the importance of this analysis in preparing the ground for our own suggestions to better link the social and physical environments in aging research, which follows in the next step, this will be done in quite an extensive manner.

EXPLORING THE LINKS AND MISSING LINKS BETWEEN THE PHYSICAL AND SOCIAL ENVIRONMENT IN MAJOR CONTEXT-RELATED THEORETICAL APPROACHES IN AGING RESEARCH

In this section, we begin with analyzing physical-social environment links (and missing links) in classic conceptual approaches and empirical work within environmental gerontology. The same will then be done with social environment research in aging and its links (and missing links) to the physical environment.

PHYSICAL ENVIRONMENT AND THE SOCIAL SURROUNDINGS IN AGING RESEARCH

Environmental gerontology or, as it sometimes has also been labeled, the ecology of aging is typically identified with the description, explanation, and modification/optimization of the relation between the elderly person and his or her physical environment (Wahl, 2001a, 2001b). Furthermore, by drawing from Lewin's (1936) basic insight that behavior has to be seen as a function of the person and his or her environment, Lawton (1982) has suggested the ecological equation as most essential for the ecology of aging. That equation considers the impact of the interaction between the aging individual and the environment on a variety of outcomes such as emotional well-being and the possible level of everyday competence. The mission of environmental gerontology within gerontology can be seen in its contributions to the understanding of prototypical environment-related tasks of the aging individual. Such tasks include preserving an as-independent-as-possible everyday life in the face of physical and mental impairments by using environmental resources within and outside the home environment ("aging in place"), initiating processes of relocation if desired or necessary, and adapting to new living environment settings (such as a nursing home or other planned housing) after relocation. It is tempting, at first glance based on these major streams of research, to identify environmental gerontology with the consideration of the physical and spatial dimension of the environment, but the picture is more complicated.

Classic Theories of Aging Addressing the Physical Domain and the Social Environment

The most widely acknowledged theory to be considered is the Press-Competence Model introduced by Lawton and Nahemow (1973). Although this theory has undergone considerable revisions across the years (e.g., Lawton, 1985, 1989a), its use of the concept of environment has remained rather stable (Lawton, 1982, 1999). In this conception, the physical component of the environment is only one element within a model of five strata of an environment:

• The physical environment: housing characteristics, the amount of seating space, and distances

- The personal environment: the number of children and number of close friends
- The small-group environment: residents of an assisted living facility and employees of a small business
- The supra-personal environment: age mix of one's neighborhood or range of health mix in a nursing home
- The mega-social environment: legislative regulations and liberal capitalism

Lawton has envisaged with this multifaceted concept of the environment, dating from 1970 (Lawton, 1970), a research challenge still under debate in gerontology. The need to consider links between the micro-, meso-, and macro-levels of person-environment analyses and thus the demand for better integration of behavioral and social science views of aging (Bengtson, Burgess, & Parrott, 1997; Hagestad & Dannefer, 2001; Marshall, 1996). Lawton has used all of these environmental elements side by side and mostly with the intention of underlining the broadness and complexity of the role of person-environment interactions in aging, although he has acknowledged the need for "linkages across environmental classes" (1999, p. 116).

This is particularly obvious when the central part of Lawton's theory, the Press-Competence idea, is also considered (Lawton & Nahemow, 1973). As is well known, Lawton has argued that variations in adaptational outcomes in old age are, as compared to younger age groups (probably with the exception of young childhood), more strongly influenced by environmental contexts. In addition, Lawton has become, in a sense, famous for his assumption (well-known as the "Environmental Docility Hypothesis") that older adults with lower competence are particularly prone to "environmental press." It deserves particular mentioning that the Environmental Docility Hypothesis was introduced at end of the 1960s and was based on an empirical study in which social relations (friendship building) *and* physical environment characteristics (physical distance) were directly linked in a nursing home setting (Lawton & Simon, 1968). As was found, friendship building was generally connected to physical distance from one's own apartment (the closer the apartment of other residents to the target person, the higher the chance of a friendship relation), but this was especially true in those being more frail. Besides, Lawton (e.g., 1982) has considered in his conceptual scholarly work a broad variety of environmental press, including physical, social, and other environmental characteristics such as the impact of specialized housing environments on adjustment, task pace, difficulty, and complexity on learning, and of relocation on longevity. In conclusion, it is hard to find any *explicit* statement in Lawton's ecology-oriented writings that in environmental gerontology priority should be given to the physical part of the environment.

There was nevertheless always an *implicit* tendency in Lawton's theoretical writings and a quite strong tendency in the majority of his empirical work on environmental issues to put more emphasis on the physical part of the environment. Particularly in his now-classic writings in this regard published during the 1970s, the beginning conceptual efforts of defining and differentiating the physical component of his five-strata model of the environment were more frequent and persisting as compared to the social environment (e.g., Lawton, 1977, 1982, 1985; Lawton & Nahemow, 1973). Also, his empirical work was mainly concerned with housing, neighborhoods, and other infrastructure phenomena mostly framed within the physical-spatial realm and much less in social terms (Lawton, 1977), but there were also some exceptions to this (see, for example, the path analysis in Lawton, 1983). In sum, although Lawton's theoretical approach has strived for the need to simultaneously consider the whole range of contextuality of aging, he has not offered much to integrate different strata of the environment, especially linking the material and social sphere, and has clearly put (predominantly in his empirical research) more attention on the material environment.

Another family of the ecology of aging approaches relevant for the present work's discussion has centered on the concept of person-environment fit. Both Kahana's (e.g., 1982) and Carp's (e.g., 1987; see also Carp & Carp, 1984) works are closely affiliated with this concept. The core idea of the person-environment fit concept is the assumption that misfits between an older person's objective competencies or subjective needs and the potential of the environment to support/fulfill these objective and/or subjective person characteristics is detrimental to using one's full developmental potential. Inversely, person-environment fit is seen as a necessary, albeit not sufficient, precondition for such development. In terms of Kahana and colleagues' theoretical and empirical work, frequently cited as a typical environmental gerontology approach, it must be emphasized that they predominantly referred to social environmental characteristics, while physical features played only a minor role. Also, all this work was very much focused on institutional settings (e.g., Kahana, Liang, & Felton, 1980). Carp's beginning ecology scholarly work commonly is linked to her now-classic study on elders relocating to Victoria Plaza in San Antonio (Carp, 1966). Again, and similarly to the early Lawton and Simon (1968) study, this truly was research addressing the role of the physical environment (especially change of the physical environment by relocation) and concomitant consequences on the social-relations level in a balanced manner. In her later writings with still referral to the person-environment fit concept (Carp, 1987; Carp & Carp, 1984), most interesting was the introduction of higher- and lower-order needs and the capability of the environment to match these needs. Empirically, it seems, however, that the physical environment has taken over again in its priority (e.g., Carp, 1994).

In sum, while obviously quite important for integrating the physical and the social environment, the use of the concept of person-environment fit in the ecology of aging research practice has more and more developed toward addressing predominantly the physical surrounding. Thus, its potential to build links between the physical and the social environment in aging research has not been played out very much yet.

More Recent Theories of Aging in the Physical Domain: Implications for Social Relations Research

Besides classic ecology of aging approaches, the additional and parallel research streams in environmental gerontology appearing since the 1980s, subsumable under the headings of subjective aging in place and social ecology of aging, deserve an analytical glance here. In the subjective aging in place scholarly work, the simultaneous consideration of ties from aging persons to his or her physical and social environment is a major feature. Typically, this kind of approach leads to more qualitative work, such as that provided by Rowles (e.g., 1983) and Rubinstein (e.g., 1989), in which processes of "making spaces into places" (Rowles & Watkins, 2003) are described and analyzed in quite a holistic manner (Oswald & Wahl, in press; see also the work of Rowles, Oswald, & Hunter in this volume). This priority has been expressed, for example, in the now-classic book *Aging and Mileu* edited by Rowles and Ohta (1983), in which each contributor was requested to "focus on the environmental context of aging, not merely considered from a physical and architectural perspective, but rather in terms of the old person's total milieu—physical, social, cultural, clinical, phenomenological, and so on" (p. xiii). In sum, the strong connectedness of the physical and the social environment has been well preserved in such work on subjective aging in place. This has, however, the disadvantage of no longer having separate entities of the person and his or her environment, as well as a tentative neglect of the objective environment, be it physical or social. Also, such theorizing tends to limit empirical research to qualitative approaches, which is at the same time valuable but also constraining in terms of using other (more quantitative) assessment options.

This is different from social ecology of aging approaches beginning with Roger Barker's sole study explicitly involving older adults and illustrating the ecology of behaviors in two places of living (Barker & Barker, 1961). Since the mid-eighties, the dependency-related work of Margret Baltes and colleagues (e.g., M. Baltes, 1996) based on a social-operant learning theoretical conception is a good example of social ecology work referring to aging. By using observational methodology aimed to detect antecedent-consequence contingencies of older persons' behaviors with the environment, there was a clear focus on the role of the social environment. As has repeatedly been found, the social environments of older persons tend to contingently support their dependent behaviors while ignoring independent behaviors. This social interaction pattern, labeled as a "dependency-support script," was assumed to have potentially negative consequences in the longer run, such as losing competencies and becoming still more dependent on others. In addition to this social environment focus, "sociophysical" setting variations, such as different kinds of nursing homes as well as private home contexts, were considered (M. Baltes & Wahl, 1992). Nevertheless, there was a tendency in this work to downplay the physical environment on the very concrete level. For example, no study in this research stream has ever addressed the question, "Is the outcome of the dependency-support social interaction script particularly detrimental in those physical environments putting particularly strong press on the aging individual?" Finally, the work of Moos is another good example for the social ecology of aging approach. Very early in his work, Rudolf Moos began to explicitly argue for the need to simultaneously consider the physical and the social context of aging (e.g., Moos, 1976). He remained a rare exception within environmental gerontology in terms of empirically addressing the social, organizational, and the physical-spatial environment based on the MEAP (Moos & Lemke, 1996). Unfortunately, this approach has been completely tailored for use in institutional settings and thus is of limited value for considering the social and physical environment in "normal" aging settings.

Social Environments and the Physical Surroundings in Aging Research

How is the physical context acknowledged in work on the social world of older people? Gerontological research on social environments is typically seeking to identify how the qualitative as well as quantitative features of an individual's social contacts and social network contribute to the individual's functioning and life quality (Lang & Carstensen, 1998; Pinquart & Sörenson, 2000; Rook, 2000). The theoretical conceptions about the role of social environments across adulthood are manifold and range from macro-theoretical approaches such as the age stratification theory (Riley, 1985) to micro-theoretical conceptions such as social exchange theory (Bengtson, Burgess, & Parrott, 1997) and socioemotional selectivity theory (Carstensen, Isaacowitz, & Charles, 1999). Theories about the social environments in later life have typically viewed the individual as a recipient or adaptive user of social resources rather than as an active person that engages him- or herself in the construal or even the production of the social environment (Lang, 2001; Steverink, Lindenberg, & Ormel, 1998). Moreover, most theories of social aging typically do not explicitly address the role of the physical and geographical surroundings for social functioning. However, a few notable and classical exceptions exist, such as social integration theory (Rosow, 1974) and the ecological research on dependency in nursing homes mentioned in the previous section (M. Baltes, 1996). Few approaches have quite explicitly acknowledged the role of the physical environment, such as geographical factors for the emergence of age-specific social roles through geographical segregation (Rosow, 1974), or the impact of institutional settings on behavioral dependency among nursing home residents (M. Baltes, 1996). Recent lifespan approaches on the development of social relationships in later life have more explicitly addressed processes that influence and gear the individual's motivations, attitudes, and behaviors toward other people throughout the lifecourse. What these theories have in common is that they are quite implicit about the possible ways in which physical surroundings might mediate or moderate specific functions and structures of the individual's social world. Most prominently among these are the social convoy model (Antonucci, Langfahl, & Akiyama, 2003), the socioemotional selectivity theory (Carstensen et al., 1999), and resource-oriented models of social behavior (e.g., Lang, 2003). Finally, research on parent-child relationships has a long tradition in highlighting the important role of geographic distance as one factor of relationship quality (Frankel & DeWit, 1989; Rosenmayr & Köckeis, 1965; Tartler, 1961). We first analyze some of the more classical theories of social aging with respect to their acknowledgment of the role of physical surroundings. Secondly, we analyze and elaborate the socio-physical implications of more recent theories on aging in the social domain.

Some "Classic" Approaches to Aging Addressing the Social and the Physical Environment

As noted above, theoretical conceptions of the social environment in later adulthood often rely on metaphors derived from features of the physical world when referring to social experiences in later adulthood. This includes concepts such as social strata, social convoy, social network, support bank, closeness, distance, or life space as metaphoric descriptions of specific aspects of an individual's social world. Such metaphors serve to keep in mind that all social relationships occur in time as well as in space. Even the now "classic" theories of social aging such as disengagement theory and activity theory have—at least implicitly—acknowledged that aspects of the physical world are relevant for a better understanding of social functioning in later life.

For example, according to disengagement theory (Cumming & Henry, 1961), older individuals are seen as limiting their social life spaces in response to societal pressures and in order to prepare for the final phase of their lives. Cumming and Henry (1961, p. 47) explicitly referred to Lewin's

(1936) notion of a psychological life space when they introduced their concept of *Social Lifespace* as reflecting the individual's decreasing social opportunities during the aging process. Activity theory emphasized that being socially engaged in a variety of social roles both within and outside the family contributes to better functioning and better life quality (Havighurst, Neugarten, & Tobin, 1968; Lemon, Bengtson, & Peterson, 1972). Keeping a physical or geographical distance from members of younger generations is seen as protecting the older individual from stressful social demands and ensuring maximal freedom to develop age-adequate and adaptive patterns of social activity that contribute to increased well-being. Tartler (1961) introduced the idea of "feeling close at a physical distance" as one adaptive feature of parent-child relationships related to a better quality of the relationship. Empirical findings could support the notion of "intimacy at a distance" (Rosenmayr & Köckeis, 1965) as an adaptive regulatory mechanism of intergenerational relationships (Frankel & DeWit, 1989; Wagner, Schütze, & Lang, 1999). For example, in a study with 454 older parents, Frankel and DeWit (1989) found that greater geographical distance was a strong predictor of reduced contact with adult children, but was significantly less strongly associated with the experience of important conversations with children. This indicates that the parent-child tie appears to remain emotionally meaningful irrespective of the physical distance. Emotional closeness in relationships may be an important compensation mechanism for overcoming a seemingly insurmountable geographic distance. This points to a critical feature of a link between social and physical environments.

In his social integration theory, Rosow (1974) argued that a loss of social roles in later life requires that individuals develop new age-specific and age-adequate social roles. According to the theory, older people who live in age-segregated environments are more likely to identify themselves with their age group and their neighborhood. Consequently, they are more likely to engage in community activities when there is no interference with the interests of the younger generation. Empirical findings are not quite consistent, though. For example, older people living in age-segregated neighborhoods were more satisfied with their living circumstances than those who lived in nonsegregated quarters (Messer, 1967; Sherman, 1975). However, it was shown that the positive effect of age segregation is mostly related to differences in socioeconomic wealth. Vaskovics (1990) reported that in regions with a good infrastructure and a high-quality living standard, age concentration in the neighborhood was unrelated to living satisfaction. Despite the lack of empirical evidence, social integration theory has made a significant contribution in linking facets of the social and the physical environment in the aging process.

Recent theories of social aging that were proposed and advanced over the past decades, such as social convoy theory, socioemotional selectivity theory, and theories about resource-congruency, have typically focused on individuals' social behaviors and activities rather than on how these social behaviors are situated in specific physical environments. However, these theories offer some implications for the role and meaning of physical surroundings in later life, which we discuss in the following section.

Recent Theories of Aging in the Social Domain: Implications for the Ecology of Aging

One of the most prominent modern theories of social aging and the lifespan development of social relationships is the social convoy model (Antonucci, 1990; Antonucci & Akiyama, 1995; Antonucci, Langfahl, & Akiyama, 2003). According to this model an individual's social world is structured hierarchically. The metaphor of a social convoy is viewed as illustrating the lifelong dynamic of social ties over one's lifespan. As an individual grows old, her or his relationships and relationship partners change synchronously while he or she moves along the time continuum of his or her life. At times, relationships drop out of the convoy while new relationship partners join the social convoy, and some partners, who were lost at times, join the social convoy again. Furthermore, the social convoy is not only moving in time and space, there is also structural change within an individual's convoy. Sometimes individuals feel close to some relationship partners, while other network partners become less important, and vice versa. The composition and functions of social convoys change depending on an individual's age, gender, culture, and physical or emotional needs, as well as depending on the specific relationship histories. There is no doubt that the social convoy has become one of the most powerful metaphors in the field of aging by elegantly capturing many of the complex and dynamic characteristics of the life-long development of social relationships. More importantly, the social convoy model has broadened the perspective on social relationships as being both outcomes of and contexts for developmental processes (Antonucci et al., 2003; Carstensen & Lang, 1997). The importance of this notion comes into mind when considering specific environments and behavior settings, such as nursing homes (M. Baltes, 1996), quality of living standards, or public places in urban cities, provide or constrain opportunities for social contact in later life. For example, in a review of research on intergenerational contacts in urban regions, Lang (1998) suggested that distinct, age-graded zones exist for children, families, and older adults in the city that do not have much overlap due to the architecture, layout, and installation of equipment in most modern urban cities. It is an open question whether social relationships follow the constraints of the physical environment or physical environments reflect the evolution of an ontogeny of social needs and motivations over the centuries.

In her socioemotional selectivity theory, Laura Carstensen and collaborators (Carstensen et al., 1999; Carstensen & Lang, 1997; Lang & Carstensen, 2002) argued that over the course of life, individuals become increasingly aware that time is a precious resource that is limited. As a consequence, when people perceive time as limited they are more eager to make the most efficient use of their time by focusing on aspects in their present lives that promise to entail meaningful experiences. According to the theory, it is expected that such experiences be related to seeking emotional meaning rather than to seeking information. This basic tenet of socioemotional selectivity theory was empirically shown to operate across different domains of cognitive and social aging. For example, in memory tasks, the proportion of recalled emotional materials from all recalled materials was largest among older adults as compared to young adults (Carstensen & Turk-Charles, 1994; Fung & Carstensen, 2003). Adults of different ages who perceived their time as limited reported a greater priority of goals related to generativity and to control of affect than adults who perceived no time limitations in their future (Lang & Carstensen, 2002). Although never made explicit, strong implications of the theory for ecology of aging exist. Over the lifecourse, individuals become attached and identify with their immediate neighborhood and living quarters (e.g., Rubinstein & Parmelee, 1992). Emotional meaning may not only be derived from those partners to which one feels close, but also from the familiarity and security of everyday routines and living circumstances. In this case, even peripheral social contacts with people known for many years, or even decades, may provide meaningful experience to the older individual (Fingerman, 2003). Going further, it can be asked whether the adaptive processes leading to changes in social motivation are not only depending on perceived time limitations, but also the individual's personal or environmental resources in general. There are great individual differences with respect to what types of social situations provide meaning to an individual. Consequently, some individuals may prefer to focus on indoor activities, while others prefer social, outdoor activities, again a hint for considering social and physical environmental phenomena in a simultaneous manner.

CONCLUSIONS II

Considering links between the physical and the social environment through the perspective of environmental gerontology and theories on social aging has led us to a mixed and partly unsatisfactory picture. Lawton has begun with a very broad conception of the environment, including both physical and social elements, but the potential of this conception in a full-blown ecological equation has not been played out. Also, social relations researchers have only rarely referred to Lawton's five-strata model of the environment and thus have not reinforced its potential from this perspective. Lang's (e.g., 2001) use of Lawton's term "proactivity" (Lawton, 1985) as a pendant concept to environmental docility in order to not only address the capacity of the aging person to shape his or her physical world, but also his or her social surrounding has remained a rare exception. The person-environment fit concept, another classic in the ecology of aging literature, seems particularly prone to integrate the physical and social environment, but similarly to the Press-Competence Model this potential has not really played out until today. Furthermore, there is a tendency in environmental gerontology to consider direct links between the physical and social environments, especially in extreme conditions such as nursing home settings, which is particularly true for the work of Kahana, Moos, and, to a certain degree, the legacy of Margret Baltes. Although it is important to note that such extreme settings are heuristically fruitful for building physical-social environment ties, limitations of such analyses in terms of generalizing to "normal" aging settings are obvious. Work done in the private home context in which bridges between the physical and social have been built, such as in the more qualitative work of Rowles and Rubinstein, has the disadvantage of remaining on the subjective level of analysis while tentatively ignoring the objective component in the physical and social environment. Social relations research, as echoed in the classic work of scholars such as Cumming and Henry (1961), Rosow (1974), or the more recent work of Antonucci (2001) and Carstensen (1995), has many physical-spatial implications, but these are, similarly to ecology theories with respect to the social environment, not spelled out yet. Another conclusion valid for both environmental gerontology and social relations theories is that when different environmental components, particularly physical and social, are targeted, it is typically done solely in a side-by-side manner, that is, without much integrative effort. Recent developments, both in the field of social relations research and the "ecology of aging," open promising ways toward a more integrative framework that allows for bridging some of these gaps of research. Some major steps of such an integrative approach will be presented next.

TOWARD A THEORETICAL FRAMEWORK TO BETTER LINK THE SOCIAL AND PHYSICAL ENVIRONMENT RESEARCH WORLDS: OUTLINING SOME MAJOR STEPS

In this section our goal is to use the insights of our analyses of the scholarly ecology and social relations literature in gerontology as a launching pad to suggest some core elements of a theoretical framework aimed to better integrate the physical with the social environment in aging research.

We begin with the introduction of a new umbrella concept intended to merge the social with the physical, namely the *Social-Physical Place Over Time* (SPOT) concept. We then use this general idea as a background to address two related issues, which we regard as basics to better understand the dynamics between the social and physical environments while persons age. First, we suggest a model of adult development that simultaneously addresses the relations to the social and physical environment. Second, we refresh some person-environment-fit ideas in order to better understand ongoing dynamics between the aging persons and their social and physical environment. In sum, we thus propose a mix of developmental and ecological approaches with equal balance on the consideration and interaction of both the social and the physical environments as a promising pathway for future research.

THE CONCEPT OF SOCIAL-PHYSICAL PLACE OVER TIME (SPOT)

In order to approach our goal to better integrate the social with the physical environment in aging, we felt that a rather general umbrella concept would be a helpful conceptual tool for navigating through the complexities inherent in any attempt toward such integration, as well as to prepare for the next, more concrete, steps of analysis. The SPOT concept is meant to serve this purpose by combining three major elements of an aging person's everyday world.

First, a central element of SPOT, namely "place," is aimed to acknowledge that every aging person's day-to-day behavior is embedded within given physical and spatial surroundings. These surroundings are meaningful only for this aging person in a variety of regards, such as long-term living at this location, long-term place attachments, ties to neighborhoods, the specifics of the physical layout of this location, and its nearer and farther surroundings in the community (Oswald & Wahl, in press). With the concept of "place," we refer to gerontology scholars such as Rowles and Watkins (2003) or Weisman, Chaudhury, and Diaz Moore (2000), but obviously also to classic environmental psychology work in more general terms (e.g., Proshansky, Fabian, & Kaminoff, 1983). It has become clear in this work that places necessarily combine both a physical-spatial as well as a social-cultural dimension.

Second, and as a consequence of our first point, we should always think of places as socially constructed, socially filled out, and socially shaped physical environments. The term "Social-Physical Place" explicitly underscores our focus on specific living places of individuals.

Third, the SPOT concept implies a developmental perspective when highlighting that places are dynamic and show both change and stability over time, as people age. Our central assumption is that "negotiating" SPOT reveals quite different dynamics across the adult lifespan that are highly relevant for the course and outcomes of aging. We will address this in the next section.

A MODEL OF THE DEVELOPMENT OF RELATIONS TO THE SOCIAL AND PHYSICAL ENVIRONMENT

Lang (2003) proposed a goal-resource-congruence model of the proactive regulation of social relationships across the lifespan. According to this model, resource changes determine changes in an individual's social motivation over the course of one's life depending on age-specific opportunity structures. The model contends that an individual's proactive regulation of social relationships consists of two basic motivations. First, one aims at maximizing a sense of belonging in one's social relationships. Second, one aims at maximizing a sense of social efficacy in social contexts. While the first type of striving to belonging may be attained through both primary control (i.e., changing the partner) and secondary control (i.e., changing oneself; see Heckhausen & Schulz, 1995, for this distinction in terms of control strategies), striving for social efficacy exclusively reflects facets of primary control strategies. Thus, the regulation of social relationships over a lifespan is expected to follow patterns of control processes as described in the lifespan theory of control (Heckhausen & Schulz, 1995). As people experience resource loss, seeking to belong to one's social world (e.g., helping other people or experiencing positive social contact) is expected to obtain greater priority, whereas individuals prioritize social efficacy goals such as autonomy or social acceptance when many resources are available. This conceptual model is consistent with recent empirical findings on age differences in social functioning (Lang, 2001; Lang & Carstensen, 2002; Lang, Rieckmann, & Baltes, 2002).

The goal-resource congruence model also applies to the regulation of physical environments that entail both meanings of belonging (e.g., familiarity of home environment) and socio-physical agency (e.g. autonomy, keeping routines, and approaching residential decisions). For example, it is a well known fact that frail older people are often reluctant to leave their community dwellings, even when it is difficult for them to manage household chores, mostly because their familiar home environment provides a strong sense of meaning and belonging for them. Losing personal resources in later life is a threatening event. Declines in physical health may lead to a heightened importance of experiencing continuity and belonging in one's immediate environment. These considerations are also consistent with socioemotional selectivity theory (Carstensen et al., 1999), which posits that as individuals perceive their future time as being limited, they are more likely to seek stimulation of positive emotions (e.g., Mather & Carstensen, in press) and positive memories (Carstensen & Turk-Charles, 1994).

As a consequence, we argue, in terms of a major integrative step of combining both a social and physical environmental perspective, that a similar adaptive dynamic, which is mainly driven by the co-occurence of decreasing competence (i.e., a lowered action potential of the individual) and the perception that future time becomes more and more limited (Table 1.1), is at work in both environmental realms from middle adulthood through early age/young old to the oldest old. A consequence is that individuals seek and benefit from an increased sense of belonging in their respective social-physical environments. This combined dynamism lies at the heart of understanding SPOT processes in development during adulthood and aging. In addition, the argument is that such a combined view provides both theoretically and empirically a stronger avenue than solely approaching aging in the context of social relations or relations with the physical environment. In particular, it means that simultaneously considering both the social and the physical environment as major resources of the aging individual adds to a more comprehensive and integrative understanding of the potential of these resources in aging in objective and subjective terms. Such thinking already has a long tradition in the developmental sciences. For example, Youniss (1980), in his classic works on social development in childhood and adolescence, coined the concept of "co-construction" in order to acknowledge that individuals share their personal control over environments with others. Objectively, the acknowledgment of the social and the physical surrounding is more comprehensive because both add at the same time to adaptive processes. Focusing on only one of these segments is too limited a view. Subjectively, aging individuals normally act within a perceived entity of environments in which both social partners and physical-spatial aspects are subjectively constructed and integrated in an ongoing, complex, and mostly inseparable manner. We regard both the objective and the subjective construction components as important elements of doing research based on the SPOT approach.

TABLE 1.1   Subjective Relevance of Socio-Physical Agency and Belonging over Adulthood and Old Age

Stage of Aging	Relevance of Social-Physical Agency	Relevance of Social-Physical Belonging
Middle Adulthood	+++	+
Early Age/"Young old"	++	++
"Old-Old"/Oldest Old	+	+++

A classic example to illustrate this SPOT dynamics is provided by relocation research, because relocation probably is the most radical process in which the physical and frequently major elements of the social environments are changed at the same time. Having lived in a specific place implies an enormous amount of implicit knowledge related to everyday routines, geographical distances inside and outside the home, distinguishing neighbors from strangers, seasonal changes of the sunlight, and community services. Seeking to enhance one's sense of belonging refers to the meaning and memories that individuals associate with their immediate home environment and that create a sense of "place identity." Not surprisingly, relocation in later adulthood may not be a question of merely finding technically more easy-going, age-adequate, comfortable, and supportive new living places. Rather it is a question of resolving the nearly impossible puzzle of keeping the meaning while simultaneously adjusting the environmental demands (Oswald, Schilling, Wahl, & Gäng, 2002). These challenges probably reveal a different dynamic at different stages of later life most directly addressed in the relocation literature by the suggestion to distinguish between first, second, and third moves (Litwak & Longino, 1987). While *first moves* are expected to predominantly appear in the early years after retirement and mainly reflect a desire to improve social-physical agency (e.g., a more comfortable home, better living conditions, shorter walks, etc.), *second moves* are expected to appear later in the course of old age and are motivated by the supportive function of the environment in terms of reducing risks or ensuring against potential needs. Relocating to be closer to one's children is a typical example. In terms of SPOT, the dynamics behind these moves are echoed in a tentative balance between social-physical agency and belonging needs. Finally, *third moves* predominantly target the supportive function of the environment and are best exemplified by moves to nursing homes or assisted living facilities quite late in life. In this situation, the need for social-physical belonging, while major competence losses frequently have occurred and future time has become quite limited, is particularly challenged and finding a new person-environment fit pattern in order to keep the meaning is a very difficult enterprise.

The example of relocation can particularly highlight the need to conceptually and empirically consider the social and physical interchange with the environment as well as address the developmental dynamics inherent in such processes as predicted by SPOT. Due to the fact that practically no (longitudinal) data on relocation are around that have given both changes in the physical and the social environment strong emphasis, SPOT dynamics cannot be addressed at this point in time even in retro-sight with already existing data. This is, however, not only true for the relatively seldom (although increasing) event of relocation, but applies also to more general research areas such as understanding the role of home and outdoor environments as people age (see also Wahl, 2001).

The relocation example also underlines that interactions between both the physical and the social environments can occur with quite different outcomes. We have decided at this stage of concept development to stay on the level of expected main effects of SPOT dynamics across the adult age range. It may, however, be very important to also address interactions such as compensatory (e.g., How long can good social networks compensate for bad physical home conditions?) or additive effects (e.g., Is the impact of both bad social networks and bad physical home conditions more negative than other, more favorable person-environment constellations in later life?) at a later stage of conceptual refinement.

PERSON-ENVIRONMENT FIT ISSUES IN SOCIAL-PHYSICAL PLACE OVER TIME PROCESSES

Importantly, the goal-resource congruence model on the regulation of social relationships builds on assumptions of person-environment fit models, thus bridging ecological research on aging (Lawton, 1989, 1998; Wahl, 2001) and social aging theories (Antonucci et al., 2003; Carstensen et al., 1999; Lang, 2001, 2003) that emphasize the individual's proactivity in regulating physical-social environments. This final section of our chapter will serve to underline substantial facets of person-environment fit or misfit in SPOT processes worth considering theoretically as well as empirically. Our argumentation has three elements:

• The first element is that person-environment fit or misfit should be addressed by use of a set of criteria simultaneously applicable to the environment and the person. This draws from Kahana (1982) and Carp and Carp (1984) as well as more recent work on important "environmental attributes" (or evaluative attributes) as suggested by Lawton, (1989b, 1999), Regnier and Pynoos (1992), and Weisman (1997). These criteria are generalized beyond institutional settings to the entire phenomenon of aging in context. Specifically, we propose the following three criteria dimensions as particularly important for the evaluation of the person-environment fit in SPOT processes:

(1) Safety and familiarity
(2) Stimulation and activation
(3) Continuity and keeping the meaning

We are not arguing that these three sets of criteria are comprehensive for SPOT, but we assume that they echo some of the most important themes to be negotiated with the environment while aging.

• The second element of our argumentation is that dimensions are in need of applying to the social and physical environment. Obviously, this is of critical importance for any attempt at striving toward integrating the physical with the social as people age. We assume that this is the case with respect to all three evaluative criteria (i.e. safety and familiarity, stimulation and activation, and continuity and keeping the meaning).

• The third element of the argument is that person-environment fit or misfit themes are differentially associated with specific life phases of adulthood and old age depending on the individual's resources, competence, and action potentials. Thus, this element further illustrates and deepens our understanding of SPOT processes.

In the following, we consider each of the three evaluative criteria of SPOT.

Safety and familiarity have been associated with barriers in the home and neighborhood environment as well as with physical hazards. The criteria of safety and familiarity represent a major dimension of the person-social environment transaction. For example, strong and close relations with children who are not living far from one's own apartment/house may strengthen feelings of safety of an aging person, even if the physical environment is demanding. Another important issue of discussing safety and familiarity with implications for person-environment fit evaluations is what Parmelee and Lawton (1990) have called the security-autonomy dialectics. For example, social partners may enhance feelings of safety, but this might become detrimental in situations when they have a tendency toward overprotection (M. Baltes & Wahl, 1992). Similarly, technology in the home environment (Wahl & Mollenkopf, in press) can provide a major tool to feel more secure, but technology might also run the risk of provoking new dependencies and questioning the full use of still-remaining competencies of an aging individual.

Stimulation and activation are criteria of person-environment fit that have often been disregarded due to a tendency in the literature to put predominant emphasis on frail older adults. Physical-spatial arrangements can facilitate or hinder social contacts. Some environments are more prone to encourage or initiate social contact than others are. The recreational functions of environments such as park areas or of spatial-related behaviors outside the home such as traveling is meanwhile widely recognized as a major resource for aging individuals (Wahl, 2001a). The interlink of stimulation to social contact and relations is obvious. Social relations serve as major stimulating functions for aging adults such as securing ongoing personal interchange and having new interpersonal experiences. Furthermore, physical constellations can stipulate new social contacts; physical-spatial behaviors outside of the home are frequently associated with seeking or caring for social contacts.

Continuity and keeping the meaning is a third set of criteria of person-environment fit in old age and is closely affiliated with the physical as well as the social environment. On the one hand, settings such as the home environment and the residential area surrounding one's home become major "landscapes of memories" (Rowles, 1983, p. 114; see also Sebba, 1991) and ecological extensions of the self (Rubinstein, 1989), and thus important material keepers of meaning. As recent research has revealed, older adults experience a whole scope of meanings associated with their home environment (Oswald & Wahl, in press). The intensity of this attachment to place becomes most obvious when the aging and particularly the very old person is challenged by a new residential decision. On the other hand, it is equally clear that continuity and meaning are also strongly bound to one's social ties and it is an important insight of the more recent research on social relations that even very old individuals are proactively able to preserve this social relations quality.

In linking such dimensions to major personal variables conditioning SPOT processes, we believe that Lawton's basic press-competence approach (e.g., Lawton, 1982, 1989a) still is the most promising approach. In particular, competence is a resource that leads to psychological adaptations. When competence is low, seeking not only low-demanding but also high-meaningful environments is adaptive. When competence is high, seeking more demanding environments even when not familiar may lead to better outcomes and new "developmental gains." In addition, it is no far stretch to link the press-competence approach of Lawton with our ideas of a developmental model that drives SPOT processes as suggested above (see again Table 1.1). Concretely, we assume that the regulation of safety and familiarity, stimulation and activation, and continuity and keeping the meaning operates differently in SPOT across different phases of the adult lifespan and that this has much to do with available, remaining, or lost action potentials related to loss of competence or the shrinkage of remaining future time in one's life (see Table 1.2).

As shown in Table 1.2, we assume in line with Lawton's press-competence model that getting older enhances the probability of lowered competence and thus the sensitivity of the aging organism to available social and physical environment constraints. On the motivational level, this comes with the challenge and task of finding new balances in terms of one's sense of social-physical agency as compared to one's sense of belonging to social-physical places.

One might also look at this in terms of what Lawton (1989a) has coined as "proactivity." To further qualify SPOT dynamics, our additional assumption is that person-environment fit processes and outcomes are mainly driven by stimulation and activation at earlier phases of the adult life span, but change toward safety and familiarity as people enter very high ages. Finally, the basic human tendency of seeking continuity and keeping the meaning is expected to operate in a parallel manner to these fit processes as people age. However, we also assume that continuity and

TABLE 1.2 Person-Environment Fit Dynamics in SPOT

Stage of Aging	Relevance of Social-Physical Agency	Relevance of Social-Physical Belonging	Person-Environment Fit Dynamics in SPOT		
			Stimulation & Activation	Safety & Familiarity	Continuity & Meaning
Middle Adulthood / High Competence	+++	+	+++	+	+
Early Age/"Young old" / Medium Competence	++	++	++	++	++
"Old-Old"/Oldest Old/ Major Loss of Competence	+	+++	+	+++	+++

keeping the meaning in SPOT become more and more important while navigating from middle adulthood and "young-old" age to the stadium of being old-old/oldest-old. This is because one of the major human strivings, namely the search for meaning, is forced to operate in very high ages within the highest constraints of the human lifespan. Although this is a general process in the human lifecourse (see Erikson, 1950), using SPOT we argue that the social and physical environment as an entity must be considered more strongly as a major and inseparable element of this existential dynamic in future conceptual and empirical work in aging research.

FINAL CONCLUSIONS

At the end of this chapter, we would like to emphasize that it is not our intention to present a finalized theoretical model on the dynamic interplay of the physical and social environments in aging research. Rather, we started with reviewing major arguments to support the need for such integration and we examined those theories on aging that explicitly have addressed development in adulthood and old age in context. We propose the Social-Physical Places Over Time (SPOT) concept as a meta-theoretical perspective that addresses both the physical and social environment of aging individuals and makes predictions in terms of the developmental dynamics inherent in person-social-physical-environment relations in the adult lifespan. We believe, though, that the SPOT concept bears the potential for a theoretical integration of social-ecological perspectives on aging. Finally, we argue that combining a developmental view (goal-resource congruence model) with an ecology view (criteria of person-environment fit dimensions) deepens our understanding of SPOT processes and simultaneously counteracts the prevalent schism in the literature toward separating the social and the physical research worlds.

The worth of such thinking for future aging research should, however, not be limited to extensions on the theoretical level. We also feel that new empirical pathways may come with the SPOT and its spelling out, which we have only begun to develop in this chapter. On the more general level, one hypothesis to be tested would be that the predicted dynamics of SPOT in terms of a tendency to switch from a sense of social-physical agency toward a sense of social-physical belonging can actually be observed in aging persons (both in their relation to the social and physical environment) (see again Table 1.1). A related general hypothesis would be that the change in importance of different person-environment processes predicted with SPOT, namely from stimulation and activation to safety, support, and familiarity in conjunction with an increasing importance of continuity and keeping the meaning is actually observable (see again Table 1.2). From a differential-gerontological perspective, one prediction deviated from

SPOT developed so far would be that older adults who focus on belonging, although capable of changing and regulating their social-physical places in accordance, may show more rapid declines and may miss important occasions to adapt their person-environment fit over time. This would be the "use it or lose it" case. We are not saying that such SPOT processes are under volitional control of the aging individual, but they do probably have different outcomes in the long run. In contrast, frail, older adults who are no longer capable of exerting much primary control in their environments, but continue to do so, may be at high risk of suffering from the many demands and eventually depression in the long run. This would be the "lose it after overusing it" case. The major and innovative potential of following such aging and developmental research avenues would be that the now typically different research worlds of focusing either on the social or physical environment would be brought into stronger coalition again. Ideas already clearly spoken out by scholars such as Margret Baltes (1996), Powell Lawton (1989a), or Leopold Rosenmayr (Rosenmayr & Köckeis, 1965) a rather long time ago may come back stronger to empirical aging research by using SPOT as a research orientation.

Obviously, questions of assessing SPOT processes, as well as the person-environment fit dimensions highlighted in this chapter, are not yet fully solved in the empirical aging literature. However, we are optimistic that a rigorous review of what already has been provided by social and environmental scholars in terms of operationalization and assessment will lead to substantial pathways and possibilities in this regard (e.g., Adams & Stevenson, 2003; Rook, 2000; Carp, 1994; Lawton, 1999). Steps in this direction would be as important as further development and differentiation of the concept of SPOT.

Two issues related to SPOT should be briefly addressed at the end. First, one might argue that disengagement theory (Cumming & Henry, 1961) served as a model for what we have described here. We do not agree, although there are some similarities between our thinking and what Henry (1964) has introduced as a revised element to the original disengagement theory, namely "intrinsic disengagement." The term disengagement is, however, misleading in this respect because we regard the person-environment regulative processes addressed in SPOT as proactive adaptational efforts. Also, we argue that concepts such as socio-physical belonging are anchored in more recent theoretical traditions with promises for future aging research. Furthermore, we feel that the ongoing strong quantitative growth of the oldest-old population as well as the research challenges coming with this (e.g., Baltes & Smith, 1999) provide an important new background for such theoretical thinking as compared to the time when disengagement theory was introduced. Second, although we believe that the social and physical environments are, in principle, inseparable, it is not our intent to state that social and physical environments should *always* be researched in combined manners in aging research. We only argue, using SPOT, that still-underused synergies to consider both the social and physical may add to a better understanding of aging. It might even be another important research option for the future, driven by SPOT, to identify those developmental dynamics in the adult lifespan in which such a combined view is or is not a necessary perspective. Finally, we clearly acknowledge that many areas have remained untouched and many questions have remained unanswered. Issues such as interactions between the social and the physical environments and the need for more differentiation (e.g., Does SPOT apply differently to different domains of competencies?) have, in many regards, only been addressed at the periphery and we have only begun with the empirical translation of SPOT.

ACKNOWLEDGEMENTS

We appreciate the excellent and invaluable comments on an earlier version of this draft provided by Laura Carstensen, Frank Oswald, and Rick Scheidt.

REFERENCES

Adams, R. G., & Stevenson, M. L. (2003). A lifetime of relationships mediated by technology. In F. R. Lang & K. L. Fingerman (Eds.), *Growing together: Personal relationships across the life span* (pp. 368-393). New York: Cambridge University Press.

Altman, I. (1975). *The environment and social behavior*. Monterey, CA: Brooks-Cole.

Antonucci, T. C. (1990). Social support and social relationships. In R. H. Binstock & L. K. George (Eds.), *Handbook of aging and the social sciences* (3rd ed., pp. 205-226). San Diego, CA: Academic Press.

Antonucci, T. C. (2001). Social relations: An examination of social networks, social support, and sense of control. In J. E. Birren & K. W. Schaie (Eds.), *Handbook of the psychology of aging* (5th ed., pp. 427-453). San Diego, CA: Academic Press.

Antonucci, T. C., & Akiyama, H. (1995). Convoys of social relations: Family and friendships within a life span context. In R. Blieszner & V. H. Bedford (Eds.), *Handbook of aging and the family* (pp. 355-371). Westport, CT: Greenwood Press.

Antonucci, T. C., Langfahl, E. S., & Akiyama, H. (2003). Relationships as outcomes and contexts. In F. R. Lang & K. L. Fingerman (Eds.), *Growing together: Personal relationships across the life span* (pp. 24-44). New York: Cambridge University Press.

Baltes, M. M. (1996). *The many faces of dependency in old age*. Cambridge, UK: Cambridge University Press.

Baltes, M. M., Maas, I., Wilms, H. U., Borchelt, M., & Little, T. (1999). Everyday competence in old and very old age: Theoretical considerations and empirical findings. In P. B. Baltes & K. U. Mayer (Eds.), *The Berlin Aging Study* (pp. 384-402). Cambridge, UK: Cambridge University Press.

Baltes, M. M., & Wahl, H. W. (1992). The dependency-support script in institutions: Generalization to community settings. *Psychology and Aging, 7*, 409-418.

Baltes, M. M., Wahl, H. W., & Schmid-Furstoss, U. (1990). The daily life of elderly Germans: Activity patterns, personal control, and functional health. *Journal of Gerontology: Psychological Sciences, 45*, 173-179.

Baltes, P. B. (1987). Theoretical propositions of life-span developmental psychology: On the dynamics between growth and decline. *Developmental Psychology, 23*, 611-626.

Baltes, P. B., & Smith, J. (1989). Multilevel and systemic analyses of old age. Theoretical and empirical evidence for the fourth age. In V. L. Bengtson, & K. W. Schaie (Eds.), *Handbook of theories of aging* (pp. 153-173). New York: Springer.

Baltes, P. B., Reese, H. W., & Lipsitt, L. P. (1980). Life-span developmental psychology. *Annual Review of Psychology, 31*, 65–110.

Barker, R. G., & Barker, L. S. (1961). The psychological ecology of old people in Midwest, Kansas, and Yoredale, Yorkshire. *Journals of Gerontology, 16*, 144-149.

Baum, A., & Paulus, P. (1987). Crowding. In D. Stokols & I. Altman (Eds.), *Handbook of environmental psychology* (pp. 533-570). New York: Wiley.

Bengtson, V. L., Burgess, E. O., & Parrot, T. M. (1997). Theory, explanation, and a third generation of theoretical development in social gerontology. *Journals of Gerontology: Psychological Sciences, 52B*, S72-S88.

Canter, D. V., & Craik, K. H. (1981). Environmental psychology. *Journal of Environmental Psychology, 1*, 1-11.

Carp, F. M. (1966). *A future for the aged*. Austin: University of Texas Press.

Carp, F. M. (1967). The impact of environment on old people. *Gerontologist, 7*, 106-108.

Carp, F. M. (1987). Environment and aging. In D. Stokols & I. Altman (Eds.), *Handbook of environmental psychology* (Vol. 1, pp. 330-360). New York: Wiley.

Carp, F. M. (1994). Assessing the environment. In M. P. Lawton & J. A. Teresi (Eds.), *Focus on assessment techniques* (Vol. 14, pp. 302-323). New York: Springer.

Carp, F. M., & Carp, A. (1984). A complementary/congruence model of well-being or mental health for the community elderly. In I. Altman, M. P. Lawton, & J. F. Wohlwill (Eds.), *Human behavior and environment* (Vol. 7, Elderly people and the environment, pp. 279-336). New York: Plenum Press.

Carstensen, L. L. (1995). Evidence for a life-span theory of socioemotional selectivity. *Current directions in Psychological Science, 5*, 151-156.

Carstensen, L. L., Isaacowitz, D. M., & Charles, S. T. (1999). Taking time seriously: A theory of socioemotional selectivity. *American Psychologist, 54*, 165-181.

Carstensen, L. L., & Lang, F. (1997). Social support in context and as context: Comments on social support and the maintenance of competence in old age. In S. Willis and K. W. Schaie (Eds.), *Societal mechanisms for maintaining competence in old age* (pp. 207-222). New York: Springer.

Carstensen, L. L., & Turk-Charles, S. (1994). The salience of emotion across the adult life course. *Psychology and Aging, 9*, 259-264.

Cumming, E., & Henry, W. E. (1961). *Growing old: The process of disengagement*. New York: Basic Books.

Dannefer, D. (1992). On the conceptualization of context in developmental discourse: Four meanings of context and their implications. In D. L. Featherman & R. M. Lerner & M. Perlmutter (Eds.), *Life-span development and behavior* (Vol. 11, pp. 83-110). Hillsdale, NJ: Erlbaum.

Erikson, E. H. (1950). *Childhood and society*. New York: Norton & Company.

Evans, G. W., & Lepore, S. J. (1993). Household crowding and social support: A quasiexperimental analysis. *Journal of Personality and Social Psychology, 65*, 308-316.

Evans, G. W., Lepore, S. J., & Schroeder, A. (1996). The role of interior design elements in human responses to crowding. *Journal of Personality and Social Psychology, 70*, 41-46.

Festinger, L., Schachter, S., & Back, K. (1950). *Social pressures in informal groups: A study of human factors in housing*. Stanford, CA: Stanford University Press.

Fingerman, K. L. (2003). The consequential stranger: Peripheral social ties across the life span. In F. R. Lang & K. L. Fingerman (Eds.), *Growing together: Personal relationships across the life span* (pp. 183-209). New York: Cambridge University Press.

Fleming, I., Baum, A., & Weiss, L. (1987). Social density and perceived control as mediators of crowding stress in high-density residential neighborhoods. *Journal of Personality and Social Psychology, 52*, 899-906.

Frankel, B. G., & DeWit, D. J. (1989). Geographic distance and intergenerational contact: An empirical examination of the relationship. *Journal of Aging Studies, 3*, 139-162.

Fung, H., & Carstensen, L. L. (2003). Sending memorable messages to the old: Age differences in preferences and memory for advertisements. *Journal of Personality and Social Psychology, 85*, 163-178.

Hagestad, G. O., & Dannefer, D. (2001). Concepts and theories of aging. Beyond microfication in social science approaches. In R. H. Binstock & L. K. George (Eds.), *Handbook of aging and the social sciences* (5th ed., pp. 3-21). San Diego, CA: Academic Press.

Havighurst, R. J., Neugarten, B., & Tobin, S. (1968). Disengagement and patterns of aging. In B. Neugarten (Ed.), *Middle age and aging* (pp. 161–172). Chicago: University of Chicago Press.

Heckhausen, J., & Schulz, R. (1995). A life span theory of control. *Psychological Review, 102*, 284-302.

Henry, W. E. (1964). The theory of intrinsic disengagement. In P. F. Hansen (Ed.), *Age with a future* (pp. 419-424). Kopenhagen, Denmark: Munksgaard.

Kahana, E. (1982). A congruence model of person-environment interaction. In M. P. Lawton, P. G. Windley, & T. O. Byerts (Eds.), *Aging and the environment: Theoretical approaches* (pp. 97-121). New York: Springer.

Kahana, E., Liang, J., & Felton, B. J. (1980). Alternative models of person-environment fit: Predicting morale in three homes for the aged. *Journal of Gerontology, 35*(4), 584-595.

Kleemeier, R. W. (1959). Behavior and the organization of the bodily and external environment. In J. E. Birren (Ed.), *Handbook of aging and the individual* (pp. 400-451). Chicago: The University of Chicago Press.

Kohli, M., & Künemund, H. (Eds.). (2000). *Die zweite Lebenshälfte. Ergebnisse des Alters-Surveys [The second half of life: Findings of the "Age-Survey"]*. Leverkusen, Germany: Leske + Budrich.

Kruse, L., & Graumann, C. F. (1998). Metamorphosen der Umwelt im Lebenslauf [Metamorphoses of the environment in the life course]. In A. Kruse (Ed.), *Psychosoziale Gerontologie: Vol. I. Grundlagen. Jahrbuch der Medizinischen Psychologie* (pp. 51-64). Göttingen, Germany: Hogrefe.

Lang, F. R. (1998). The young and the old in the city: Developing intergenerational relationships in urban environments. In D. Görlitz, H. J. Harloff, G. Mey, & J. Valsiner (Eds.), *Children, cities, and psychological theories: Developing relationships* (pp. 598-628). Berlin, Germany: DeGruyter.

Lang, F. R. (2001). Regulation of social relationships in later adulthood. *Journal of Gerontology: Psychological Sciences, 56B*, P321-P326.

Lang, F. R. (2003). Social motivation across the lifespan: Developmental perspectives on the regulation of personal relationships and networks. In F. R. Lang & K. L. Fingerman (Eds.), *Growing together: Personal relationships across the life span* (pp. 341-367). New York: Cambridge University Press.

Lang, F. R., & Carstensen, L. L. (1998). Social relationships and adaptation in late life. In B. Edelstein (Ed.), *Comprehensive clinical psychology: Vol. 7. Clinical geropsychology*. Oxford, UK: Elsevier.

Lang, F. R., & Carstensen, L. L. (2002). Time counts: Future time perspective, goals, and social relationships. *Psychology and Aging, 17*, 125-139.

Lang, F. R., Rieckmann, N., & Baltes, M. M. (2002). Adapting to aging losses: Do resources facilitate strategies of selection, compensation, and optimization in everyday functioning? *Journal of Gerontology: Psychological Sciences, 57B*, P501-P509.

Lawton, M. P. (1970). Ecology and aging. In L. A. Pastalan & D. H. Carson (Eds.), *Spatial behaviour of older people* (pp. 40-67). Ann Arbor: University of Michigan — Wayne State University.

Lawton, M. P. (1976). Contextual perspectives: Psychosocial influences. In L. W. Poon & T. Crook (Eds.), *Handbook for clinical memory assessment of older adults* (pp. 32-42). Washington, DC: American Psychological Association.

Lawton, M. P. (1977). The impact of the environment on aging and behavior. In J. E. Birren & K. W. Schaie (Eds.), *Handbook of the psychology of aging* (pp. 276-301). New York: Van Nostrand.

Lawton, M. P. (1982). Competence, environmental press, and the adaption of older people. In M. P. Lawton, P. G. Windley, & T. O. Byerts (Eds.), *Aging and the environment* (pp. 33-59). New York: Springer.

Lawton, M. P. (1983). Environment and other determinants of well-being in older people. *The Gerontologist, 23*(4), 349-357.

Lawton, M. P. (1985). The elderly in context: Perspectives from environmental psychology and gerontology. *Environment and Behavior, 17*, 501–519.

Lawton, M. P. (1989a). Environmental proactivity in older people. In V. L. Bengtson & K. W. Schaie (Eds.), *The course of later life* (pp. 15-23). New York: Springer.

Lawton, M. P. (1989b). Three functions of the residential environment. In L. A. Pastalan & M. E. Cowart (Eds.), *Lifestyles and housing of older adults: The Florida experience* (pp. 35-50). New York: Haworth.

Lawton, M. P. (1999). Environmental taxonomy: Generalizations from research with older adults. In S. L. Friedman & T. D. Wachs (Eds.), *Measuring environment across the life span* (pp. 91-124). Washington, DC: American Psychological Association.

Lawton, M. P., & Nahemow, L. (1973). Ecology and the aging process. In C. Eisdorfer & M. P. Lawton (Eds.), *The psychology of adult development and aging* (pp. 619-674). Washington, DC: American Psychological Association.

Lawton, M. P., & Simon, B. B. (1968). The ecology of social relationships in housing for the elderly. *The Gerontologist, 8*, 108-115.

Lemon, B. W., Bengtson, V. L., & Peterson, I. A. (1972). An exploration of the activity theory of aging: Activity types and life satisfaction among in-movers to a retirement community. *Journal of Gerontology, 27,* 511–523.

Lewin, K. (1936). *Principles of topological psychology.* New York: McGraw-Hill.

Litwak, E., & Longino, C. F., Jr. (1987). Migration patterns among the elderly: A developmental perspective. *The Gerontologist, 27*(3), 266-272.

Marshall, V. W. (1996). The state of theory on aging and the social sciences. In R. Binstock & L. George (Eds.), *Handbook of aging and the social sciences* (4th ed., pp. 12-30). San Diego, CA: Academic Press.

Mather, M., & Carstensen, L. L. (in press). Aging and attentional biases for emotional faces. *Psychological Science.*

Messer, M. (1967). The possibility of an age concentrated environment becoming a normative system. *The Gerontologist, 7,* 247-251.

Moos, R. H. (1976). Conceptualizations of human environments. In R. Moos (Ed.), *The human context: Environmental determinants of behavior* (pp. 3-35). New York: Wiley.

Moos, R. H., & Lemke, S. (1996). *Evaluating residential facilities: The multiphasic environmental assessment procedure.* Thousand Oaks, CA: Sage.

Moss, M. S., & Lawton, M. P. (1982). Time budgets of older people: A window of four lifestyles. *Journal of Gerontology, 37,* 115-123.

Oswald, F., Schilling, O., Wahl, H. W., & Gäng, K. (2002). Trouble in paradise? Reasons to relocate and objective environmental changes among well-off older adults. *Journal of Environmental Psychology, 22*(3), 273-288.

Oswald, F., & Wahl, H. W. (in press). Place attachment across the life span. In J. R. Miller, R. M. Lerner, & L. B. Schiamberg (Eds.), *Human ecology: An encyclopedia of children, families, communities, and environments.* Santa Barbara, CA: ABC-Clio Press.

Parmelee, P. A., & Lawton, M. P. (1990). The design of special environment for the aged. In J. E. Birren & K. W. Schaie (Eds.), *Handbook of the psychology of aging* (3rd ed., pp. 465-489). New York: Academic Press.

Pinquart, M., & Sörensen, S. (2000). Influences of socioeconomic status, social network, and competence on subjective well-being in later life: A meta-analysis. *Psychology and Aging, 15,* 187-224.

Proshansky, H. M., Fabian, A. K., & Kaminoff, R. (1983). Place-identity. *Journal of Environmental Psychology, 3,* 57-83.

Rebok, G. W., & Hoyer, W. J. (1977). The functional context of elderly behavior. *Gerontologist, 17,* 27-34.

Regnier, V., & Pynoos, J. (1992). Environmental intervention for cognitively impaired older persons. In J. E. Birren, R. B. Sloane, & G. D. Cohen (Eds.), *Handbook of mental health and aging* (2nd ed., pp. 763-792). San Diego, CA: Academic Press.

Riley, M. W. (1985). Age strata in social systems. In R. H. Binstock & E. Shanas (Eds.), *Handbook of aging and the social sciences* (2nd ed., pp. 369–411). New York: Van Nostrand Reinhold.

Rook, K. S. (2000). The evolution of social relationships in later adulthood. In S. H. Qualls & N. Abeles (Eds.), *Psychology and the aging revolution: How we adapt to longer life* (pp. 173-191). Washington, DC: American Psychological Association.

Rosenmayr, L., & Köckeis, E. (1965). *Umwelt und Familie alter Menschen* (*Environment and Family in old age*). Neuwied, Germany: Luchterhand.

Rosow, I. (1974). *Socialization to old age*. Berkeley: University of California Press.

Rowles, G. D. (1983). Geographical dimensions of social support in rural Appalachia. In G. D. Rowles & R. J. Ohta (Eds.), *Aging and milieu: Environmental perspectives on growing old* (pp. 111-130). New York: Academic Press.

Rowles, G. D., & Ohta, R. J. (1983). Emergent themes and new directions: Reflection on aging and milieu research. In G. D. Rowles & R. J. Ohta (Eds.), *Aging and milieu: Environmental perspectives on growing old* (pp. 231-239). New York: Academic Press.

Rowles, G. D., & Watkins, J. F. (2003). History, habit, heart and hearth: On making spaces into places. In K. W. Schaie, H. W. Wahl, H. Mollenkopf, & F. Oswald (Eds.), *Aging independently: Living arrangements and mobility* (pp. 77-96). New York: Springer.

Rubinstein, R. L. (1989). The home environments of older people: A description of the psychosocial processes linking person to place. *Journal of Gerontology: Social Sciences, 44*(2), S45-53.

Rubinstein, R. L., & Parmelee, P. A. (1992). Attachment to place and the representation of the life course by the elderly. In I. Altman & S. M. Low (Eds.), *Place attachment* (pp. 139-163). New York: Plenum.

Sebba, R. (1991). The landscapes of childhood: The reflection of childhood's environment in adult memories and in children's attitudes. *Environment and Behavior, 23*, 395-422.

Sherman, S. R. (1975). Patterns of contacts for residents of age-segregated and age-integrated housing. *Journal of Gerontology, 30*, 103–107.

Steverink, N., Lindenberg, S., & Ormel, J. (1998). Towards understanding successful aging: Patterned change in resources and goals. *Aging and Society, 18*, 441-467.

Tartler, R. (1961). *Das Alter in der modernen Gesellschaft* (*Aging in modern society*). Stuttgart, Germany: Enke.

Vaskovics, L. A. (1990). Soziale Folgen der Segregation alter Menscher in der Stadt (Social consequences of segregating older people in the city). In L. Bertels & U. Herlyn (Eds.), *Lebenslauf und Raumerfahrungen* (pp. 35-58). Opladen, Germany: Leske + Budrich.

Wagner, M., Schütze, Y., & Lang, F. R. (1999). Social relationships in old age. In P. B. Baltes & K. U. Mayer (Eds.), *The Berlin Aging Study: Aging from 70 to 100* (pp. 282-301). New York: Cambridge University Press.

Wahl, H. W. (2001a). Environmental influences on aging and behavior. In J. E. Birren & K. W. Schaie (Eds.), *Handbook of the psychology of aging* (5th ed., pp. 215-237). San Diego, CA: Academic Press.

Wahl, H. W. (2001b). Ecology of aging. In N. J. Smelser & P. B. Baltes (Eds.), *International encyclopedia of the social and behavioral sciences* (Vol. 6, pp. 4045-4048). Amsterdam: Elsevier.

Wahl, H. W., & Mollenkopf, H. (in press). Impact of everyday technology in the home environment on older adults' quality of life. In K. W. Schaie & N. Charness (Eds.), *Impact of technology on successful aging*. New York: Springer.

Wahl, H. W., & Weisman, J. (in press). Environmental gerontology at the beginning of the new millennium: Reflections on its historical, empirical, and theoretical development. *The Gerontologist*.

Weisman, G. D. (1997). Environments for older persons with cognitive impairments. In G. Moore & R. Marans (Eds.), *Environment, behavior and design* (Vol. 4, pp. 315-346). New York: Plenum Press.
Weisman, G. D., Chaudhury, H., & Diaz Moore, K. (2000). Theory and practice of place: Toward an integrative model. In R. L. Rubinstein, M. Moss, & M. Kleban (Eds.), *The many dimensions of aging: Essays in honor of M. Powell Lawton* (pp. 3-21). New York: Springer.
Youniss, J. (1980). *Parents and peers in social development: A Sullivan-Piaget perspective.* Chicago: University of Chicago Press.

CHAPTER 2

The General Ecological Model Revisited: Evolution, Current Status, and Continuing Challenges

RICK J. SCHEIDT AND CAROLYN NORRIS-BAKER
KANSAS STATE UNIVERSITY

It emerged 25 years ago from an integrative review of a new field called "ecology and aging" (Lawton & Nahemow, 1973) as a chapter in an edited volume on adult development and aging. After discussing for "hours and days of how best to conceptualize the field," Powell Lawton and Lucille Nahemow "in desperation decided to draw what we were talking" (Lawton, 1990, p. 348). The final drawing was done in about three minutes and became widely known as the "competence-press" model or, as we refer to it here, *the general ecological model of aging* (Lawton, 2000; Nahemow, 2000). It stands as the most influential model to date of person-environment relations in environmental gerontology.

This chapter revisits the general ecological model, reviews evolutionary changes in its major dimensions, and evaluates its capacity for guiding current and future research in environmental gerontology. Readers interested in the relatively sparse literature dealing with empirical tests of the model are advised to see Nahemow (2000). We have chosen to discuss features of the model that have affected research on its testability, as well as its future usefulness. While recognizing thoughtful reviews by others, the review portion of the chapter is drawn primarily from the work of the model's creators, Lawton and Nahemow, who continued to reflect upon it until their deaths in recent years.

THE GENERAL ECOLOGICAL MODEL: ORIGINAL INCARNATION

Figure 2.1 displays the now-classic components of the general ecological model, often referred to as the competence-press model. The model

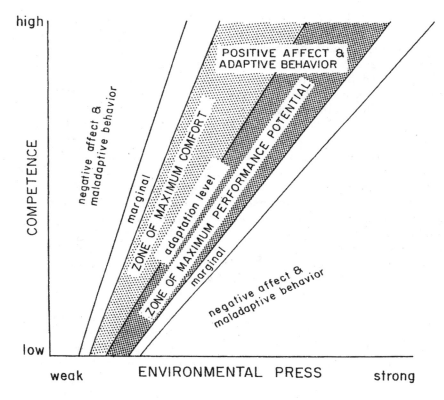

FIGURE 2.1   The general ecological model (frequently referred to as competence-press model).

"explores the interplay between individuals and their environments" (Nahemow, 2000, p. 23). The surface shows alternative adaptive outcomes (behavior and affect) resulting from the degree of match "between a person, characterized in terms of competence, and an environment of a given level of press (Murray's term for environmental demand)" (Lawton, 1999, p. 92). Competence is defined globally by "relatively stable capacities of biological health, sensory and motor skills, and cognitive function" that could exhibit marked changes in varying "trajectories of illness and health" (Lawton, 1999, p. 92). The capacities possess a functional value for the individual when dealing with demands posed by tasks of everyday life. Environmental press consists of forces appraised by the individual as possessing a demand or supporting quality. Press is perceived oftentimes as problematic and stress-evoking; may vary in kind, intensity, and complexity; and as with competencies, may fluctuate over time (Lawton & Nahemow, 1973). Though rarely occurring as an enduring outcome, the "adaptation level" represents all points at which competence and environmental press are exactly matched. A mild excess of press over competence is called "the zone of maximum performance potential" (or "challenge zone" [Nahemow, 2000]), where stimulation, motivation, and learning occur. A mild deficit of environmental press is called the "zone of maximum comfort," where relaxation of effort occurs (Lawton, 2000, pp. 190-191).

Lawton believed there were benefits to the person "who flirts with these borderline zones" (2000, p. 191), a point of significance for our later discussion.

Though derived originally from a research study on older adults (Lawton & Simon, 1968), both Lawton (2000) and Nahemow (2000) believe the model applied to diverse vulnerable populations that may experience departures from normal competence and normal press levels. The model, however, was targeted at elderly populations, particularly focusing on vulnerable elders. An integral and important feature purposely embedded within the original model was the "environmental docility" hypothesis, which informed the efforts of both community planners and architects who worked with elders. As Lawton observed in retrospect,

> I framed the "environmental docility" hypothesis to suggest that decreased personal competence led to a greater likelihood that one's behavior or subjective state would be controlled by environmental factors, or alternatively, that a greater proportion of explanation for personal outcomes was due to environmental influence for less competence people. (Lawton, 1990, p. 345)

A later review by Lawton (1982) upheld the validity of the hypothesis for more impaired elders.

In the following section, we briefly review major changes and revisions to the major conceptual components—environment, competence, and adaptation—of the general ecological model since its inception.

EVOLUTION AND THE CURRENT CONFIGURATION OF THE GENERAL ECOLOGICAL MODEL: BEYOND COMPETENCE

Lawton was keenly sensitive to the meanings of psychological constructs, particularly to the theoretical and empirical problems they pose when poorly distinguished. In 1982, he revisited the general ecological model, modifying "the central processing by which the external environment is given meaning by the person" (Lawton, 1982; 1998, p. 4). He believed that *environmental appraisal* processes within the individual might exert causal effects on behavior and affect, over and above those effects derived from the purely physical environment. Thus, he modified Lewin's (1935) now classic ecological equation [Behavior = (f) Person, Environment] to include

an interaction term: Behavior = (f) Person, Environment, *Person* ×
Environment. Second, he distinguished key constructs comprising competence (biological health, sensory and perceptual capacities, motor skills,
cognitive capacity, and ego strength) from constructs that were less useful
in describing the range of adaptive activity (i.e., needs, traits, and personal
style). Third, Lawton allowed that more complex "transactional attributes"
(e.g., social status, cognitive performance, effectance, and social behavior)
may, at times, serve empirical purposes as both competencies as well as
adaptive outcomes (when predicted by less complex competences).

In response to criticisms raised by Carp and Carp (1984) that the general ecological model was environmentally deterministic, that it placed the
person in *a passive-receptive* mode, and that it did not deal with needs and
preferences (Lawton, 1989a, 1998), Lawton derived the "environmental
proactivity" hypothesis (Lawton, 1989a, 1989b), which held that

> as competence increases, a greater proportion of environmental resources
> becomes available with which the person may interact. Thus, a differential
> interactional hypothesis is set up whereby the less competent are controlled by,
> and the more competent are in control of, the environment. (Lawton, 1998, p. 4)

In this revision, both environmental docility and environmental proactivity may lead to psychological well-being and, in turn, enhance competence. However, only proactivity shapes the environment.

The proactivity hypothesis required Lawton to insert additional "terms
of the organism" within the model. With "personal competences" already
in place, Lawton now posited two types of "personal resources," namely,
effectance and *affective self-regulation*. Effectance is a much more environmentally linked characteristic than is competence, according to Lawton. It
is the normatively judged quality of the behaviors developed to deal with
the environment. "Competence is necessary for effectance and it is competence expressed through effectance that leads to one's more general ability to respond to environmental press" (Lawton, 1989b, p. 60). Effectance
has a subjective aspect as well, as when one expects to respond successfully to an environmental challenge. Efficacious responses can be triggered
by personal needs, desires, preferences, or by environmental demands.
Affective self-regulation describes the degree of success one experiences in
"keeping the type, amount, quality, and conditions of affective stimulation
[and one's responsiveness to these] within the bounds of one's personal
needs, preferences, and ability to manage" (Lawton, 1989b, p. 61). It gov-
erns the active search for specific affective experiences inside and outside
of the person. Lawton (1989b) believed that effectance represented "successfully directed behavior," whereas affective self-regulation promoted
"successfully directed emotion" (p. 61).

The complimentary representation of both personal resources and
environmental resources is displayed in Figure 2.2. The critical distinc-

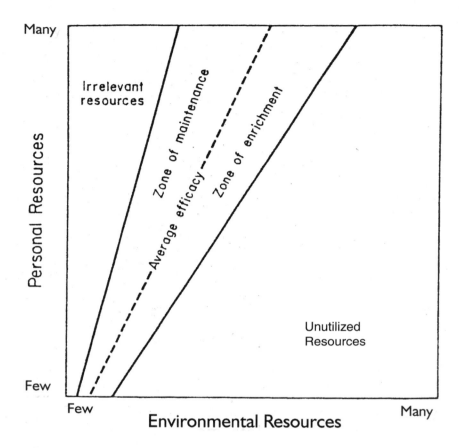

FIGURE 2.2   Extension of the general ecological model: personal and environmental resources, environmental docility, and environmental proactivity.

tions between the original model (Figure 2.1) and this revised one are that "(1) the environment is differentiated into resources and demands and (b) the stance of the person may be either passive or active" (Lawton, 1989b, p. 66).

Lawton posed a number of hypotheses predicting when proactivity might occur, its neural origins in affective arousal and cognitive/motor activation, and its relations to competence. The interested reader should see Lawton, 1989b. We return to the issue of hypothesis testing in later pages.

In a sweeping 1998 book chapter, Lawton paid his last significant, formal visit to the P (person) dimension of the general ecological model (Lawton, 1998). It was prompted by his belief that "advances in environmental knowledge have *not* been matched by advances in knowledge regarding the person and individual differences in the person-environment transaction" (Lawton, 1998, p. 2). He considered this chapter and its environmental counterpart (Lawton, 1999) as complementary updates on his thinking about both P and E components and their transactions within the general ecological model (Lawton, personal communication, May, 1998). Lawton evaluated research on three traditional aspects of the person —motivation, cognition, and effect—and their concrete representations (temperament, personality, and preferences, respectively) to explore gaps in knowledge related to individual differences in environmental transactions. He speculated on the opportunities that such information might afford for personal and behavioral change, particularly for improving person-environment congruence in housing environments.

In this treatise, Lawton reviewed the status of the general ecological model, reaffirming its role as a heuristic (as opposed to a formal) theory. He acknowledged that all existing theoretical frameworks, including those of Kahana (1982), Schooler (1982), Rowles (1984), and Carp and Carp (1984), as well as his own, "fall short as theoretical statements, however, because none of them makes a systematic attempt to account for all the major examples of each concept or to make sufficiently clear how to operationalize the concepts" (Lawton, 1998, p. 2). He expressed his disappointment that, in recent years, the frameworks had a declining influence in directing policy and practice, an ironic observation when one considers that early ecological frameworks were criticized for contributing more to application than to science (Scheidt & Windley, 1985).

Lawton was fascinated with links between neural functioning and environmental transactions. He gave considerable attention to the "inseparable" link between emotion and cognition, exploring neuropsychological relations between cognitive-affective processes and the two major components of mental health—positive and negative affect. He reviewed the environmental relevance of the "Big 5" personality factors (Costa & McCrae, 1992), concluding that these second-order factors, although useful for exploring linkages to positive and negative affect, are, overall, less explanatory and mutable than first-order surface traits (e.g., sociability) for understanding and modifying *individual differences* in person-environment adaptation. With respect to the person as a point of intervention, Lawton held that while "most people, regardless of age, do not require changing" (Lawton, 1998, p. 24), preferences (learned wishes for environmental objects) are much more changeable than personality and temperament needs; those who target preferences must recognize the greater resistance to change posed by the latter, particularly in long-term interventions.

Perhaps the most fitting summary of this evolving aspect of the general ecological model is Lawton's observation that "there is a great deal more to the P component of the ecological equation than competence, and there is a great deal more to the P × E interactional term than environmental cognition" (Lawton, 1998, p. 17).

THE ENVIRONMENTAL COMPONENT:
EVOLVING CONSIDERATIONS

The initial presentation of environmental press in the ecological model seemed deceptively simple. The x-axis of the model (see Figure 2-1) represents "The strength with which the environment demands a response from the person" (Lawton, 1989c, p. 38), ". . . characterized as Murray did, in terms of 'alpha press' (objective, externally observable criteria) and 'beta press' (demand as perceived by the person)" (Lawton, 1999, p. 92). The amount of press increases from low to high as one moves toward the right on the axis. Lawton and Nahemow conceived of this press as a "statistical construct expressing the probability that a specified environmental stimulus or context would elicit some response among all people" (Lawton, 1998, p. 2). Whether or not a response occurred is determined by an individual's level of personal competence. As part of the evolution of the model and the development of the environmental proactivity hypothesis, opportunities or resources have been added to demands to expand the definition of environmental press (Lawton, 1998).

How "environment" can be defined, however, is far from simple. Over the course of more than 30 years of refinement, Lawton's conceptualizations of environment (and thus environmental press) became increasingly complex, ultimately encompassing the three dimensions of environmental classes, the objective/subjective dimensions, and attributes (Lawton, 1999). One of the foundations of the ecological model, Lawton's taxonomy of five broad environmental classes, can be traced back even earlier than the first dissemination of the model in 1973. In 1970, he suggested basic distinctions between

1. the physical environment, including both natural and human-built dimensions
2. the personal environment
3. the small-group environment
4. the suprapersonal environment
5. the social or megasocial environment

Although the definitions of these classes have changed little, one of the last refinements of the descriptions of these classes can be found in Lawton's reconsideration of environmental taxonomies in Friedman and Wach's (1999) *Measuring Environment Across the Lifespan*. (See also Wahl and Lang, present volume.) There, he defines the five classes as follows (Lawton, 1999, Table 1 p. 96):

- **Physical environment:** Objective (alpha press): what can be counted, measured in centimeters, grams, or seconds or consensually evaluated. Subjective (beta press): personally ascribed meaning, salience, or evaluation of the objective environment.
- **Personal environment:** One-on-one relationships; friends, family, and support networks.
- **Small-group environment:** The dynamics that determine the mutual relationships among people in a small group in which all members have some one-on-one relationship or interaction.
- **Suprapersonal environment:** Modal characteristics of people in geographic proximity to the subject (as in social area analysis).
- **Social (megasocial) environment:** Organizational character, social norms, cultural values, legal system, regulations, political ideology, and psychosocial milieu.

The original competence-press model also incorporates a second, orthogonal dimension that reflected the distinction between alpha and beta presses—each class can have components that are subjective as well as objective. As noted, Lawton's elaboration of the model in the 1980s added an interactive $P \times E$ term, recognizing the causal behavioral impact of the subjective as well as the objective environment (Lawton, 1982). Lawton believed it was essential to separate the objective environment (about which one could typically expect some consensus) from the ways in which the individual experiences the environment. "Although common cultural definitions may move some such subjective assessments toward consensus, a person's view of the physical environment remains unique and unknowable from the outside" (Lawton, 1999, p. 106). In fact, in his discussions of the *good-life* model, he places the subjective environment "as perceived by the person" within the domain of perceived quality of life, not the objective environment (Lawton, 1983). (In this model, four interrelated but relatively autonomous sectors:

- Behavioral competence,
- Psychological well-being
- Perceived quality of life
- Objective environment

channel into the *self*, which in turn reenergizes the sectors.) If we consider the graphical representations of these two models together (see Figure 2.3), then environmental press must exist on the surface of the good-life model that is the circle representing the objective environment and the overlapping area of the circle that represents perceived quality of life.

Another critical, and often overlooked, dimension of environmental press is that it is dynamic. Environments change over time, as does press. As Nahemow points out, "Environmental press decreases as a direct

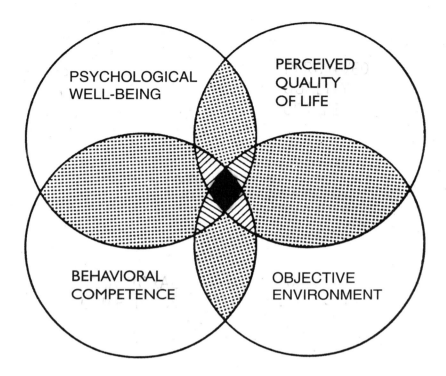

FIGURE 2.3 The good-life model.

function of time spent within 'environments.' All novel environments, no matter how 'simple' they may be objectively, require new learning and adjustment to their demands" (2000, p. 25). At this point, it should be clear that the graphic representation of environmental press (or competence for that matter) as a single line must have been a default position; it is impossible to truly portray these complexly related dimensions in any graphically meaningful way.

This dilemma may also provide one explanation for what Lawton himself acknowledged about the ecological model—that "despite a number of empirical confirmations, [it] has not led to very productive operationalizations of environmental press" (Lawton, 1999, pp. 94-95).Or, as Gitlin recently observed, "This aspect of the model remained the least developed conceptually and with regard to the advancement of assessment tools" (Gitlin, in press-a, p. 4). The overwhelming majority of research using the ecological model has employed what is best characterized as single-variable research, albeit selecting these variables from different taxonomic classes. In reflecting on this phenomenon, Lawton suggested that Roger

Barker's (1968) term, "tesserae"—or traditionally fractionated units for measuring person and environment separately—was appropriate to describe the majority of research growing out of the ecological model of aging. "The tessera is a convenient metaphor for each of a very long list of highly specific aspects of the environment that cannot be ignored in the real world of environmental planning and design" (Lawton, 1999, p. 95).

Several ways of collecting tesserae into more conceptually meaningful and comprehensive dimensions have been attempted. Lawton characterized these as "bottom-up" approaches, such as Carp and Carp's (1984) use of factor analytic strategies, and "top-down" approaches, beginning with global explanatory concepts, such as needs or goals, and searching for their components. The goals of these top-down "mosaic strategies" are "to define major dimensions that explain broader phenomena than tesserae while still maintaining close ties to observable reality" (Lawton, 1999, p. 98). According to Lawton, creating better mosaics will require concepts and measures that link mosaics with their tessarae as well as linking the physical and nonphysical dimensions of environment.

The third (and most recently elaborated) dimension of Lawton's conceptualization of environment is environmental attributes—characteristics by which the cells formed by the matrix of environmental classes and objective/subjective dimensions can be described. Although classes and objective/subjective dimensions apply universally to environments, attributes may describe some and not others (Lawton, 1999). Lawton's rationale in elaborating the taxonomy of the environment in this tripartite way is that the combination of the dimensions "affords the opportunity to characterize environments in their great diversity while still providing a uniform structure into which other investigators may locate the specific environments of concern in their research" (1999, p. 111). There are two groups of attributes: evaluative ones, with presumed effects on outcomes that are neither positive nor negative, and descriptive ones, where the effects on outcomes are neither good nor bad. The connotative dimensions of evaluative attributes may result from empirical evidence, individual judgments, or consensus. Among descriptive attributes are quantitative ones that can be measured in physical units or subjective judgments. They include environmental scale, intensity of stimulation, and temporal qualities such as duration and frequency. Also characterized as descriptive are structural attributes that relate disparate parts of the environment to each other: patterned versus random; distal versus proximate, predictability, diversity, and complexity; and contextual attributes that identify transactional relationships between P and E. Lawton conceptualized these contextual attributes as interactive quality (requiring reciprocity), environmental responsiveness, activity versus passivity, and novelty versus familiarity. Finally, the realm of evaluative attributes includes the often-used environmental satisfaction and environmental preference, as well as affective and general qualities.

Lawton readily admitted that neither the mosaic that describes a milieu nor the three-dimensional structure of environmental classes, attributes, and objective/subjective dimension adequately reflected the complexity and integrated nature of the person-environment system. However, he suggested that this framework does provide a useful rubric for organizing research and it is desirable to "view the measurement of milieu as a profile of separately measured dimensions, in any combination of classes" (Lawton, 1999, p. 117). It is clear that Lawton's concepts of environment and the press it creates were very much a work in progress. He left us with many unresolved issues, but also many directions to pursue in the future —including integrative ways we might "blend" components and/or create linkages across environmental classes, ways in which the objective and subjective dimensions might become a continuum, ways of identifying mechanisms of influences across environmental elements, and, perhaps most challenging of all, ways of empirically determining the relationships among dimensions, milieu, and ambience—a "holistic, subjective term for characterizing entire environments" (p. 117).

ADAPTATION AS THE OUTCOME DOMAIN: SELECTED "SURFACE" CHANGES

The *evaluation* of person-environment transactions is guided by the hypothetical boundaries between adaptation and maladaptation on the surface of the general ecological model. The relative "success" of adaptive efforts is judged using subjective criteria for functional behavior and affective states, most often translated into normative terms within specific person-environment studies. This normative approach, as opposed to an ipsative approach that uses self-comparative standards, affords greater generalizability of outcomes and is undoubtedly responsible for the significant appeal that the model holds for policy and design professionals.

Lawton's extensive and varied research interests led him to revisit a number of conceptual and empirical "surface"-relevant issues over the years. We highlight a few of the issues that have major relevance for current definitions and uses of the model.

Because it inserted "environment" so freshly and prominently into the behavioral equation, the model served as both a rationale and a guide for the emerging field of environmental gerontology. Empirically, early use of the model was characterized by a *style of research* that continues today,

> a style whereby we typically defined psychological and social outcomes (for example, psychological well-being, housing satisfaction, or amount of social interaction) and sought environmental correlates of these outcomes that remained significant after controlling for the usual background and other personal factors that might be associated with outcome. Such empirical find-

ings from our research were in demand by the gerontological services community. (Lawton, 1990, p. 348)

This style of research not only characterizes the early functional view of the outcome domain, but also illustrates the interactionist paradigm that stimulated it. Lawton expressed disappointment that environmental gerontologists still seem content with using the model to show that "environment counts" but have done little advanced research to "establish rules to predict when that effect will be observed and when it will not" (Lawton, 1990, p. 348).

Conceptually, the introduction of the "environmental proactivity" hypothesis (Lawton, 1989c) necessitated the specification of ranges of efficacious behavior for persons displaying varying levels of personal resources against varying utilizations of environmental resources, as Figure 2.2 illustrates. At a broader level, Lawton stressed the "open system" features of the model, hypothesizing that person-environment transactions represented by environmental docility and proactivity may affect the P domain (perceived resources and competence) as well as E domain components (press and resources), which, in turn, have reverberative effects on psychological well being. Thus, the adaptive surface of the model is intended to reflect the dynamic nature of person-environment transactions represented both as possible outcomes *and* causes.

The consideration of how to conduct research on this kind of system forced Lawton to reflect on the value of alternative paradigms within environmental psychology—interactionist and transactional approaches, in particular (Lawton, 1990, 1998; Parmalee & Lawton, 1990). The general ecological model is decidedly interactionist. Personal and environmental attributes are assumed to be conceptually and empirically distinguishable. In this approach, unique and interactive "causally prior" influences of personal and environmental factors on behavioral and psychological outcomes are both assumed and sought. Lawton held that "virtually all empirical research in environmental psychology that has related the person and the environment to some outcome has utilized the interaction paradigm" (1990, p. 358). Within the past two decades, however, research in environmental gerontology has increasingly utilized a transactional approach that "has no focus on outcomes or causal determination but has focus on multiple features of person and context" (Lawton, 1990, p. 358). More qualitative approaches (Norris-Baker & Scheidt, 1994; Rowles, 1987; Rowles, Oswald, & Hunter, this volume; Rubinstein, 1998; Rubinstein & de Medeiros, this volume) are used to depict the meaning of person-environment transactions at various levels and across environments varying in scale (e.g., proximal to neighborhood to community). Indeed, Lawton (1985; Parmelee & Lawton, 1990) conducted research inspired by the transactional approach (e.g., revealing the "control center" that older residents used to monitor everyday activities). Parmelee and Lawton (1990) concluded that it should be possible to use the same data to explore both transactional issues as well as "traditional linear hypotheses," urging a greater use of longitudinal designs that employ both qualitative and quantitative strategies. He believed that concepts derived from qualitative data could be subjected to quantitative use. In one of his final statements, Lawton acknowledged the philosophical inseparability of person and environment, but for heuristic purposes, he believed "it is necessary to speak of, and attempt to measure, them separately" (Lawton, 1998, p. 1).

Deserving greater space than we afford here, Lawton's later research focused extensively on emotion in older adulthood (Lawton, 1990; 1998). This research has implications for the general ecological model, given the role of affect as an outcome domain on the surface of the model. In the 1970s and 1980s, affective outcomes were often assessed using various measures generally referred to as "psychological well-being." Though conceptually distinct, their fuller meanings and distinctions often occurred only in conjunction with their empirical use (Scheidt, 1985, 1998). They included measures of life satisfaction, morale, happiness, affect balance, field measures of "demoralization," and more specific assessments of depression.

During the 1990s, *positive and negative affect* (Bradburn, 1969) became Lawton's critical representatives of mental health in the adaptive model.

> What is needed to advance our knowledge is to look again through a chain going from temperament to personality to preferences to environmental resources and ending with the two major affective facets of mental health as outcomes. (Lawton, 1998, p. 22)

He sorted out long-lasting affective outcomes (largely associated with temperaments such as extroversion and neuroticism) from those more short-lived outcomes, recognizing that there are "happy and unhappy" people, certainly partly determined by temperament, but also happy and unhappy periods of life (partially independent of temperament), as well as good days and bad days (Lawton, 1998).

He believed that happy and sad feelings had different antecedents, the former being more highly affected by social, leisure-time, and environmental attributes, whereas the latter by "physical health and self-sentiments" (Lawton, 1998, p. 11). Lawton believed that people search for emotional experiences to satisfy personal needs for enjoyment, relief from pain, and security. He believed "the synchrony of personal need and environmental resources is the condition associated with favorable affective outcomes" (p. 11). Although this argument is indirectly relevant to the general ecological model, he did not link his thoughts about the structural features of affect or its antecedents to the specific dynamics of the model. He was aware that affect served powerful motivational and moderating functions, inseparable from cognition and imbuing environment with stimulus value.

Interestingly, as originally presented, the general ecological model contained a model for targeting "passive responders" and "active intiators" at either individual or environmental levels (Lawton & Nahemow, 1973). Lawton (1998) returned to this issue in a much more sophisticated way, exploring *which* features of the person (e.g., preferences and surface traits) could be most readily changed to reduce person-environment incongruities. On the environmental side, he explored the effectance of "place therapies" championed by others (Scheidt & Windley, 1985; Scheidt & Norris-Baker, 1999). The present point is that Lawton advised evaluation of the effectance of these interventions based almost solely upon their success in increasing positive and reducing negative affect.

CURRENT STATUS AND FUTURE CHALLENGES: SELECTED ISSUES

Clearly, the general ecological model of aging has evolved much over the past 30 years. Nahemow (2000) cites the many influences of the model on both research and policy, including its stimulus value for generating new hypotheses, for developing environmental assessment procedures, for advancing research in the wider field of psychological gerontology and beyond (e.g., health psychology), and for showcasing other ideas. The hypothesis-testing functions of the model have been more modest by comparison. Even toward the end of his career, Lawton was hesitant to refer to the model as a formal theory, holding that it had not been "worked out in sufficient detail and with requisite vigor to qualify" as a formal theory (Lawton, 1998, p. 2). Lawton added to its conceptual differentiation but never seriously pursued its formal testing. He seemed more interested in broader conceptions of environment-behavior relations. In his gerontological autobiography, Lawton reveals, "cutting wood and brush and walking through the changing forest is my type of outdoor work, not small-plot gardening or lawn manicure" (2000, p. 186). Metaphorically speaking, we believe the same preferences describe his research interests. It is possible that the detailed and lengthy demands of model refinement and testing required manicuring activity that failed to inspire his interest in this way. Nahemow (2000) acknowledges that research on the basic assumptions of the model and its hypotheses is sparse and that limited research based on predictions of the model has produced "mixed" results. The model has contributed little to measurement (Lawton, 1999) and, when it has, these measures have left much to be desired (Wahl & Weisman, in press).

BAROMETRIC FUNCTIONS: CROSSING TO SAFETY?

We believe the model also has served a less formal function. From its inception to the present day, researchers have revisited the model, using it to assay the state of theory development and theory testing in environmental gerontology. This chapter is no exception. At times, the evaluation of the model itself is used to draw conclusions about the state of health of theorizing in environmental gerontology as a whole. Lawton himself was perhaps the first to do this. For example, a dozen years after it was originally proposed, Lawton paused to assess the status of the general ecological model. After noting a number of conceptual gaps in its central components, he concluded that "the net message to be derived from these gaps is that the study of the ecology of aging is still emerging from a pre-scientific phase" (1985, p. 57). Thus, conceptual and empirical progress with the model was considered highly reflective of progress in the field as a whole.

At the time, of course, the model stood at the heart of theorizing in environmental gerontology, along with the alternative models of Carp and Carp (1984), Kahana (1982), and Schooler (1982). The general ecological model and Kahana's Person-Environment Congruence Model reached back to Murray's (1938) need-press theory for foundational elements, while Schooler's Stress-Theoretical Model borrowed heavily from Lazarus's Stress Theory. The Carps elaborated on subjective and objective aspects of the environment and, in particular, distinguished between lower- and higher-order needs. As with the other models, the Complementary/Congruence Model proposed by the Carps owed much to the work of Murray and Lewin, and, according to Lawton (1998), to the general ecological model itself.

Over the past two decades, it has become boilerplate practice for those reviewing the status of environmental gerontology to cite almost rhetorically these same four models (Lawton, 1977; Scheidt & Windley, 1985; Wahl, 2001) while noting and decrying the languid state of theory development. More recently, some researchers have stated the belief that a revivified general ecological model might stimulate more general theory development and testing in the field (Gitlin, in press-b; Golant, in press; Wahl & Weisman, in press). Hence, there appears to be a continuing tendency to equate its untapped empirical capabilities with the theoretical potential of environmental gerontology as a broader area of study. It may be predicated on the belief that the general ecological model can serve as a vehicle to take us to new theoretical territory. To some extent, this expectation is a function of the unrealized empirical promise of the model. It is also due partially to the legacy of expectations placed by environment-behavior researchers upon Lawton himself, who contributed so much to the field during his remarkable career. We wonder, however, whether these expectations form the heart of a "rescue wish" for those seeking fresh perspectives in environmental gerontology and whether the continuing unparalleled preoccupation with the general ecological model may have actually constricted theory development by drawing energy and attention away from new theoretical pursuits. We will return to this point in our closing comment.

OF "VISION AND GRAND SCALE"

Wahl (2001) broke with past boilerplate practice in his review in the *Handbook of the Psychology of Aging* by classifying the general ecological model among the "classic theoretical accounts" in environmental gerontology. He states that most of the new conceptual models in the field "lack the vision and grand scale found among the classic theoretical approaches in the field" (Wahl, 2001, p. 231), yet acknowledges that "classic theories are too entrenched in the well-worn concepts from yesterday's gerontology and psychology and tend to neglect individual differences in behavior-environment links" (p. 231).

There is danger, of course, in suggestions that new conceptions or models in environmental gerontology should return to the grander scale. The sweeping range of such theories makes it difficult, if not impossible, to translate the vision into a meaningful empirical enterprise. Grand scale theory is not theory per se; rather, it is "a formulation lying between a taxonomy and a conceptual framework" (Denzin, 1970, p. 67), orienting researchers to specific problems. One need only to turn to classic, grand scale theories of human development or of personality theories in general psychology to appreciate this point. Few have generated hypothesis-testing research that would support or refute their own internal tenets. Hypotheses from grand scale theory often have the appearance of axioms and may be less likely to be subjected to an empirical test for this reason. In our view, this may apply to the general ecological model as well. At this level, the relations it specifies seem almost axiomatic. One may be less likely to think of the "environmental docility" and "environmental proactivity" hypotheses as requiring empirical support, particularly if intervention-based programs informed by the model produce positive outcomes.

The "vision and grand scale" of the general ecological model is conceptually alluring but empirically constrictive. As originally presented and as currently configured, the general ecological model resides someplace between "grand systems theory" and "middle range theory" (Merton, 1967). It stimulates action-oriented programs and policies, but, as a research tool, serves largely categorical or taxonomic functions. Modifications attempting to make the model more general or to address its perceived shortcomings have increased its complexity exponentially. To design research that can test the model in its entirety is beyond the reach of current methods. Further, at an operational level, it is difficult to do comparative research on broad person-environment-adaptation interactions given the myriad choices that exist for representing these terms in hypothesis-testing research.

TWO MODELS?

The original general ecological model was embraced heartily because it filled a significant void in theorizing. But, despite revisions of the original model, it is burdened with expectations that may now exceed its intent and structure as an empirical rubric. In our view, the primary reason that the general ecological model has generated so little self-reflecting hypothesis-testing research (Nahemow, 2000) rises from its inherent generality as a *theory type*, as stated above. Those interested in using the general ecological model to frame such research should focus on developing specific, lower-level models using standard, relevant variables to represent its major components.

In addition, there is confusion at times about which incarnation of the model might offer the most to hypothesis-testing research and to future theory development. We believe that *two* ecological models have emerged from the work of Lawton and Nahemow over the past 30 years—the original, relatively circumscribed model of competence-press and the more complex, largely taxonomic articulation that emerged from its revisions. It may be functional to separate the two, distinguishing the more modest (or at least more applicable for action research) interactionist competence-press framework from the more differentiated and more transactional person-environment model of recent years. Compared to the original model, the latter model includes both personal and environmental resources (as opposed to docility and press alone), diverse categories of the environment (as opposed to a vaguer emphasis on press), and a larger number of personal components (beyond the dimensions of competence). Each model has the potential to inform our understanding of environment-aging issues at both programmatic and basic empirical levels. We believe, however, that fundamental revision in the nature of expectations or in depicted uses of the model (in both forms) may be in order. In the remaining space, we offer a couple of suggestions that may aid this process.

TEMPUS FUGIT

One of the greatest future challenges for the continued use of the general ecological model is incorporating appropriate temporal dimensions into the competence, environmental, and outcome domains of the model, rather than treating it as a cross-sectional "snapshot." More completely acknowledging this dimension would allow the model to function in a transactional, rather than a solely interactionist, way. We know that individual characteristics and competencies change over time both gradually and abruptly. For example, slow transformations, such as the yellowing of the lens in the eye, may go virtually unnoticed, but the change over time in the ways in which the physical environment is perceived impacts not only the experience of color, but may create safety risks that are not recognized as increased environmental press. Past experiences also shape the competencies of individuals, from ego-strength to chronic disease resulting from lifestyle choices. Similarly, the positive or negative nature of both psychological and behavior outcomes of changes in the balance of competence and press accumulate over the life cycle of each individual.

Although the temporal influences in both of these domains tend to vary by individual, changes in environmental press represent complex combinations of individual, societal changes, and cohort effects. Some are inevitable. As mentioned earlier, press decreases as a function of time spent within them (Nahemow, 2000). At the same time, the environment is in constant transition around all of us, regardless of age. Some of these changes, however, may have greater consequences for elders. Changes in the suprapersonal and societal environments are largely beyond the control of the individual, limiting people's ability to be "active initiators." Examples include changes in social and economic policies, such as those that impact the length of time spent in health care and rehabilitation settings, growth in the availability of assisted living options, or demographic changes in neighborhoods and small rural communities that lead to declines in services, property values (critical for the high percentage of elders who own their homes), and even stigmatization of place. Changes in small group and personal environments typically accompany the aging process: widowhood, loss of friends and support networks due to moves, or relocating to a different (and more communal) type of residential environment, such as a *Continuing Care Retirement Center* (CCRC) or an assisted living residence. The ability to target elders who are "passive responders" versus "active initiators" could play a key role in facilitating adaptation to new environments with their many sources of additional (even if temporary) press. Here the distinction between locus of control for an event and locus of control for handling/responding to the event (Gatz, Siegler, & Tyler, 1986) may be helpful in extending the model. Many changes in press may be beyond the control of the individual, but the perception of where the locus of control lies for responding to the event may shape outcomes more than the event itself.

The physical environment has received the greatest attention as a source of both alpha and beta press, but not with regard to time as a dimension. When we think of changes in press, most often they are those that occur at a single point in time—from relocation (which may reflect a passive or active response to change) to installing a ramp at the front door because of loss of mobility, or even changing the wattage of a light bulb in a reading lamp. What seems to remain relatively unexplored are the feedback loops, through outcomes and changes in competence, that extend adaptive (or maladaptive) processes over time. Although Lawton (1985) did not highlight this characteristic, it is likely that the development of a "control center" has a temporal dimension that includes a feedback loop from positive and negative outcomes. The negative consequences of too little press clearly imply a time dimension, since decreases in competencies from too-low demands typically reflect the atrophy of specific abilities. It is also true that environments may gradually transform over time without a noticeable change in press. The treasured house of a lifetime may begin to fall into disrepair because the elder cannot afford to make repairs, is sufficiently habituated to the environment that he or she does not recognize the need, and/or the intensity of the attachment to home precludes seeing the changing press.

PROCESS: A MISSING FOCUS

Nahemow (2000) believed that the failure of the original competence-press model to focus on the temporal dimension was due partly to the difficulty of working with four dimensions at once (i.e., competence, environment, adaptation, and time). There are at least two other reasons as well. First, much of the appeal of the original competence-press model was its central defining focus on short-term adaptation. More immediate behavioral and affective outcomes were the primary concern of interventionists seeking relief for less competent elders residing within ill-fitting physical and program environments. Second, due to its inherent partitive nature, the model has failed to focus on the *processes* (e.g., feedback loops discussed) of adaptation. This feature made program, policy, and design targeting more conveniently applied to individual and environmental *states* and *traits*. Unfortunately, it offered little to researchers interested in understanding the basic dynamics—the *how* and *why*—of adaptation. The behavioral sequelae of adaptation require time to unfold.

Developmental theorists, of course, must necessarily work with four dimensions (i.e., charting the flow of person-environment interactions in behavioral outcomes across periods of years). Several posit direct study of person-environment interactions across the lifespan (Baltes, Lindenberger, & Staudinger, 1998; Bronfenbrenner & Morris, 1998; Elder, 1998; Magnusson & Stattin, 1998). Gitlin (in press-b) has suggested that theory development efforts in environmental gerontology might benefit from the use of existing models designed to explain broad phenomena (e.g., health and quality of life). In this spirit, it may be possible to use existing lifespan developmental models to inform more specifically the general ecological model, particularly with respect to process orientation.

Baltes & Baltes' (1990) *selective optimization with compensation* (SOC) model is an attractive candidate, having the advantages of being "rather open as to its deployability and domain-specific refinement" (Baltes,

Lindenberger, & Staudinger, 1998, p. 1054) as well as focusing on the *processes* of both short-term and long-term adaptation. The model assumes that behavioral adaptation is characterized by "the maximization of gains and the minimization of losses" occurring within the same individual. Individuals specify or select goals (either through preference or as required by loss), optimizing their realization using a wide set of "means-end resources." The loss of means-end resources requires compensatory efforts, either through enlisting "new means as strategies of compensation" or through changing the goals themselves (Baltes et al., 1998, p. 1057). Environmental (institutional) relocation, for example, "may involve a loss in environment-based resources (means) or make some acquired personal means dysfunctional" (Baltes et al., 1998, p. 1057). As applied to the general ecological model, compensatory strategies for dealing with these losses may be initiated at the individual level both psychologically (e.g., altering equity comparisons) and behaviorally (drawing upon developmental "reserve" capacity in the zone of marginally tolerant affect) or at both individual and environmental levels (e.g., selecting a facility with alternative programs congruent with one's needs, such as a medical model versus a regenerative model for long-term care environments). At its origin, of course, the general ecological model targeted vulnerable elders more "controlled by" the environment (i.e., the "environmental docility" hypothesis). Later, Lawton modified the model to deal with those possessing greater resources, those who are more "in control" of the environment (i.e., the "environmental proactivity" hypothesis; Lawton, 1998). However, there is little in the model to date that affords the study of adaptive decision-making within or between individuals who *simultaneously* exhibit both of these aspects across coexisting, perhaps competing, types and levels of environments that bring both gains and losses. The orchestration of these resource-deficit control tendencies is a function that might be hosted by the general ecological model if it had a more formal focus on process as well as a transactional core that recognized individual differences among elders in their ongoing modulation of needs and resources.

It is not our intent, of course, to suggest that developmental models such as SOC should replace ecological models; rather, they serve to remind us that short-term person-environment interactions may be in the service of long-term developmental dynamics that prompt and moderate person-environment transactions across the lifecourse. It is surprising, however, that few ecologically oriented longitudinal studies exist to date. This may be prompted by the rather "mission-oriented" purposes of ecological research toward the amelioration of acute problems associated with environmental incongruence (Scheidt & Windley, 1985). Given the agenda of interests, it is also surprising that so few experimental environment-aging studies have been conducted to date, despite early urgings to do so (Willems, 1973). Illustratively, experimental strategies may be useful for establishing performance set-point thresholds and plasticity boundaries for dimensions on physical environmental assessment instruments, as well as for discerning behaviors under developmental and non-developmental control (Baer, 1973).

The temporal dimension has additional relevance here as well. Since its inception, significant socio-historical changes have occurred that have implications for the general ecological model. For example, time lag studies indicate general improvements in the health status of older adults over the past 25 years (Rowe & Kahn, 1998). Technological innovations have enhanced everyday environmental adaptations for many older adults, particularly in terms of communication and household technology (Wahl & Mollenkopf, in press). Although Lawton did not discuss *changes* in personal and environmental resources as they affect the general ecological model, those who work with the model should be aware that specific time-of-measurement and cohort-related events may affect specific person and environment components chosen for study.

In this respect, the recent work of Wahl and Mollenkopf (in press) on "historical trajectories" for household technology is illustrative and useful, charting "technology period effects" that may have explanatory as well as descriptive values for understanding $P \times E$ dynamics, particularly when contrasting older and younger cohorts (Scheidt, in press). Wahl and Mollenkopf (in press) believe that understanding the impact of changes in the technology environment requires consideration of both micro- and macro-level variables, including social structure, individual coping strategies, personal interests, individual attitudes, and societal trends. A virtue of the general ecological model is the flexibility it affords for targeting population- and context-specific personal and environmental components, with varying outcome criteria. This means that there are necessarily a number of potential *extra*-personal and environmental factors—newly emergent across time—that may affect the observed dynamics in each application. It would be a rather ironic error if ecological researchers failed to take these into account when employing the model, particularly across longer time periods.

QUO VADIS

Lewin's oft-quoted observation that "there is nothing so practical as a good theory" certainly applies to the general ecological model, particularly to its original formulation. Lawton noted that the model was forwarded as a rubric to orient environmental gerontologists to a "manner of thinking [that] may help us define which personal characteristics of a user group are relevant to a design problem and which environmental features are most central to the user's ability to have a good life" (2000, p. 191). Lawton's modifications to the model enriched our understanding of both individual and environmental attributes that enter into the interaction equation for "good life" outcomes.

What role might the general ecological model have in theory development efforts in future years? We believe that it will continue to serve valuable orienting functions for professionals, particularly in sensitizing new generations of gerontologists to the fact that environment is more than simply a background "surround" against which behavior is enacted and sensitizing new generations of designers to the importance of the individual and one's adaptive or maladaptive responses. Environmental gerontologists may continue to draw upon the practical, almost axiomatic, relations specified by the original model and appreciate the complexity of person-environment interactions specified through its revisions. However, we believe that although it is important to revisit the essential issues and missions specified by the model, it is time for environmental gerontologists to release the model itself from loftier expectations that, by virtue of its theoretical level and paradigmatic nature, it simply cannot fulfill.

As to the future, we believe that contextually embedded, problem-focused models that preserve both the immediacy and holistic nature of person-environment transactions could yield a greater empirical understanding of the ecology of adaptive processes than the classic predecessors afforded. See Golant (in press) for suggestions regarding a refreshing alternative focus on environmental behaviors and activities as theoretical constructs in person-environment models. Establishing contextual validity for such models might be possible across adaptive contexts posing similar challenges that place elders at risk. However, such higher-level generalizations may no longer represent critical elements of the original phenomena of interest (Stokols, 1987). Perhaps we should be satisfied with an environmental science of both problem-posing and palliative contexts, one that affords, at best, "petite" or limited generalizations (Stake, 1995) that preserve a focus on individual differences in context and fosters a differential gerontology of person-environment relations. At the same time, the general ecological model in its more evolved form may continue to provide a valuable heuristic for conceptualizing broader fundamental elements and outcomes of environmental adaptation.

REFERENCES

Baer, D. (1973). Control of developmental process: Why wait? In J. Nesselroade & H. Reese (Eds.), *Life-span developmental psychology: Methodological issues* (pp. 185-193). New York: Academic Press.

Baltes, P., & Baltes, M. (1990). *Successful aging: Perspectives from the behavioral sciences.* New York: Cambridge University Press.

Baltes, P., Lindenberger, U., & Staudinger, U. (1998). Life-span theory in developmental psychology. In W. Damon & R. Lerner (Eds.), *Handbook of Child Psychology: Vol 1. Theoretical models of human development* (5th ed., pp. 1029-1144). New York: John Wiley & Sons.

Barker, R. G. (1968). *Ecological psychology.* Stanford, CA: Stanford University Press.

Bradburn, N. (1969). *The structure of psychological well-being.* Chicago: Aldine.

Bronfenbrenner, U., & Morris, P. (1998). The ecology of developmental processes. In W. Damon & R. Lerner (Eds.), *Handbook of Child Psychology: Vol 1. Theoretical models of human development* (5th ed., pp. 992-1028). New York: John Wiley & Sons.

Carp, F., & Carp, A. (1984). A complementary/congruence model of well-being on mental health for the community elderly. In I. Altman, M. P. Lawton, & J. F. Wohlwill (Eds.), *Elderly people and their environment* (pp. 279-336). New York: Plenum Press.

Costa, P., & McCrae, R. (1992). Four ways five factors are basic. *Personality and Individual Differences, 13,* 653-665.

Denzin, N. (1970). *The research act.* Chicago: Aldine Publishing Company.

Elder, G. (1998). The life course and human development. In W. Damon & R. Lerner (Eds.), *Handbook of Child Psychology: Vol. 1. Theoretical models of human development* (5th ed., pp. 939-992). New York: John Wiley & Sons.

Friedman, S., & Wachs, T. (Eds.). (1999). *Measuring environment across the life span.* Washington, DC: American Psychological Association.

Gatz, M., Siegler, I., & Tyler, F. (1986). Attributional components of locus of control: Longitudinal, retrospective, and contemporaneous analyses. In M. Baltes & P. Baltes (Eds.), *The psychology of control and aging* (pp. 237-263). Hillsdale, NJ: Lawrence Erlbaum Associates.

Gitlin, L. N. (in press-a). M. Powell Lawton's vision of the role of the environment in aging processes and outcomes: A glance backward to move us forward. In K. W. Schaie, H. W. Wahl, H. Mollenkopf, & F. Oswald (Eds.), *Aging in the community: Living arrangements and mobility.* New York: Springer.

Gitlin, L. N. (in press-b). Conducting research on home environments: lessons learned and new directions. *The Gerontologist.*

Golant, S. (in press). Conceptualizing time and behavior in environmental gerontology: A pair of old issues deserving new thought. *The Gerontologist.*

Kahana, E. (1982). A congruence model of person-environment interaction. In M. P. Lawton, P. G. Windley, & T. O. Byerts (Eds.), *Aging and the environment: Theoretical approaches* (pp. 97-121). New York: Springer.

Lawton, M. P. (1982). Competence, environmental press, and the adaptation of older people. In M. P. Lawton, P. Windley, & T. O. Byerts (Eds.), *Aging and the environment: Theoretical approaches* (pp. 33-59). New York: Springer.

Lawton, M. P. (1983). Environment and other determinants of well-being in older people. *The Gerontologist, 23*(4), 349-357.

Lawton, M. P. (1985). The elderly in context: Perspectives from environmental psychology and gerontology. *Environment and Behavior, 17,* 501–519.

Lawton, M. P. (1989a). Environmental proactivity and affect in older people. In S. Spacapan & S. Oskamp (Eds.), *Social psychology of aging* (pp. 135-164). Newbury Park, CA: Sage Publications.

Lawton, M. P. (1989b). Behavior relevant ecological factors. In K. W. Schaie & C. Schooler (Eds.), *Social structure and aging: Psychological processes* (pp. 57-77). Hillsdale, NJ: Erlbaum.

Lawton, M. P. (1989c). Three functions of the residential environment. *Journal of Housing for the Elderly, 5*, 35-50.

Lawton, M. P. (1990). An environmental psychologist ages. In I. Altman & K. Christensen (Eds.), *Environment and behavior studies: Emergent intellectual traditions* (pp. 339-363). New York: Plenum Press.

Lawton, M. P. (1999). Environmental taxonomy: Generalizations from research with older adults. In S. Friedman & T. Wachs (Eds.), *Measuring environment across the life span* (pp. 91-124). Washington, DC: American Psychological Association.

Lawton, M. P. (2000). Chance and choice make a good life. In J. Birren & J. Schroots (Eds.), *A history of geropsychology in autobiography* (pp. 185-196). Washington, DC: American Psychological Association.

Lawton, M. P., & Nahemow, L. (1973). Ecology and the aging process. In C. Eisdorfer & M. P. Lawton (Eds.), *The psychology of adult development and aging* (pp. 619-674). Washington, DC: American Psychological Association.

Lawton, M. P., & Simon, B. (1968). The ecology of social relationships in housing for the elderly. *The Gerontologist, 8*, 108-115.

Lewin, K. (1935). *Dynamic theory of personality*. New York: McGraw-Hill.

Magnusson, D., & Stattin, H. (1998). Person-context interaction theories. In W. Damon & R. Lerner (Eds.), *Handbook of Child Psychology: Vol 1. Theoretical models of human development* (5th ed., pp. 685-760). New York: John Wiley & Sons.

Merton, R. (1967). *On theoretical sociology*. New York: The Free Press.

Murray, H. A. (1938). *Explorations in personality*. New York: Oxford.

Nahemow, L. (2000). The ecological theory of aging: Powell Lawton's legacy. In R. Rubinstein, M. Moss, & M. Kleban (Eds.), *The many dimensions of aging*. New York: Springer.

Norris-Baker, C., & Scheidt, R. (1994). From "Our Town" to "Ghost Town"?: The changing context of home for rural elders. *International Journal of Aging and Human Development, 38*, 181-202.

Parmalee, P., & Lawton, M. P. (1990). The design of special environments for the aged. In J. Birren & K. W. Schaie (Eds.), *Handbook of the psychology of aging* (pp. 464-488). New York: Academic Press.

Rowe, J., & Kahn, R. (1998). *Successful aging*. New York: Random House.

Rowles, G. (1984). Aging in rural environments. In I. Altman, M. P. Lawton, & J. F. Wohlwill (Eds.), *Elderly people and the environment* (pp. 129-157). New York: Plenum Press.

Rowles, G. (1987). A place to call home. In L. L. Carstensen & B. A. Edelstein (Eds.), *Handbook of clinical gerontology* (pp.335-35). New York: Pergamon Press.

Rubinstein, R. (1998). The phenomenology of housing for older people. In R. Scheidt & P. Windley (Eds.), *Environment and aging theory: A focus on housing* (pp. 89-110). Westport, CT: Greenwood Press.

Scheidt, R. (1985). The mental health of the aged in rural environments. In R. Coward & G. Lee (Eds.), *The elderly in rural society* (pp. 105-127). New York: Springer.

Scheidt, R. (1998). The mental health of the elderly in rural environments. In R. Coward & J. Krout (Eds.), *Aging in rural settings: Life circumstances and distinctive features.* New York: Springer.

Scheidt, R. (in press). The nested context of technology: A response to Wahl and Mollenkopf. In N. Charness & K. W. Schaie (Eds.), *Impact of technology on older persons.* New York: Springer.

Scheidt, R., & Norris-Baker, L. (1999). Place therapies for older adults: Conceptual and interventive approaches. *International Journal of Aging and Human Development, 48,* 1-15.

Scheidt, R., & Windley, P. (1985). The ecology of aging. In J. Birren & K. W. Schaie (Eds.), *Handbook of the psychology of aging* (pp. 245-260). New York: Van Nostrand Reinhold.

Schooler, K. (1982). Response of the elderly to environment: A stress-theoretic perspective. In M. P. Lawton, P. G. Windley, & T. O. Byerts (Eds.), *Aging and the environment: Theoretical approaches* (pp. 80-96). New York: Springer.

Stake, R. (1995). *The art of case study research.* Thousand Oaks, CA: Sage Publications.

Stokols, D. (1987). Conceptual strategies of environmental psychology. In D. Stokols & I. Altman (Eds.), *Handbook of environmental psychology* (pp. 41-70). New York: Wiley & Sons.

Wahl, H. W. (2001). Environmental influences on aging and behavior. In J. Birren & K. W. Schaie (Eds.), *Handbook of the psychology of aging* (5th ed.) (pp. 215-237). New York: Academic Press.

Wahl, H. W., & Mollenkopf, H. (in press). Impact of technological changes on the quality of living environments for the elderly. In N. Charness & K. W. Schaie (Eds.), *The impact of technology on older persons.* New York: Springer.

Wahl, H. W., & Weisman, G. (in press). Environmental gerontology at the beginning of the new millennium: Reflections on its historical, empirical, and theoretical development. *The Gerontologist.*

Willems, E. (1973). Behavioral ecology and experimental analysis: Courtship is not enough. In J. Nesselroade and H. Reese (Eds.), *Life-span developmental psychology: Methodological issues* (pp. 195-217). New York: Academic Press.

CHAPTER 3

Ecology and the Aging Self

ROBERT L. RUBINSTEIN
DEPARTMENT OF SOCIOLOGY AND ANTHROPOLOGY
UNIVERSITY OF MARYLAND

KATE DE MEDEIROS
DOCTORAL PROGRAM IN GERONTOLOGY
UMBC: UNIVERSITY OF MARYLAND BALTIMORE COUNTY

In this chapter we examine the relationship of *the self* and the ecology of later life. We review literature about the self and the ecology of later life and present an argument that reshapes some of this literature. More specifically, we will examine the "fit" between the self—a cultural and psychological entity—and the environment as constructed through ecological theory. The chapter finds that there is a significant failure in theory to incorporate the self, leading to some unrealized consequences and lack of appropriate richness. In evaluating this theory we suggest an alternative point of view based on the symbolic nature of human culture and its representation in narrative and language. This we believe incorporates more of the vitality of the self.

Development of the self in later life occurs in both sociocultural and eco-environmental contexts. In the sociocultural domain, both powerful social forces and cultural meanings dramatically affect and construct the life course. At the present time the older self is changing dramatically in its conceptualization due to new economic, health, social, cultural, and political circumstances (Giddens, 1991; Taylor, 1989), the political economy, the body, lifestyle, and culture (Featherstone & Hepworth, 1991; Turner, 1996). How these two domains—the sociocultural and the eco-environmental—intersect is of great interest. At some point, the cultural merges with the ecological in a way that tends toward the recreation and maintenance of the self in later life. A very simple example of this merger is this: Living alone is quite different than living with others and calls for both a differing arrangement of selves and ecological relationships within space and place (Ewing, 1990).

Although there are many social and cultural theories about aging, one set of eco-environmental perspectives that we will address is particularly manifest in theories of *person-environment* (P-E) fit. In examining theories of P-E fit, one notices the nearly complete absence of sociocultural meaning in regard to the self, meaning, and the environment. In fact, P-E theories include very limited social and psychological factors or variables and are also based around the many functional issues that elders may face. This largely limits these theories from taking the self more seriously (see below). How might meaning work out in theories of P-E fit and how might such a relationship evolve between the varieties of settings that elders inhabit? This is a point that we will address in some detail later.

The main goal of this chapter is to outline factors that affect lack of meaning in ecological models and to show how a focus on meaning might complement them. A variety of works have approached this task and will be reviewed here. In so doing, we will examine cultural meaning and P-E fit as these conceptually move outward from the self as embodied in the person to the larger domains of surveillance zones (Rowles, 1981), personal surround-spaces, communities, and special environments for the aged.

We will then examine the idea of meaning as it is arranged in larger conceptual environments around the person. This will be an ecological view of the aging self—by looking at where the self, meaning, and embodiment might fall. We will explore in more detail the notion of the self, its relationship to the environment, and the dynamics of culture—both inside and outside the self. We will discuss the symbolic nature of ecological process and the role of narrative as broadly defined as a representation and construction of personal and cultural meaning. Finally, we will suggest how a narrative approach to the environment may better satisfy the inclusion of meaning in any model (Hazan & Raz, 1998; Raz, 1995).

SOCIOCULTURAL DOMAIN

Our first step in examining the fit between self and environment in old age is to explore the sociocultural domain through three concepts: the self, cultural and personal meaning, and embodiment (or the body as a seat of a culturalized ecology).

THE SELF

Fundamental to defining the self is a notion of what constitutes the self. There is certainly a long history of research and writing on the nature of the self from a variety of disciplinary perspectives, including a growing literature on the aging self itself (Brandstädter & Greve, 1994; Ewing, 1990;

George, 1999; Herzog & Markus, 1999; Kaufman, 1986). Recent work in anthropology, for example, has illuminated the self as a culturally constituted personhood; that is, the process by which a self is defined and made in a cultural space. The question of what it means to be a person in a given setting also varies from place to place (Lindholm, 2001). This literature cannot be fully discussed here. For our purposes, we draw on work by both Brandstädter and Greve (1994), and Herzog and Markus (1999), whose work on the aging self has been important in gerontological literature, to situate the self as the interpreter and mediator of personal experience within the individual.

In the West, and in the United States in particular, the self rests within the individual, and within a larger ethos of individualism (Bellah et al., 1985). Although various external events, identities, expectations, and other factors no doubt influence the self, selfhood is primarily contained within the subjective realm of the person—the *culturally* constituted individual. In framing our definition of self in this respect, we would also include the selves of the demented or cognitively impaired, which may be experienced in a different way than the unimpaired. This is an idea about which very little research has been conducted, but may have profound implications on the self and the environment (Jervis, 2001).

Although Herzog and Markus (1999) distinguish the "self" from "self concept," the two are related. Herzog and Markus define self-concept narratively as "the socio-culturally appropriate stories we learn to tell about ourselves," which are the "understandings of the self that are enduring and recurrent" (p. 231). Herzog and Markus' view suggests that self-narrative is an important aspect of selfhood. Much work suggests the need for outside validation of the self (Erikson, 1980/1959; Goffman, 1969; Mead, 1993). But here we are concerned more with the cultural and personal constitution of selfhood.

Brandstädter and Greve (1994) state that their use of self corresponds closely to Erikson's (1980) understanding of the self-concept, specifically to include only self-protective processes "which are central or relevant to the person's self-conception" (p. 53). They list three essential aspects to self-concept:

- continuity and permanence,
- discriminative relevance (e.g., in which one distinguishes one's self from others, in one's own view), and
- biographical meaningfulness (only those things which the person considers important in his or her biography).

Problems arise when internal inconsistencies, "personally valued aptitudes, traits, or dispositions" affect discriminative relevance, and internal or external events affect continuity. Achieving congruence between present and future states is important. Discrepancies are reduced through "problem-directed action" in self-reference activities, adjustments to self-evaluation, and "immunizing" processes to defend against discrepancies. Brandstädter and Greve propose an Assimilated Mode consisting of "instrumental and self-corrective activities," "compensatory activities," and "confirming actions." The Assimilated Mode occurs through accommodation of goals and standards, such as disengaging from "blocked goals," "adjustment of aspirations and self-evaluative standards," and using "self-enhancing comparisons."

Unlike Kaufman (1986) who described an elder's sense of an "ageless self," Brandstädter and Greve (1994) propose that the elder's past self is closer to his or her desired self. Ultimately, they suggest that the stable self-esteem many older people have in advanced age is due to accommodative processes that help compensate for loss. In addition, they argue that older people may use "fuzzy and malleable" self-referential concepts, which lend themselves well to the positive effects of immunizing behaviors. Their conclusion is that a balance between assimilative, accommodative, and immunizing modes is key to positive experiences of the aging self (cf. Carstensen & Freund, 1994). Brandstädter and Greve also note that individuals themselves have been shown to have views on what comprises the optimal experience of aging, and that they are based on how people replace or substitute goals over time to best meet their present needs. Although Brandstädter and Greve's approach outlines some of the processes of selfhood, their approach does not treat the issues of personal meaning and how personal meaning changes over time.

CULTURAL AND PERSONAL MEANING

In previous work, we have attempted to develop the notion of meaning as significant throughout the gerontological terrain (Rubinstein, 1989). Cultural meaning concerns the shared and not-so-shared ways in which reality is symbolically constituted. Both cultural systems and persons constitute their realities differently. For example, the meaning of space and place are not human universals, but depend on the larger cultural systems of which they are a part (Basso, 1996; Diaz-Moore, 2000; Kane, 1994; Rapoport, 1969, 1990; Rodman, 2001). Personal meaning is that component of culturally constituted meaning that is utilized by the person to construct personal reality. For example, whereas home has a generic cultural meaning for us (e.g., a place where one lives), "home" is known and individually appropriated through personal use, routines, and local meanings (e.g., the house fitting like a glove, where things are at hand, known and usable). For example, an elder may live in a house but only occupy two rooms (i.e., personal use). Routines may include cleaning rituals, eating breakfast at the kitchen table, watching television in a particular room at a particular time, and others. Local meanings can include the significance of the house to the elder (e.g., it was built by a spouse, it belonged to a parent, it was the first house on the street, and so on). The meaning of home is also worked out dialogically or transactionally through ongoing conversations and narratives to oneself and to others. Finally, meaning can also refer to physical, social, and personal components affecting the dynamics between an individual and his or her living space (Oswald & Wahl, 2001; Rubinstein, 1987, 1989, 2002; Wahl, 2001).

EMBODIMENT

Csordas (1988) has described embodiment in this way: "the body is not an *object* to be studied in relation to culture, but is to be considered as the *subject* of culture" (p. 5). In other words, embodiment comprises a continuing negotiation and reinterpretation between the self, a myriad of externally placed identities relative to the physical body, and the relationship between the body (past, present, and future) to the environment (Csordas, 1988). We use the term "embodiment" to refer to the complex set of meanings and physical realities associated with one's body. For example, weight, height, health, comfort, pain, mobility, and attractiveness, all comprise the larger notion of embodiment—the physical and emotional sensations and conceptions associated with one's body. To reduce embodiment to a single, objectified variable would be to severely minimize the importance of the ongoing self-body-environment interaction (Waskel, Douglass, & Edgely, 2000). One example of what we mean here concerns functional decline. Culture constructs decline as the major metaphor for old age itself. In a sense, this deep cultural theme is the same as the way in which we socioculturally experience functional loss, through internalization within the person. A difficulty in rising from a chair, for example, implicates the entire cultural apparatus of decline, a metaphor that runs throughout our cultural life as well as self-esteem and personal competence (discussed later). Similarly, elements such as bodily focus or place attachment also are embodied relative to their experience (Oswald & Wahl, 2001; Rubinstein, 1989; Wahl, 2001). Embodiment is also experienced through the positioning of the body within routines of everyday life (Spencer et al., 2001).

ECO-ENVIRONMENTAL PERSPECTIVES

Having described three sociocultural concepts central to our position, our next step is to closely examine ecological models of aging. The ecological model of aging, in its various forms, as P-E "fit," congruence and similar terms, has had an important place in gerontology and in the study of P-E

interaction in later life. More than the usual psychosocial theory in gerontology, this set of models has practical implications for the design of living
settings in later life (Zeisel, 1997). These related theories provide a functional, ecological, and psychosocial scheme for understanding the fit
between the aging person and his or her environment at a variety of levels. Following this set of theories, design of living settings for the aged has
often tried to balance an appropriate match of environmental access that is
both challenging and rewarding to the elder (Parmelee & Lawton, 1990).
With physical decline, illness, or increasing functional or neurological disability, environments must be altered, or persons "re-placed" immediately
or gradually, to recalibrate the fit.

Although both physical and social fit may be ecologically maximal in a
given setting, P-E fit can be altered by the elder's consciousness of the life
world, by how the older person experiences the self, by how a person individually interprets cultural meaning and the importance of place in later
life, and by a person's self-knowledge of bodily experience (Howell, 1983).
Consequently, P-E fit theories compromise what Geertz (2000) might have
sardonically called "thin description;" at best P-E fit theories clearly show
the interaction of variables and measure press and competence, but they
don't say much about the self, the person, or his or her life. Nevertheless,
it is important to recognize the role of environmental fit theories in shaping thought about the elderly and in shaping real-world solutions to physical and mental challenges among the aged.

The ecological model of aging (Lawton & Nahemow, 1973) and the congruence model of P-E (Kahana, 1982) have become key theoretical corner-
stones for research on the ecological interplay between older individuals
and their environments (Cvitkovich & Wister, 2001; Knipscheer et al., 2000;
Lawton, 1998; Wahl, Oswald, & Zimprich, 1999). Each identifies key measurable characteristics of individuals and their environments and suggests
how levels of variables within one may affect levels within the other.
However, we argue that through a misconceptualization of selves, both
models diminish or exclude some of the most compelling yet least mod-
eled aspects of the relationship of aging and environment. It is important
to note as well that although personality has been considered a key P-E fit
variable in some approaches, we define the self differently from personality and view it as a more central sociocultural constant. The three elements
we discussed earlier—the self within its cultural environment (Hallowell,
1955); personal meaning (Howell, 1983; Rubinstein, Kilbride, & Nagy,
1992); and the role of embodiment—are significant lacunae. We are not
suggesting that the concepts self, embodiment, and meaning are *completely*
absent from either model, but they are nearly absent or fragmentary. Their
fragmentation masks their overall importance as whole entities by reducing a sense of their effects. Moreover, self, meaning, and embodiment are
not accounted for by the implicit theories these models represent (see

below). In short, elements of meaning are too scattered throughout and too difficult to isolate as individual components to emphasize in their own right in P-E theories. Yet the everyday experiences of the elderly suggest that these components constitute an important part of the P-E fit (Basso, 1996; Diehl, 1998; Kilbride & Nagy, 1992; Lawton, 1999; Rubinstein, Ryff, Marshall, & Clarke, 1999; Wahl, 2001).

In essence, these on-paper P-E models presuppose a more hidden model, namely that ecology and environment directly influence *an organism,* rather than a person who lives in a world of meaning. This means that in the models, the relationship between environment and the person is *unmediated by culture.* It is a significantly incomplete and impossible view. Human life *is* based on meaning and meaning systems (Geertz, 2000). In our view, P-E models must be based on another implicit model: that environment influences the person in ways mediated by cultural and personal meaning. To push this concept a bit further, one might say that although some ecological stressors—such as temperature—may be "purely objective" in nature, both the person and the stressor are constructed through the same meaning system that acts as the mediator not only of "objective" phenomena but all others as well (Sahlins, 1976). Thus, eco-environmental factors *engage and* are situated in a complex meaning system.

Among the many domains explored by theories of P-E fit, competence, adaptability, and well-being stand out as both key features in general and key components through which the ideas of self, meaning, and embodiment are scattered. With regards to the study of competence, Diehl (1998) has suggested that, "Competence should be seen as the result of the transactions between an active human individual and his or her physical and social environment" (p. 423), and "competence does not exist in a vacuum but involves [older adults'] active adaptation of a variety of environmental conditions" (p. 429). Diehl's insights are important, but can be pushed further when we consider the "human individual", or self, as culturally (that is, meaningfully) constructed. Thus, we must consider person-ecological interface as symbolic and meaningful.

Nahemow (2000) describes the *Ecological Theory of Aging* (ETA) as exploring, "the interplay between individuals and their environments," (p. 23) with key focus on the individual's adaptation to the external environment relative to the "environmental press," or the objective and subjective environmental forces that evoke a response by the individual (p. 24), and his or her level of competence (Lawton, 1989, 1998). Similarly, the congruence model of P-E interaction suggests that salient "personal life space" dimensions within an environment play a strong role in predicting overall well-being (Kahana, 1982, p. 98). Lawton (1998) provides an excellent critical discussion of each theory. Since the 1970s, several approaches to understanding the P-E relationship in old age have been developed and studied (Cvitkovich & Wister, 2001; Lawton, 1998; Nahemow, 2000; Scheidt, 1998;

Wahl, 2001; Windley & Scheidt, 1980). Besides the two models, Lawton's ETA and Kahana's congruence model that will be discussed here, there are other P-E theories. These include Moos's (1976) social ecological approach, which emphasized the importance of choice, social climate, policy, and personal control within a given environment (Maddox, 2001; Parr, 1980; Scheidt, 1998; Timko & Moos, 1991); Carp and Carp's (1984) "environmental proactivity" hypothesis, which broadened the domain of "environmental press" to include positive opportunities that may impact the P-E relationship (Cvitkovich & Wister, 2001; Lawton, 1998; Windley & Scheidt, 1980); and Rowles's (1980) "transactional view," which linked "insideness," or the present and autobiographical selves, with the present physical and social environments (Lawton, 1998; Wahl, 2001). Although these and other theories have made important contributions to environmental research, they may lack the simple, linear structure and discrete, measurable variables, which have made the ETA and congruence models more easily applied and more often used (Cvitkovich & Wister, 2001; Lawton, 1998; Wahl, 2001). We will therefore provide a more in-depth overview of these models, specifically looking at where and how the aging self, personal meaning and the role of embodiment fit into each.

THE ECOLOGICAL THEORY OF AGING (ETA)

The ETA describes behavior and affect as the function of personal competence level (y axis) and strength of environmental press (x axis), mediated by adaptation level as the point of balance (Lawton, 1982, 1989, 1998; Nahemow, 2000). In the model, competence is "low" and environmental press is "weak" at the origin point, increasing along the axes. Adaptation level comprises the balance point. The zones of maximum comfort, marginal and negative affect, and maladapted behavior appear to the left of the adaptation level; maximum performance potential, marginal and negative affect, and maladaptive behavior to the right. The well-known schema, simple yet rich, provides an effective way for considering the P-E relationship. To take a closer look at the model's components, we will consider its key terms and associated methods of assessment. "Competence" in the model refers to "the theoretical upper limit of capacity of the individual to function in the areas of biological health, sensation and perception, motor behavior, and cognition" (Lawton, 1983, p. 350; Lawton, 1982). There is nothing here at all about how persons interpret the environment, leading to an emic assessment of upper limits. Domains of competence include physical, psychological, social, and emotional areas and are often assessed through measures of health behaviors, self-maintaining and instrumental activities of daily living, mental status, enrichment activities, interpersonal interactions with friends and family, and health conditions

(Diehl, 1998; Lawton, 1982; Lawton, 1983; Nahemow, 2000). However, as Diehl (1998) and others have suggested, limiting "competence" to measurable tasks fails to capture "everyday competence" or the complex way in which people use a broad and overlapping array of strategies and skills in real-life situations (Schaie & Willis, 1999; Wahl, Oswald, & Zimprich, 1999). In effect, the performance-focused measures provide only an "X-ray" view of the self without the distinguishable qualities unique to the whole person or the ways in which they interpret the world. Consequently, competence in the ETA does not include direct assessment of the aging self, personal meaning, or embodiment, (nor does it consider any temporal component, either through daily variations of everyday routines or over longer periods of time) although this triad may be partially inferred through self-reporting scales of health status, personal relationships, personal enrichment activities, or others.

"Environmental press" in the ETA describes the objective (alpha) and subjective (beta) environmental forces that evoke a response by the individual (Lawton, 1989, 1998; Nahemow, 2000). Press is, therefore, the main stimulus that places a demand on an individual leading to a specific behavioral outcome (Lawton, 1982). Measures used to assess the strength of environmental press include self-report scales on safety of neighborhood and home, proximity of the environment to needed services and ability to access those services, ability to communicate needs to others, and environmental predictability (Nahemow, 2000). Missing from the environmental press assessments are key subjective measures of autobiographical and personal meaning of place, physical and social comfort, attitudes toward the specific environment, homelikeness, and others (Cvitkovich & Wister, 2001; Howell, 1980, 1983; Nahemow, 2000; Namazi et al., 1989). It is likely that this personal sense of, and attachment to, place *extends or shapes* personal competence and the perception of press through a variety of techniques including the pure disregard of stressors ("immunization") due to a greater personal sense of attachment to place and the segmentation of an activity to a process over time by creating smaller, more manageable units.

The relation between competence and environmental press leads to overall adaptation level, demonstrated through behavior and affect. The absolute adaptation level refers to the "indifference point," when competence and press have neither a positive nor negative effect on behavior or affect (Lawton, 1989, p. 3.). The two zones surrounding adaptation level—the comfort zone and the challenge zone—comprise the adaptation range and represent the individual's ability to respond to weaker or stronger environmental press through strategies, which are dependent upon one's level of competence. In this model, adaptation is the psychologist's attempt to dimensionalize human experience as well as more distally the self, meaning, and embodiment (see below). Adaptation, though, does not account for how selves apply meaningful understandings of their life-world to the process of "adaptation." Given the narrow scope of assessment tools for competence and environment, it is difficult to determine from the model what effect more subjective, deeply personal aspects of the aging individual in a given environment have in determining adaptation level and, ultimately, whether positive adaptation equals well-being in a holistic sense.

THE CONGRUENCE MODEL OF PERSON-ENVIRONMENT FIT

In response to some of the person-centered issues not addressed by the ETA, Kahana's (1982) congruence model describes the fit between salient, "personal life space" (p. 98) dimensions and environmental influences. In this model, congruence or a positive fit is thought to contribute to overall well being, whereas incongruence or negative fit results in either adaptive compensation strategies to achieve congruence or, when compensation is not possible, to impaired psychological health (Cvitkovich & Wister, 2001; Kahana, 1982; Lawton, 1998). It should be noted that a major limitation of the congruence model is its focus on nursing home residents, which may prove inapplicable to community-based settings.

The congruence model proposes seven dimensions, with corresponding subdimensions, for congruence to occur between the environment and individual. The seven are as follows:

- segregate
- congregate
- institutional control
- structure
- stimulation/engagement
- affect
- impulse control

(Kahana, 1982)

Unlike the structure of the ETA, which proposes an overall relationship between environment and competence, the congruence model presents environmental-individual pairings within each dimension; this means that each subdimension has an environmental and individual component through which congruence occurs (or does not occur). Overall congruence is therefore the function of several smaller congruence-incongruence relationships that influence overall well-being.

The first dimension of the congruence model, the segregate domain, presents components of sameness and change for both environment and individual. Congruence is determined by the degree to which the environment is homogeneously composed and similar to a previous environment, and the degree to which the individual prefers sameness to change and continuity. The congregate dimension deals with how much the environment supports privacy, individual expression, and autonomy and whether the individual desires these. Institutional control looks at staff's expectations toward conformity and dependency in light of the individual's need for support and personal control. Structure is centered on the environment and individual's need for order and ambiguity. Stimulation includes the level of input from the physical and social environment and the person's desired engagement level. Affect addresses the mechanism in place for emotional display and experiences (e.g., excitement, calm) in relation to individual needs. Finally, impulse control describes the environment's rules for impulse and motor expression versus the individual's control level (Kahana, 1982; Kahana & Kahana, 1983, 1996). In our view, these dimensions, although significant, tend to overpsychologize the realm of personal and biographic meaning that is so important to the aged in everyday life. These dimensions, we believe, capture little of the ways in which the person actually interprets the environment or understands her or his ecological relationships.

Further, although the interrelationship between the seven dimensions presents a different way of examining the P-E relationship than the ETA, it essentially doesn't directly address attitudes that comprise the larger notion of self or meaning within and toward an environment. For example, "structure" might be more complex in many ways. Instead, it breaks down some of the larger ideas expressed in the ETA into smaller couplings to allow a finer assessment of P-E phenomena. If the ETA is an "X-Ray view," then the congruence model perhaps is more like a CAT scan, which can examine interrelationships more closely within the overall body but is still unable to capture the essence of the individual. Neither of these theories, the ETA or the congruence model, tell us much about the person who, in fact, lives in a world of meaning.

Concerning the models we have described above, Lawton (1983) has noted, "The self . . . is indicated only indirectly and in a glancing fashion by the many measurable attributes from the sectors of the good life. The self is inaccessible to measurement directly . . . but it may be thought of as the repository of the most meaningful aspects of the good life" (p. 356). In other words, the self may be inaccessible to measurements in a quantitative sense, but not inaccessible to research.

INTERSECTION OF THE SOCIOCULTURAL AND ECO-ENVIRONMENTAL

There are many ways in which the ETA and congruence theory fail to identify and utilize a variety of important personal activities that are highlighted through a focus on the self, meaning, and embodiment. First, the "ecological" reality is that people do not live their lives with reference to these models, but to others that are implicit personally and culturally. Implicit models of the self involve the nature of experience, temporal phenomena, and "the habitus" (Bourdieu, 1977, 1990). For example, everyday life, including eco-environmental relations, is *experienced* phenomenologically (Bachelard, 1992; Rowles, 1987). In the everyday experience of elders, environmental relationships are micronegotiated through constant monitoring of bodily states, activity demands in the context of time and ever changing situations, and the meaning world of the self.

Figure 3.1 presents a conceptual diagram of the complex interplay between environment, person, and culture.

In our diagram, "environment" represents the physical space surrounding the person. "Person" includes self, meaning, and embodiment. Culture intercedes as a powerful mediator as well as originating impetus. Originating culture refers to the overall cultural ideals that frame the reference point for both the outsider (e.g., the researcher and the individual); it includes our assumptions about space (e.g., what a house should be composed of), language (as a string of meaningful cultural symbols), narration (or the appropriate way to string events together), the concept of self, and many others. Mediating culture encompasses the realm of cultural interpretations unique to the individual. Although rooted in the overall originating culture, mediating culture includes personal influences like past experiences, marginalized (or empowered) status, and other interpretive realms. Through our figure, we also suggest that all approaches to the understanding of P-E begin from a preconceived base (originating culture), which influences how environment and person are conceptualized. In addition, the boundaries between environment, culture, and person are

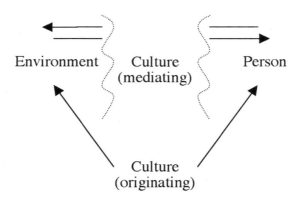

FIGURE 3.1   Interplay between environment, person, and culture.

fluid to suggest an influencing flow between the three as opposed to a pre-dictable linear relationship.

PERSON COMPETENCE

The demand characteristics of everyday life derive their sense of necessity not from bodily competence, but from the level of self-competence that is culturally required for standards of selfhood. This is a second kind of competence that has not been addressed in the eco-environmental aging literature and needs to be considered. Anthropologists have discussed the idea of cultural competence—in one sense the minimum necessary one would have to know and feel to be a member of a culture—for decades. Similarly, as part of a system of personal meaning, elders abstract from the general cultural level (originating culture), altering it through personal experience and interpretation standards for personal competence (mediating culture). This is a kind of personal morality—things one needs to do to feel oneself to be a full person. Although eco-environmental competence is physical, functional, and psychosocial, these are mediated by cultural standards for and personal views of what it means to be a person culturally. Thus, the activities of home or self-maintenance, for example, do not merely respond to "environmental press" or "environmental affordances," but rather respond to the (at least) minimal definition of a personally inculcated set of standards for what one does to be a "person." Embodiment itself is a process by which such cultural standards are in part felt and experienced. *Activities of daily living* (ADLs) and *instrumental activities of daily living* (IADLs) are about competences, environmental press, and objective bodily status, but they are also about what it is to be a person, to be in "decline," to be "ok," and similar issues as defined within a cultural context.

The issue of competence also directly affects those with neurological disease. Although measurement of mental and physical functioning is important, there is another process that has not been addressed much in the literature. This is how others (next-of-kin, care workers) become increasingly responsible for the selfhood of the demented. This selfhood is not functional, but is cultural and personal, referring to who the person is and who the person was. Increasingly, as persons become more and more impaired and move through the long term care system, responsibility for the selfhood of the person is shifted—especially in cases of dementia—from the person to others who may not be knowledgeable or who may not desire this responsibility.

In our view, these are not trivial points. Rather they are an important way to reconstitute our measured view of the aging self in eco-environmental context. Although clearly important and well validated through many studies (Nahemow, 2000), notions of press and ecological competence fail to account for *what it is to be a person*, that is, what it means to have a self. If, in my history, I always make tea at three o'clock in the afternoon and my competence to do so diminishes, this is not so much an environmental issue as one of selfhood; this aspect has been unmodelled. The temporal component is important here as well. As noted by many informants in our previous work, a day may have texture that adds to the qualities of personal experience. An ability to do certain tasks in the morning, or at a certain time of the year, that is, to micromanage competence or press on the basis of personal identity and personal meaning, has not been accounted for in environmental theory, even though it is a primary means through which elders adapt, especially those with diminishing functional abilities. Moreover, these activities and routines are at the core of the self and are symbolically significant to the person; they are what the person does and who she is. Routines and activities are embodied within the person through their unconscious nature and the habitus (Bourdieu, 1977, 1990). Again, it is not so much the environmental issues that are important (although they are); it is the local definition of selfhood that is important: How can I manage to do the things I need to do in order to remain, as best as possible, myself?

BODILY CHANGES: AGING AND ILLNESS

With age, selves and bodies take on important characteristics that affect the dynamic relationship with the environment. Because some form of functional decline is common in advanced age, the embodied self must take into account these changes. Given the particular American cultural construction of the person, two outcomes have been suggested. The first is that the self remains more or less constant, that it is "ageless" (Kaufman, 1986). The self does this through the present-day reworking of present and past material to conform to a given self-concept. In this process, changes in cultural competence or in the embodied self have meaningful ramifications for environmental relations. Life-space may further shrink, which aids in retaining the constancy of the self, because it must face fewer external environmental challenges (Weisman, 1997). The home itself may become a support for the self in a number of ways (see below).

The second possibility is that there is a cutoff or discontinuity in the self, due to severe illness, trauma, relocation, or functional decline (Becker, 1997; Hiatt, 1990). The dramatic event that causes one to redefine the self in later life is traumatic and may be catalytic. Redefinition means both a new relationship with one's body and with one's environment. Such may be seen as examples of increased press or declining competence, a mismatch between "fit" and ability that requires some kind of ecological adjustment. Certainly this is true, but the meaning of this change in environmental relations derives from how the person defines and experiences the embodied self, and is not merely the unmediated outcome of press on the organism. Declining ability to walk or to lift certainly requires adjustments in routine and object relations, but the origin of these changes comes from the culturally constituted embodied self.

Cognitive decline presents another adjustment to these relationships. Unfortunately, there is very little research that deals with the environmental relations of demented elders. How these elders view home or adjust abilities to environments waits to be more thoroughly examined (Aud, 2002; Chaudhury, 1997, 2002; Regnier & Pynoos, 1992; Young, 1998; Zeisel, 1997).

ENVIRONMENT PLACE

Space has no meaning unless it is culturalized. We make constant inferences and interpretations about the nature of space based on who we are as cultural beings; indeed, space is culturally constituted and defined in some way prior to our arrival on it. Place concerns how we individualize or define for a community or for ourselves the meaning of space. Phenomenological studies of space and place have emphasized relationship and experience as key components of the intersection of selves and spaces or places. This literature is important because it focuses on the nature of experience, which is the end product of cultural meaning, the self, and embodiment. We often experience things with emotionality or sensuality that are tied to the self and the historical or biographical experiences of the self.

Rowles (1987) and others (Rubinstein, Kilbride, & Nagy, 1992) have shown that, with aging and its discontents (illness, cognitive impairment, functional decline) comes a miniaturization of space—a decline in the degree of space to which one has or wishes access. During this spatial shift comes a lesser focus on "away places"—except through geographic fantasy—and, in many cases, an increased focus on home and the self. In terms of "the Third Age" (Weiss & Bass, 2002), (a phrase coined to refer to healthy and financially stable elders who, upon retirement, begin a new period of education, volunteerism, sensory cultivation, or travel), the miniaturization of space may be preceded by a period of spatial expansion, through travel and new local activities. Environmental themes change in importance and emphasis under reduced living space and increased press.

There has been some work on the personal surrounds or older persons (Fisher & Giloth, 1999). In the view taken here, these are extensions of the self (see the following sections). Lawton (1985) has described "the control center" a small area, such as a kitchen table, that exemplifies miniaturization. This is an activity center that may include close access to a radio or television, storage of bills, market circulars, store coupons, and a place to sit. The world is addressed from this nook. A similar concept concerning space around the self is the "surveillance zone," Rowles's (1981) well-known notion of the range of vision through a window or from a porch. This is both a geographic interface as well as a social and cultural one, as elders can watch goings-on in the outer world.

Works on the meaning of home (see below) and of personal surrounds have suggested an idea about meaning that has been virtually unaddressed in the literature, and is certainly missed by competence and press models. That is, that every activity and object that involves a habitual, rather unconscious procedure can be considered part of the self (Bourdieu, 1977, 1990). This is an approach that builds on the notion of "behavior setting" (Barker, 1968), which combines both place and activity (Norris-Baker, 1998, 1999). While this phenomenological view would be at odds with standard psychological perspectives on the person, which see the person ending at the skin, this idea would suggest that the *object-activity set* to which a person relates unconsciously be regarded, for lack of a better means of expression, as part of the self. There are several arguments for this.

First, this view would better account for the totality of change in later life; that is that adaptation of the person with age is in fact a larger entity, as the self extends into the world around it. Second, this would reveal a truer picture of the elder through actively constituting the nature of embodiment and habitus as cultural processes such that routines and usual objects enter into a close relationship with the body and through to the self. Third, this might more actively portray the self as both a cultural subject and object, and both as mutually constitutive of eco-environmental relations. Becker, (1997) and others who are concerned with the process of reinventing a life through or after chronic illness, have suggested that the change in embedded bodily and daily unconscious routines is a representation of profound changes in the self as part of both changing (Becker, 1997) and re authored (Kaufman) identities. As Kaufman has noted, despite change, the self appears ageless since it is constantly reinterpreted in the present on the basis of raw materials of the past and present.

THE BUILT ENVIRONMENT

In this chapter, we are pushing towards the notion that what is seen as largely "objective" in models of fit could also be looked at—we feel in a deeper and more productive way—as signs and symbols within a large, complex system of meanings. There is nothing "natural" or "objective" about the natural environment. It is largely understood through cultural and personal meaning. Many indigenous people understand and experience the environment through the meanings that are culturally attached to significant places, land-ideas, and movements. Similarly, there is nothing "natural" or "objective" about the built environment. The way cultural persons interact with the built environment is through this larger system of personal and cultural meaning (Lawrence & Low, 1990).

THE HOME AND PERSONAL POSSESSIONS

There has been a great deal of research on home environments of elders and the meaning of home, its objects, and its surround spaces (McHugh & Mings, 1996; Rowles, 1981; Wagnild, 2001). Some of this work has dealt with the centrality of home and its objects in functioning as a site of embodied meaning, as an extension of the self or person, and as a setting that helps to maintain the self (Kalymun, 1985; Morris, O'Bryant & Nocera, 1985; Paton & Cram, 1992, 1992; Savashinsky, 2001). Certainly, homes can present considerable challenge to elders, who may reside in spaces that are too big, or with environmental obstacles that are dangerous or currently cannot be handled. Because of this, many elders downsize their homes and relocate, leaving a long inhabited home for something smaller and transporting elements of environmental meaning—their possessions and objects—with them (O'Bryant & Murray, 1986; Rowles & Ravdal, 2002; Schwarz, Brent & Barry, 1996; Sixsmith & Sixsmith, 1991). Because of the closeness of the home to the body and the home's role as a kind of "second skin" for the self, it is perhaps easier to see the home in its symbolic dimensions and as a medium for narration about the person. Further, the sense of being-in-place (Rowles, 2000), unconsciously personally establishes another form of relationship of self to environment. Assistive technology and the prosthetic environment (Gitlin, 2002; Pinto et al., 2000), home modification (Tabarrah, Silverstein, & Seeman, 2000), aging in place (Fisher & Gilroth, 1999; Rojo et al., 2001), and personal care (Spencer et al., 2001) are phenomena which display and construct both the embodied self and narrate the story of the person.

OTHER SPACES

With respect to places outside the home, the self can permeate three sorts of environments, places that are the object of fantasy (Rowles, 1978; Scott-Weber & Koebel, 2001), spaces of engagement, such as those with which one interacts on a daily, weekly, or monthly basis, and places of attachment. Places of fantasy include those with which one has a biographical relationship and therefore engage memory of the past (Blokland, 2000); even others' descriptions of places *they* have visited may be called up here. These are places one may never see again or that one has never seen. Places of engagement expand out from the home and involve the self in routines reoccurring over periods of time. Places of attachment include those with an environmental or cognitive valence, often in the past (Altman & Low, 1992; Proshansky, Fabian, & Kaminoff, 1983). Although persons may have different attitudes to such places, their engagement, whether conscious or unconscious, depends on a world experienced and constructed by the self (Perkins Taylor, 2001). Streets, neighbors' homes, communities, and sites of amenities all come into play here. Relations with "other places" also have been described as "transactional" by some (Howell, 1994; Oxley et al., 1986; Scheidt & Norris-Baker, 1990) and involve personal and family relations with streets, locales, communities, and neighborhoods (LaGory, Ward, & Sherman, 1983). Issues of the narration of self in specialized environments such as assisted living, nursing homes, Alzheimer's disease units, congregate house, and board and care are complex and not fully investigated (Hazen & McCree, 2001; Mardsen, 2001; Yee et al., 1999; Young, 1998).

THE NARRATION OF "FIT"

Narrative, or telling somebody about something, is one of the most important human endeavors. The use of narrative approaches offers another way to better understand P-E fit. Cultural elements (such as the self, meaning, and embodiment) are critical in this relationship. In a sense, a person in place—regardless of which approach to competence is used—is also telling a story about himself or herself, using environmental objects, experiences, capacities, understandings, and relationships as a particular language of expression (Howell, 1983; Rubinstein, 1987).

In some sense, because the environment is objectified, the language used to express it is an action language, that is, the act of expression is itself an act of doing. A desire to move or to stay in a long occupied home, the inability to rise from a chair some of the time, difficulty or success in making meals, and a routine need for tea at three o'clock in the afternoon are part of the story of the self that unfolds over time. They are a function of negotiated selfhood over time. In this sense, such concepts as adaptation, when applied to humans, are symbolic in nature; elders make something of the adaptation event, with little reference to the "objective" forces that "necessitate" adaptation. It is important to note that we do not yet have a complete understanding of either this environmental language or its symbol system. The audience for this language appears to be other significant people as well as elders themselves. In later life, an important function of environmental relations may be to "speak" to the person and to others about one's self and one's life. We would argue that narrative in its broadest sense as story, environment, and their subjective fit is a more "ecologically valid," "on-the-ground" approach to P-E relations. It is also rooted in a variety of theories about human action, cognition, narration, and meaning systems, which are beyond the scope of this chapter. To dismiss this perspective would be to dishonor the ways in which the aged define competence and press for themselves. This theory would also eliminate the significant problem in P-E theory of the lack of mediation between the environment and "the organism," which is more clearly defined in this chapter as a cultural entity (cf. Krampen, 1991).

CONCLUSION

We would suggest a number of points that would better explain the relationship of person to place if one takes as given the reality that people live first and foremost in worlds of meaning through which they assess and experience the world and through which they themselves are constructed. The most important of these points is that the notion of the person employed in the ETA and other eco-environmental models, while predictive in many ways, has nothing much to say about people, as Lawton (1993) said (noted earlier). Such models purport to be about only "objective" phenomena and to venture only very little into the subjective. However, they are not objective because any human or psychosocial category they contain, at least in a small way, refers to the complex nature of human life. Nevertheless, they miss some very important components, as we have described here. They also miss the element of time, including the micro time of daily-lived experience. They miss the myriad of strategies and understanding that people use or undertake to manage eco-environmental relations. Accordingly, they miss elements of the self, of meaning, and of embodiment. Moreover, they miss the rich systems of meaning that structure relationships with press and competence. To have press and competence unmediated by cultural and personal meaning raises serious problems that affect in a unique way much work in environment and aging.

We are suggesting that ecological "theory" would benefit from conceptualization with two aims. First, the ecological model must be based on the rich set of meanings with which persons actually engage the environment. Taking this as given, there is much in the way of flow between the person and the environment, a subjective erasure of the boundary between subject and object at times, and a large number of both implicit and explicit meanings. Second, the model must incorporate the way in which the body (as part of the overall person) and the environment relate. More important, it must revise a view of the self to include the acts of personal and cultural interpretation and ecological relations and understandings.

One of the most important elements of cultural life is narrative, or storytelling. In different cultural contexts, people tell stories as a way of constructing and communicating experience. In a sense, the environment and personal ecology may be thought of as a type of symbol system that narrates something. And, the relation of the self and the environment may be thought of as a story, a narrative of sorts that tells, in situated terms, what is happening to the person. This story is based on the ongoing set of interpretations the person makes of the environment and the state of the body at any time. The story may change frequently or hardly at all.

REFERENCES

Altman, I., & Low, S. M. (1992). *Place attachment.* New York: Plenum Press.

Aud, M. (2002). Interactions of behavior and environment as contributing factors in the discharge of residents with dementia from assisted living facilities. *Journal of Housing for the Elderly, 16*(1/2), 61-83.

Bachelard, G. (1992 [1964]). *The poetics of space.* Boston: Beacon Press.

Barker, R. (1968). *Ecological psychology: Concepts and methods for studying the environment of human behavior.* Stanford, CA: Stanford University Press.

Basso, K. (1996). *Wisdom sits in places: Landscape and language among the Western Apache.* Albuquerque: University of New Mexico Press.

Becker, G. (1997). *Disrupted lives: How people create meaning in a chaotic world.* Berkeley: University of California Press.

Bellah, R. N., Madsen, R., Sullivan, W. M., Swidler, A., & Tipton, S. M. (1986). *Habits of the heart: Individualism and commitment in American life.* New York: Harper and Row.

Blockland, T. (2001). Bricks, mortar memories: Neighbourhood and networks in collective acts of remembering. *International Journal of Urban and Regional Research, 25*(2), 268-283.

Bourdieu, P. (1977). *Outline of a theory of practice.* New York: Cambridge University Press.

Bourdieu, P. (1990 [1980]). *The logic of practice.* New York: Cambridge University Press.

Brandstädter, J., & Greve, W. (1994). The aging self: Stabilizing and protective processes. *Developmental Review, 14,* 52-80.

Carp, F. M., & Carp, A. (1984). A complementary/congruence model of well-being on mental health for the community elderly. In I. Altman, M. P. Lawton, & J.F. Wohlwill (Eds.), *Elderly people and their environment* (pp. 279-336). New York: Plenum Press.

Carstensen, L. L., & Freund, A. (1994). The resilience of the aging self. *Developmental Review, 14,* 81-92.

Chaudhury, H. (1997). Self and reminiscence of place: Toward a theory of (re)discovering selfhood in place-based reminiscence for people with dementia. *Environmental Design Research Association, 28,* 79-88.

Chaudhury, H. (2002). Journey back home: Recollecting past places by people with dementia. *Journal of Housing for the Elderly, 16*(1/2), 85-106.

Csordas, T. J. (1988). Embodiment as a paradigm for anthropology. *Ethos,* 5-47.

Cvitkovich, Y., & Wister, A. (2001). A comparison of four person-environment fit models applied to older adults. *Journal of Housing for the Elderly, 14*(1/2), 1-25.

Diaz-Moore, K. (2000). *Culture-meaning-architecture: Critical reflections on the work of Amos Rapoport.* Burlington, VT: Ashgate.

Diehl, M. (1998). Everyday competence in later life: Current status and future directions. *Gerontologist, 38*(4), 422-433.

Erikson, E. (1980). *Identity and the life cycle.* New York: W.W. Norton & Company. (Reprinted from 1959, International Universities Press.)

Ewing, K. (1990). The illusion of wholeness: Culture, self and the experience of inconsistency. *Ethos, 18,* 251-278.

Featherstone, M., & Hepworth, M. (1991). *The mask of aging and the postmodern life course.* Thousand Oaks, CA: Sage Publications.

Fisher, J., & Giloch, R. (1999). Adapting rowhomes for aging in place: The story of Baltimore's "our idea house." *Journal of Housing for the Elderly, 13*(1/2), 3–18.

Geertz, C. (2000 [1973]). *The interpretation of cultures.* New York: Basic Books.

George, L. (1999). Social perspectives on the self in later life. In C. D. Ryff & V. W. Marshall (Eds.), *The self and society in aging processes* (pp. 42-66). New York: Springer.

Giddens, A. (1991). *Modernity and self-identity: Self and society in the late modern age.* Stanford, CA: Stanford University Press.

Gitlin, L. N. (2002). Assistive technology in the home and community for older people: Psychological and social considerations. In M. J. Scherer (Ed.), *Assistive technology: Matching device and consumer for successful rehabilitation* (pp. 109-122). Washington, DC: American Psychological Association.

Goffman, E. (1969). *The presentation of self in everyday life.* London: Allen Lane.

Hallowell, A. I. (1955). *Culture and experience.* New York: Schocken Books.

Hazan, H., & Raz, A. (1998). The authorized self: How middle age defines old age in the postmodern. *Semiotica, 113*(3/4), 257-276.

Hazen, M., & McCree, S. (2001). Environmental support to assist an older adult with independent living: Safety and activity accommodation in senior's housing. *Journal of Housing for the Elderly, 14*(1/2), 27-52.

Herzog, A. R., & Markus, H. R. (1999). The self-concept in life span and aging research. In V. Bengston & K. Warner Schaie (Eds.), *Handbook of theories on aging* (pp. 227-252). New York: Springer.

Hiatt, L. G. (1990). Design of the home environment for the cognitively impaired person. In N. L. Mace (Ed.), *Dementia care: Patient, family and community* (pp. 231-141). Baltimore, MD: The Johns Hopkins University Press.

Howell, S. (1980). Environments as hypotheses in human aging research. In L. W. Poon (Ed.), *Aging in the 1980s: Psychological issues* (pp. 424-432). Washington, DC: American Psychological Association.

Howell, S. C. (1983). The meaning of place in old age. In G. D. Rowles & R. J. Ohta (Eds.), *Aging and milieu: Environmental perspectives on growing old* (pp. 97-107). New York: Academic Press.

Howell, S. C. (1996). Environment and the aging woman: Domains of choice. In I. Altman and A. Churchman (Eds.) *Women and the environment: Vol. 13. Human behavior and environment: Advances in theory and research* (pp. 105-131). New York: Plenum Press.

Jervis, J. L. (2001). Nursing home satisfaction, biography and the life worlds of psychiatrically disabled residents. *Journal of Aging Studies, 15*(3), 237-252.

Kahana, E. (1982). A congruence model of person-environment interaction. In M. P. Lawton, P. G. Windley, & T. O. Byerts (Eds.), *Aging and the environment: Theoretical approaches* (pp. 97-121). New York: Springer.

Kahana, E., & Kahana, B. (1983). Environmental continuity, futurity, and adaptation of the aged. In G. D. Rowles & R. J. Ohta. *Aging and milieu: Environmental perspectives on growing old* (pp. 205-228). New York: Academic Press.

Kahana, E., & Kahana, B. (1996). Conceptual and empirical advances in understanding aging well through proactive adaptation. In V. L. Bengston (Ed.), *Adulthood and aging: Research on continuities and discontinuities* (pp. 18-40). New York: Springer.

Kalymen, M. (1985). The prevalence of factors influencing decisions among elderly women concerning household possessions during relocation. *Journal of Housing for the Elderly*, 3(3-4), 81-99.

Kane, S. C. (1994). *The phantom gringo boat: Shamanic discourse and development in Panama.* Washington, DC: Smithsonian Institution Press.

Kaufman, S. (1986). *The ageless self: Sources of meaning in late life.* Madison: The University of Wisconsin Press.

Knipscheer, C. P. M., Broese van Groenou, M. I., Leene, G. J. F., Beekman, A. T. F., & Deeg, D. J. H. (2000). The effects of environmental context and personal resources on depressive symptomatology in older age: A test of the Lawton model. *Ageing and Society*, 20(2), 183-202.

Krampen, M. (1991). Environmental meaning. In E. H. Zube and G. T. Moore (Eds.), *Advances in environment, behavior, and design* (Vol. 3, pp. 231-268). New York: Plenum Press.

La Gory, M., Ward, R., & Sherman, S. (1983). The ecology of aging: The significance of the neighborhood for elderly populations. (Paper) North Central Sociological Association.

Lawrence, D. L., & Low, S. M. (1990). The built environment and spatial form. *Annual review of anthropology*, 19, 453-505.

Lawton, M. P. (1982). Competence, environmental press, and the adaptation of older people. In M. P. Lawton, P. G. Windley, & T. O. Byerts (Eds.), *Aging and the environment: Theoretical approaches* (pp. 33-59). New York: Springer.

Lawton, M. P. (1983). Environment and other determinants of well-being in older people. *The Gerontologist*, 23(4), 349-357.

Lawton, M. P. (1989). Environmental proactivity and affect in older people. In S. Scpacapan & S. Oskamp (Eds.), *The social psychology of aging* (pp. 135-163). Newbury Park: Sage.

Lawton, M. P. (1998). Environment and aging: Theory revisited. In R. J. Scheidt and P. G. Windley. *Environment and aging theory: A focus on housing* (pp. 1-31). Westport, CT: Greenwood Press.

Lawton, M. P. (1999). Environmental taxonomy: Generalizations from research with older adults. In S. L. Friedman and T. D. Wachs (Eds.), *Measuring environment across the life span: Emerging methods and concepts* (pp. 91-124.) Washington, DC: American Psychological Association.

Lawton, M. P., & Nahemow, L. (1973). Ecology and the aging process. In C. Eisdorfer & M. P. Lawton (Eds.), *The psychology of adult development and aging.* Washington, DC: American Psychological Association.

Lindholm, C. (2001). *Culture and identity: The history, theory and practice of psychological anthropology.* Boston: McGraw-Hill.

Maddox, G. L. (2001). Housing and living arrangements: A transactional perspective. In R. H. Binstock & L. K. George, *Handbook of aging and the social sciences* (5th ed., pp. 426-443). San Diego, CA: Academic Press.

Marsden, J. P. (2001). A framework for understanding homelike character in the context of assisted living housing. In D. Schwarz (Ed.), *Assisted living: sobering realities* (pp. 79-96). New York: Hayworth Press.

McHugh, K. E., & Mings, R. C. (1996). The circle of migration: Attachment to place in aging. *Annals of the Association of American Geographers, 86*(3), 530-550.

Mead, G. H. (1993). *The social self.* Reprint series in sociology, Irvington.

Moos, R. H. (1976). Conceptualizations of human environments. In R. Moos (Ed.), *The human context: Environmental determinants of behavior* (pp. 3-35). New York: John Wiley & Sons.

Morris, B. R. (1992). Reducing inventory: Divestiture of personal possessions. *Journal of Women and Aging, 4*(2), 79-92.

Nahemow, L. (2000). The ecological theory of aging: Powell Lawton's legacy. In R. Rubinstein, M. Moss, & M. Kleban (Eds.), *The many dimensions of aging* (pp. 22-40). New York: Springer.

Namazi, K. H., Eckert, J. K., Kahana, E., & Lyon, S. (1989). Psychological well-being of elderly board and care home residents. *The Gerontologist, 29*(4), 511-516.

Norris-Baker, C. (1998). The evolving concept of behavior settings: Implications for housing older adults. In R. J. Scheidt & P. G. Windley (Eds.), *Environment and aging theory: A focus on housing* (pp 141-160). Westport, CT: Greenwood Press.

Norris-Baker, C. (1999). Aging on the old frontier and the new: A behavior setting approach to the declining small towns of the Midwest. *Journal of Aging Studies, 5,* 333-346.

O'Bryant, S. L., & Murray, C. I. (1986). "Attachment to home" and other factors related to widows' relocation decisions. *Journal of Housing for the Elderly, 4*(1), 53-72.

O'Bryant, S. L., & Nocera, D. (1985). The psychological significance of "home" to older widows. *Psychology of Women Quarterly, 9*(3), 403-411.

Oswald, F., & Wahl, H. (2001). *Place attachment and the meaning of home in older adults in Germany.* Symposium on "International Perspectives on the Meaning of Place" at the meeting of the International Association of Gerontology, Vancouver, Canada.

Oxley, D., Haggard, L. M., Werner, C. M., & Altman, I. (1986). Transactional qualities of neighborhood social networks: A case study of "Christmas Street." *Environment and Behavior, 18*(5), 640-677.

Parmelee, P. A., & Lawton, M. P. (1990). The design of special environments for the aged. In J. E. Birren & K. W. Schaie. *Handbook of the psychology of aging* (3rd ed., pp. 464-488). San Diego, CA: Academic Press, Inc.

Parr, J. (1980). The interaction of persons and living environments. In L. W. Poon (Ed.), *Aging in the 1980s: Psychological issues* (pp. 393-406). Washington, D.C.: American Psychological Association.

Paton, H., and Cram, F. (1992). Personal possessions and environmental control: The experiences of elderly women in three residential settings. *Journal of Women and Aging, 4*(2), 61-78.

Perkins Taylor, S. A. (2001). Place identification and positive realities of aging. *Journal of Cross-Cultural Gerontology, 16*(1), 5-20.

Pinto, M. R., De Medici, S., Van Sant, C., Bianchi, A., Zlotnicki, A., & Napoli, C. (2000). Ergonomics, gerotechnology and design for the home-environment. *Applied Ergonomics, 31,* 317-322.

Proshansky, H. M., Fabvian, A. K., & Kaminoff, R. (1983). Place identity: Physical world socialization of the self. *Journal of Environmental Psychology, 3,* 57-83.

Rapoport, A. (1969). *House form and culture.* Englewood Cliffs, NJ: Prentice-Hall.

Rapoport, A. (1990). *The meaning of the built environment: A nonverbal communication approach.* Tuscon: University of Arizona Press.

Raz, A. (1995). The discourse of aging and other age-related languages: How selves are authorized in the postmodern. *Studies in Symbolic Interaction, 18,* 23-57.

Regnier, V., & Pynoos, J. (1992). Environmental interventions for cognitively impaired older people. In J. Birren, R. B. Sloane, & G. D. Cohen, (Eds.), *Handbook of mental health and aging.*

Rodman, M. (2001). *Houses far from home: British colonial space in the New Hebrides.* Honolulu: University of Hawaii Press.

Rojo Perez, F., Fernandez-Mayoralas, G., Pozo Rivera, F. E., & Rojo Abuin, J. M. (2001). Ageing in place: Predictors of resident satisfaction of elderly. *Social Indicators Research, 54*(2), 173-208.

Rowles, G. D. (1978). *Prisoners of space? Exploring the geographic experience of older people.* Boulder, CO: Westview Press.

Rowles, G. D. (1980). Growing old "inside:" Aging and attachment to place in an Appalachian community. In N. Datan & N. Lohmann (Eds.), *Transitions of aging* (pp. 153-170). New York: Academic Press.

Rowles, G. D. (1981). The surveillance zone as meaningful space for the aged. *Gerontologist, 21*(3), 304-311.

Rowles, G. D. (1987). A place to call home. In L. L. Carstensen and B. A. Edelstein (Eds.), *Handbook of clinical gerontology* (pp. 335-353). New York: Pergamon.

Rowles, G. D. (2000). Habituation and being in place. *Occupational Therapy Journal of Research, 20* (suppl. 1), 52S-67S.

Rowles, G. D., & Ravdal, H. (2002). Aging, place and meaning in the face of changing circumstances. In R. S. Weiss, and S. A. Bass, *Challenges of the third age: Meaning and purpose in later life* (pp. 81-114). London: Oxford University Press.

Rubinstein, R. (1987). The significance of personal objects to older people. *Journal of Aging Studies, 1*(3), 225-238.

Rubinstein, R. (1989). The home environments of older people: A description of the psychosocial processes linking person to place. *Journal of Gerontology: Social Sciences, 44*(2), S45-S53.

Rubinstein, R. (2002). Reminiscence, personal meaning, themes, and the "object relations" of older people. In J. D. Webster & B. K. Haight (Eds.), *Critical advances in reminiscence work: Form theory to application* (pp. 153-165). New York: Springer.

Rubinstein, R. L., Kilbride, J. C., & Nagy, S. (1992). *Elders living alone: Frailty and the perception of choice.* New York: Aldine de Gruyter.

Ryff, C., Marshall, V., & Clarke, P. (1999). Linking the self and society in social gerontology: Crossing new territory via old questions. In C. D. Ryff & V. W.

Marshall (Eds.), *The self and society in aging processes* (pp. 3-41). New York: Springer.

Sahlins, M. (1976). *Culture and practical reason.* Chicago: University of Chicago Press.

Savishinsky, J. (2001). Lonesome in the saddle, or how to feel at home in later life. *Journal of Housing for the Elderly, 14*(1/2), 85-96.

Schaie, K. W., & Willis, S. L. (1999). Theories of everyday competence and aging. In V. L. Bengtson & K. W. Schaie (Eds.), *Handbook of theories of aging* (pp. 174-195). New York: Springer.

Scheidt, R. J. (1998). The social ecological approach of Rudolf Moos. In R. J. Scheidt & P. G. Windley, *Environment and aging theory: A focus on housing* (pp. 111-139). Westport, CT: Greenwood Press.

Scheidt, R. J. & Norris-Baker, C. (1990). A transactional approach to environmental stress among older residents of rural communities. *Journal of Rural Community Psychology, 11,* 5-30.

Schwarz, B., Brent, R., & Barry, D. (1996). Priceless, meaningful and idiosyncratic: Attachment to possessions. *Environmental Design Research Association, 27,* 92-97.

Scott-Webber, L., & Koebel, T. (2001). Life-span design in the near environment. *Journal of Housing for the Elderly, 14*(1/2), 97-122.

Sixsmith, A., & Sixsmith, J. A. (1991). Transitions in home experience in later life. *Journal of Architecture and Planning Research, 8*(3), 181-191.

Spencer, J., Hersch, G., Aldridge, J., Anderson, L., & Ulbrich, A. (2001). Daily life and forms of "communitas" in a personal care home for elders. *Research on Aging, 23*(6), 611-632.

Tabbarah, M., Silverstein, M., & Seeman, T. (2000). A health and demographic profile of noninstitutionalized older Americans residing in environments with home modifications. *Journal of Aging and Health 2000, 12*(2), 204-228.

Taylor, C. (1989). *Sources of the self: The making of modern identity.* Cambridge, MA: Harvard University Press.

Timko, C., & Moos, R. H. (1991). A typology of social climates in group residential facilities for older people. *Journal of Gerontology: Social Sciences, 46*(3), S160-S169.

Turner, B. S. (1996). *The body and society: Explorations in social theory.* Thousand Oaks, CA: Sage.

Wagnild, G. (2001). Growing old at home. *Journal of Housing for the Elderly, 14*(1/2), 71-84.

Wahl, H. (2001). Environmental influences on aging and behavior. In J. Birren and K. W. Schaie (Eds.), *Handbook of the psychology of aging* (5th ed., pp. 215-237). San Diego, CA: Academic Press.

Wahl, H., Oswald, F., & Zimprich, D. (1999). Everyday competence in visually impaired older adults: A case for person-environment perspectives. *The Gerontologist, 39*(2), 140-149.

Weisman, G.D. (1997). Environments for older persons with cognitive impairments: Toward an integration of research and practice. In G. T. Moore and R. W. Marans (Eds.) *Advances in environment, behavior and design: Vol. 4. Toward the integration of theory, methods, research and utilization* (pp. 317-346). New York: Plenum Press.

Weiss, R. S. & Bass, S. A. (Eds.). (2002). *Challenges of the third age: Meaning and purpose in later life.* New York: Oxford University Press.

Windley, P. G., & Scheidt, R. J. (1980). Person-Environment dialectics: Implications for competent functioning in old age. In L. W. Poon (Ed.), *Aging in the 1980s: Psychological issues* (pp. 407-432). Washington, DC: American Psychological Association.

Yee, D. L., Captiman, J. A., Leutz, W. N., & Sceigai, M. (1999). Resident-centered care in assisted living. *Journal of Aging and Social Policy, 10*(3), 7–26.

Young, H. (1998). Moving to congregate housing: The last chosen home. *Journal of Aging Studies, 12*(2), 149-165.

Zeisel, J. (1997). Space design and management for people with dementia. *Environmental Design Research Association, 28,* 18-22.

CHAPTER 4

Assessing the Fit Between Older People and Their Physical Home Environments: An Occupational Therapy Research Perspective

SUSANNE IWARSSON
DEPARTMENT OF CLINICAL NEUROSCIENCE:
DIVISION OF OCCUPATIONAL THERAPY, LUND UNIVERSITY, SWEDEN

The study of home environments has long been one important research domain within the field of environmental gerontology, but there are few recent studies in this area. Furthermore, there is still a paucity of adequate theoretical foundations and appropriate methodology for this kind of research (Gitlin, 2003). The frequently cited idea of *person-environment* fit (P-E fit) is obviously applicable to research concerning elderly people's housing situation (Steinfeld & Danford, 1999). Much literature concerned with environmental gerontology theories, as well as empirical findings, has been published (see, e.g., Gitlin, 1998), whereas this chapter approaches assessment of the fit between older people and their physical home environments from an occupational therapy research perspective. The concept of P-E fit is broad and complex, comprising different dimensions of the personal as well as the environmental components. Covering all aspects of the personal component requires research attention to physical, cognitive, social, psychological, and spiritual aspects, whereas physical, spatial, psychosocial, and cultural aspects must be taken into account in order to embrace the environmental component in full. However, this chapter is principally confined to assessing P-E fit in terms of the physical capacity aspect of the personal component and the physical aspect of the environmental component in housing.

An important goal in health promotion is to create environments supporting healthy living and subjective well-being (World Health Organization [WHO], 1991). Particularly in old age, much time is spent in the home and many daily activities are performed in this arena (Gitlin, 2003). Following a line of thought proceeding from the fact that independence in daily activities is an important health indicator, a physical home environment supporting daily activity independence is most likely health-promotive (Iwarsson, 1997).

Accessibility to the physical environment is an issue that has increasingly come into focus in the public debate in recent years (Regeringens proposition, 2000; United Nations [UN], 1993), targeting people with functional limitations due to disease, injury, or the normal process of aging. Basic accessibility is of vital importance to all citizens' participation in society (UN, 1993). Even though legislation in many Western countries regulates physical accessibility in housing, there are still accessibility problems in many environments in society (Handikappombudsmannen, 1997; Preiser & Ostroff, 2001). Guidelines and standards have been gradually developed, especially in the last 25 years (Steinfeld & Danford, 1999), but the built environment still shows serious deficiencies with regard to accessibility (Iwarsson, 1997; Regeringens proposition, 2000). This is a multifaceted problem and there are many interacting factors leading to the rise of obstacles to accessibility. One basic problem in research on accessibility is the lack of reliable methods for assessing and analyzing accessibility problems (Iwarsson, 1997; Steinfeld & Danford, 1999).

Presumably because the topic originated in the field of rehabilitation (Steinfeld & Tauke, 2002), accessibility issues have long been of explicit interest in occupational therapy (Iwarsson, 1997). For decades, architects, public planners, and geographers with a specific interest in promoting possibilities for persons with disabilities to participate in society have advocated accessibility and universal design, and the need for intensified teaching and research endeavors in this field (see, e.g., Christophersen, 2002; Steinfeld & Danford, 1999). Relating accessibility to research on home environments within the field of environmental gerontology, this aspect of housing has been of interest in terms of descriptions of living arrangements and home modifications, representing what Lawton (1989a) denoted as the support function of the home environment (Wahl, 2003). Having said this, it is obvious that the kind of research at target for this chapter has much to gain from multidisciplinary collaboration. However, whenever engaging in literature searches in this field, it becomes evident that different disciplines use different vocabularies. Thus, efficient knowledge transaction between disciplines would benefit from explicit discussions on vocabulary and definitions.

Disability in old age is complicated because many factors, such as medical conditions, functional capacity, physical and social environmental aspects, motivation, coping skills, et cetera, contribute. This still increases the difficulty of determining the cause and effect of different factors in individual patients as well as in epidemiological studies (Campbell, Busby,

Robertson, Lum, Langlois, & Morgan, 1994). For example, co-morbidity in old age is a problem rendering difficulties in describing levels of functioning in the elderly population (Carlsson, Iwarsson, & Ståhl, 2002). When it comes to the physical home environment, only a few detailed descriptions of environmental barriers in older people's homes exist (Iwarsson, 1997).

Recent literature on the way the physical environment influences the aging process based on population-directed surveys is rare (Gitlin, 2003), but there are examples. In one Swedish study, Lundh (1992) concluded that housing standards, the degree of continuity in home help, the opportunities for the recipients to form close relationships, health, and functional ability influence health status and elderly people's potential to live independently. Some evidence was demonstrated in gerontological population studies in Germany, where analyses of the relationship between objective housing conditions and patterns of capacity confirmed that reduced ability to perform *activities of daily living* (ADL) was due to unfavorable conditions in the physical environment in the home (Schmitt, Kruse, & Olbrich, 1994). In another German study, Wahl, Oswald, and Zimprich (1999) demonstrated that in contrast to among older adults without visual impairments, unfavorable P-E fit affected persons with impairments negatively. If at all addressed in medical literature, the physical home environment has mainly been targeted in terms of risks of falling. Physical environmental evaluations of patient groups have thus been reported, focusing on fall prevention (see, e.g., El-Faizy & Reinsch, 1994; Steinfeld & Shea, 1993). To summarize this, even if representing important aspects of the physical home environment, housing standards, objective housing conditions in general, or environmental details identified as potential risks for falling are not equivalent to housing accessibility.

In general, in research targeting home environments, there is a lack of psychometrically sound measures (Gitlin, 2003). Regardless of the scope of the few studies published focusing on physical accessibility, in most cases the methods used for assessing P-E fit in terms of physical accessibility are study-specific with unknown reliability and validity. In order to gain knowledge on the role of P-E fit in terms of physical housing accessibility, valid and reliable assessment methods are imperative. For more than one decade Iwarsson et al. have engaged in developing assessment tools for accessibility research, and in addition substantial efforts for practical implementation have been effectuated (Iwarsson & Slaug, 2001). Applying our assessment tools in empirical research, we explored and confirmed relationships between functional capacity, environmental factors, accessibility problems, everyday activity, and subjective well-being among older people. In addition, we showed that disability rates are affected by environmental factors (Iwarsson, 1997; Iwarsson & Isacsson, 1997a; Iwarsson, Isacsson, & Lanke, 1998). In this chapter, our research efforts on how to operationalize accessibility to the physical home environment, or in other words P-E fit, will be summarized, along with considerations on future research challenges. Furthermore, reflections on the need to incorporate assessments covering related concepts will be communicated (Carlsson, 2002; Fänge & Iwarsson, 2003).

CONCEPTUAL DEFINITIONS AND TECHNICAL REFLECTIONS

Environmental gerontology represents pluralism as regards to theoretical approaches (Wahl, 2003), and placing the study of home environments within a theoretical framework is a major challenge for future research (Gitlin, 2003). In order to make valid operationalization possible, an analysis and critique of the conceptual definitions used in accessibility research and practice is a first and necessary step. A basic problem regarding accessibility is the fact that different societal stakeholders, people in general, researchers of different disciplines, and persons with functional limitations themselves use different definitions of the concept. In fact, most people do not use any explicit definitions at all, neither in practice nor in research. A first prerequisite for assessment is to define what accessibility to the physical environment means.

Like many other words, accessibility has a common, everyday meaning as well as having specific meanings in different contexts (Iwarsson & Ståhl, 2003). According to the *Oxford Popular Dictionary and Thesaurus* (1998), "accessible" is an adjective synonymous with "approachable, at hand, attainable, available, close, convenient, handy, and within reach." In its specific meaning in this chapter, accessibility is a relative concept because it expresses the relationship between the capacity of the individual and the demands from the environment (Iwarsson, 1997). In objective terms, accessibility can be assessed reliably and validly by professionals (Iwarsson & Slaug, 2001) in relation to existing norms and guidelines (Iwarsson & Ståhl, 2003; Preiser & Ostroff, 2001).

A word often used in parallel to accessibility is usability, i.e., perceptions of how well the design of the environment enables functioning and well-being, mainly from the user's perspective (Fänge & Iwarsson, 1999; Steinfeld & Danford, 1999). For example, for many years, Swedish building and planning legislation required that all housing, work premises, or other premises open to the public must be accessible and usable for persons with restricted mobility or restricted sense of locality. In this legal framework, usability was interpreted and defined as follows: "The built environment has to allow any individual, in spite of impairments, to be able to perform daily activities within it" (Didón, Magnusson, Millgård, & Molander, 1987). When it comes to the word in itself, "usable" is an adjective synonymous with "fit to use, functioning, operational, serviceable, valid, and working" (*Oxford Popular Dictionary and Thesaurus*, 1998), that is, it is not synonymous with accessibility.

Even if the words accessibility and usability have different definitions, Steinfeld and Danford (1999), for example, use them in parallel, stating that they are both usually defined in terms of observed task performance. According to a recent paper by Golant (2003), the conceptualization of environmental behaviors or activities, describing how people use, manipulate, or perform tasks in their settings, represents an important area for P-E fit research that could explain and predict the appropriateness of older people's home settings. Thus, because accessibility and usability are closely connected to the performance of everyday activities, both concepts need to be defined and deserve to be highlighted in P-E fit research.

In occupational therapy, the term occupational performance is used to represent "doing" in everyday life and is the experience of a person engaged in activity within an environment (Canadian Association of Occupational Therapists [CAOT], 1997). Occupation is close to the term activity as used in other disciplines (Clark, 2002), but in the context of this chapter the definition of occupation is fruitful. The concept of occupation refers to groups of activities and tasks of everyday life, named, organized, and given value and meaning by individuals and a culture. Occupations are often classified into self-care, productivity, and leisure activities, for example. Some key features of occupations are that they represent a basic human need, a determinant of health, and a source of meaning, choice, and control. Through occupations people organize their daily lives (CAOT, 1997). People, their activities and roles, and the environments in which they live, work, and play over their lifespans, are in dynamic interaction. In order to stick to more common vocabulary, in this chapter the word activity will be used henceforth, but defined in the same way as the concept of occupation as described above.

Concluding on definitions, accessibility as well as usability is an aspect of P-E fit, but the distinction Steinfeld and Danford made is that usability is based on individual interpretations. Applying definitions underlying the research of Iwarsson et al., the concept of activity as defined above (CAOT, 1997; Clark, 2002) must be reflected upon as well. Thus, the following definitions of accessibility and usability are suggested (Iwarsson & Ståhl, 2003):

• Accessibility is a relative concept, implying that accessibility problems should be expressed as a P-E relationship. In other words, accessibility is the encounter between the person's, or target group's, functional capacity and the design and demands of the physical environment. Accessibility refers to compliance with official norms and standards, thus being mainly objective in nature. Thus, accessibility comprises two components; the personal component and the environmental component.

• The concept of usability implies that a person should be able to use, that is, to move around, be in, and use, the environment on equal terms with other citizens. Accessibility is a necessary precondition for usability, implying that information on P-E fit (personal component and environmental component) is imperative. However, usability is not only based on compliance with official norms and standards; it is mainly subjective in nature, taking into account user evaluations and subjective expressions. It means that when included in usability, the personal and environmental components have other characteristics than when included in accessibility; that is, they are more subjectively oriented. Most important, there is a third component distinguishing usability from accessibility, vis-a-vis the activity component. Further, usability is explicitly transactional in nature, implying that the components are less distinct and more interwoven than in accessibility (Fänge & Iwarsson, 2003). Thus, taking all its different aspects into account, usability is a wider concept (Carlsson, 2002), approaching the concept of performance including aspects such as values, interests, et cetera (Steinfeld & Danford, 1999).

Keeping the focus on the fit between older people and their physical home environments, empirical research, as well as implementation of practical solutions for more accessible environments, has increased, but, as in other fields of P-E research, the theoretical foundations are weak (Preiser & Ostroff, 2001; Steinfeld & Danford, 1999). Lewin's early definition (1951) of behavior as a function of the person and the environment is often referred to as the basis for P-E fit research. Several decades later, Carp and Kahana published a body of literature representing important foundations for research into this field (for a summary, see Stokols & Altman, 1987). However, the model most often referred to in many different disciplines (Gitlin, 1998; Iwarsson, 1997; Iwarsson & Ståhl, 1999; Steinfeld & Danford, 1999; Svensson, 1996) is Lawton and Nahemow's (1973) ecological model, representing a landmark of environmental gerontology (Golant, 2003; Wahl, 2003). In the ecological model the person is defined in terms of a set of competencies, and the environment is defined in terms of its demands, labeled environmental press. Persons with lower competence are much more sensitive to the demands of the environment than persons with higher competence, as stated by Lawton and Simon (1968; Lawton, 1986) in the docility hypothesis. Later on, as a supplement or contrast, Lawton introduced the proactivity hypothesis (Lawton, 1989b, 1989c), stating that persons with greater competence are more likely to search the environment for resources to satisfy their needs.

A conceptual framework of interest in this context is the *International Classification of Functioning, Disability and Health* (ICF) (WHO, 2001). Originally it was developed in order to complement the *World Health Organization* (WHO's) *International Classification of Diseases* (ICD) (WHO, 1992), i.e., it emanated from the medical context. Components defined in the current version of the ICF are body function and structures, activities and participation, environmental factors, and personal factors. The environmental factors are divided into two levels: individual and societal. In order to explain the relationships between the components of the classification, a model is presented in which all the components interact with each other (WHO, 2001).

In the theory of occupational therapy, human activity and the relationship between individual and environment are central concepts (CAOT, 1997). Through meaningful, goal-directed activity in interaction with the surrounding environment, the individual develops his or her skills throughout the life cycle. By means of occupational therapy, individuals with impaired functional capacity can be given the necessary conditions for continued development, with the aid of measures geared to both the individual and the environment. The individual is in constant interaction with the environment, adapting his or her activity to the changed demands that arise (Miller, Sieg, Ludwig, Shortridge, & Van Deusen, 1988). A recent occupational therapy model including the outcome of P-E relationships is the *Canadian Model of Occupational Performance* (CMOP) (CAOT, 1997), focusing on the performance of daily activities, which the CMOP labels occupational performance. As described in the CMOP, transactions between person, environment, and activity result in performance of daily activities (Law, Cooper, Strong, Stewart, Rigby, & Letts, 1996). Since the concept of activity is of interest for disciplines outside occupational therapy as well, such as for environmental gerontology, Law et al.'s work should be of interest, because explicitly introducing activity to future research on P-E fit might result in novel insights (Golant, 2003).

So far, Iwarsson's research team has presented theoretical reflections of importance for accessibility research. Most of all we were inspired by the CMOP (CAOT, 1997) and Law et al.'s work (1996), but Lawton's theories as well as the ICF (WHO, 2001) have served as additional sources of inspiration. A tentative model outlined in Carlsson (2002) focuses on the complex dynamics of *person-environment-activity* (P-E-A) transactions. The model for future accessibility research presented was outlined with the inspiration of occupational performance as described in the CMOP (CAOT, 1997; Law et al., 1996). Inspired by Law et al. (1996), the circles in Figure 4.1 represent a person with all his or her characteristics and capacities (P), the entire environment with all its different dimensions (E), and the broad repertoire of possible activities (A). The person–activity intersection is the repertoire of current activities a single person performs, the activity–environment intersection is the environments in which current activities are performed, and the person–environment intersection represents the environments the person interacts within. The result of the dynamic, transactional relationship between the three components—person, environment, and activity—represents the actual "doing" of activities, that is, performance (CAOT, 1997; Law et al., 1996; WHO, 2001).

The model outline (Figure 4.1) can be used in order to move further toward a theory on accessibility-usability-performance. Because accessibility and usability only represent part of the complex dynamics of P-E-A transactions, the approach requires clear-cut delimitation. That is, the personal component is delimited to functional capacity, the environmental component to physical environmental demands, and the activity component is delimited to activities defined for the situation at target, such as household chores or personal maintenance. It should be noted that even after having stated these delimitations, each component is still comprehensive and complex. For example, the body of literature and assessment instruments targeting ADL, applying different measurement levels, is substantial (see Wade, 1994). Nevertheless, the definitions of the three components serve well as a basis for operationalization for accessibility research (Carlsson, 2002), not only in housing, but also in other arenas, such as in public outdoor environments.

Delineating the conceptual definitions further, the personal component in accessibility, that is, functional capacity, focuses on functional limitations, when necessarily classified in the performance components as defined in CMOP: physical, cognitive, and affective dimensions (CAOT, 1997; Figure 4.1). In relation to housing accessibility, the environmental

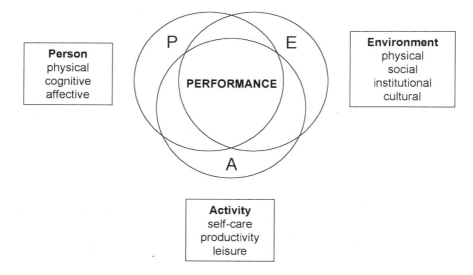

FIGURE 4.1   Performance — a dynamic, transactional relationship between person, environment and activity. With inspiration from "Occupational Performance" as described in the CMOP (CAOT, 1997). From "Catching the bus in old age. Methodological aspects of accessibility assessments in public transport" by G. Carlsson, 2002. Copyright 2002 by G. Carlsson.

component is confined to aspects of the built environment (Figure 4.2), although more environmental dimensions such as social, institutional, and cultural dimensions, of course, are included in the environmental component when regarded in full (Figure 4.1; Carlsson , 2002).

The relationship between functional capacity and environmental demands, i.e., accessibility (Figure 4.2), is one of the first issues to take into consideration when deciding to perform any activity, since an accessible environment is one precondition for performance (Carlsson, 2002). However, information about the nature of the activity to be performed in the environment must be included as well (Iwarsson & Ståhl, 2003). In the suggested model (Figure 4.2), usability is represented by the area where functional capacity, environmental demands, and activity intersect. Thus, the suggested model elucidates the activity component in the concept of

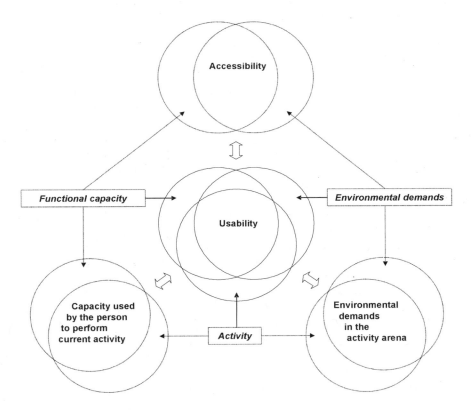

FIGURE 4.2 Preconditions for performance: accessibility and usability. From "Catching the bus in old age. Methodological aspects of accessibility assessments in public transport" by G. Carlsson, 2002. Copyright 2002 by G. Carlsson.

usability, implying that a person should be able to use, that is, to move around, be in, and use the physical environment, on equal terms with other citizens (Iwarsson & Ståhl, 2003).

The suggested model is applicable to individual as well as societal levels, but the contents of the P-E-A components differ depending on the level in focus. That is, at the individual level information on a specific individual's functional capacity and the demands of his or her specific environment, and information on his or her activity repertoire is needed (Carlsson, 2002). On the societal level, the personal component is represented by epidemiological data on functional capacity at group or population level (Carlsson et al., 2002), whereas the environmental component is represented by aggregated data on environmental demands as described by Iwarsson and Isacsson (1996). The activity component is represented by knowledge on activity repertoires in the group or population at target (see Bränholm & Fugl-Meyer, 1994).

METHODOLOGY

Accessibility problems may be considered from a number of different perspectives. A common situation is that accessibility problems need to be dealt with as a part of individual rehabilitation processes (Steinfeld & Tauke, 2002), such as, in the form of an individual housing adaptation (Gitlin, 1998; Iwarsson, 1997). From another perspective, accessibility problems must be tackled at the societal level, in connection with the building or renovation of houses and public places (Steinfeld & Danford, 1999). This means that there is a need for reliable and valid methods for assessing and analyzing the accessibility problems that arise when a given individual or group/population meets a given environment. Methods for assessing accessibility problems should give a measure of the degree to which a particular physical environment prevents or supports daily activity and participation in society (Steinfeld & Danford, 1999). Given the definition of accessibility suggested by Iwarsson & Ståhl (2003), accessibility assessments should be based on norms and regulations, and they should be objectively and professionally administered.

When it comes to assessment of usability, another approach is necessary because such assessments should capture the person's own perceptions of his or her physical home environment (Fänge & Iwarsson, 1999), including the activity component (Fänge & Iwarsson, 2003). Thus, the only way to gather information about the usability of the environment is to ask the individual (Baum & Law, 1997; Feinstein, Josephy, & Wells, 1986; Pollock, 1993). No outside observer can be so familiar with the individual's physical and social environment, lifestyle, and needs that a valid assessment of usability can be made solely from an external perspective (Pollock, 1993).

Because activity is one of the components underlying the concept of usability, methods for assessing ADL performance could well be used in combination with assessments targeting the usability of the home environment.

Applying an interactional paradigm (Golant, 2003; Wahl, 2003), Lawton and Nahemow's ecological model (1973) and the docility hypothesis (Lawton & Simon, 1968; Lawton, 1986) work well as a theoretical explanation for accessibility assessments (Iwarsson, 1997, 1999). However, as outlined earlier, we suggest a new model as the basis for P-E fit research targeting accessibility and usability from a transactional perspective (Carlsson, 2002). Input from occupational therapy scholars as described in this chapter offers a new and complementary dimension of potential interest to environmental gerontology research. The presented approach positions the concepts of accessibility and usability in relation to each other as well as in relation to the concept of activity; that is, it elucidates P-E-A transactions of importance for future environmental gerontology research on home environments.

THE ENABLER CONCEPT AND THE HOUSING ENABLER

The Enabler Concept is originally an American idea, with a design (Steinfeld et al., 1979) operationalizing P-E fit in terms of functional capacity (personal component) and environmental demands (environmental component from references [Iwarsson, 1997; Jensen, Iwarsson, & Ståhl, 2002]). It can be applied with great flexibility and is thus suitable for assessment tasks from various perspectives. Iwarsson et al. gradually developed methodology for assessment and analysis of housing accessibility based on the Enabler Concept (Steinfeld et al., 1979). This methodology enables a *predictive, objective,* and *norm-based* assessment and analysis of accessibility problems in the physical home environment. It allows analysis from individual as well as group/population perspectives.

The Housing Enabler instrument is intended for housing accessibility assessment and comprises an introductory descriptive part concerning individual or group data and housing standards. Inter-rater reliability and content validity have been established (Iwarsson & Isacsson, 1996; Iwarsson & Slaug, 2001). The assessment is administered in three steps, as detailed in Figure 4.3. In the first and second steps the assessment is conducted according to checklists for functional limitations and dependence on mobility devices as well as for physical environmental barriers. In the third step, an analysis of accessibility problems is undertaken by relating functional limitations and dependence on mobility devices to environmental barriers. The result of this analysis is a quantification of the accessibility problems anticipated in each case, in terms of a total score.

1. Assessment of functional limitations: This first step of the assessment is a combination of interview and observation, in order to dichotomously assess the person's functional limitations (13 items) and dependence on mobility devices (2 items; Figure 4.3). Thus the personal component of accessibility is operationalized primarily in terms of physical functional capacity, though four of the items concern perception or cognition. This section of the instrument fulfills very high inter-rater reliability requirements, kappa=0.87 (Iwarsson & Isacsson, 1996). Alternatively, if the assessment targets societal level and not individual cases, i.e., if the descrip-

First mark the functional limitations and dependence on mobility aids that have been observed. Then copy the crosses to all the rating forms for environmental barriers.

DIFFICULTY INTERPRETING INFORMATION	A
SEVERE LOSS OF SIGHT	B1
COMPLETE LOSS OF SIGHT	B2
SEVERE LOSS OF HEARING	X
PREVALENCE OF POOR BALANCE	X
INCOORDINATION	E
LIMITATIONS OF STAMINA	F
DIFFICULTY IN MOVING HEAD	G
DIFFICULTY IN REACHING WITH ARMS	H
DIFFICULTY IN HANDLING AND FINGERING	X
LOSS OF UPPER EXTREMITY SKILLS	J
DIFFICULTY BENDING, KNEELING, ETC.	K
RELIANCE ON WALKING AIDS	X
INABILITY TO USE LOWER EXTREMITIES	M
EXTREMES OF SIZE AND WEIGHT	N

Mark the observed environmental barriers with a cross. Then put a circle around the points (1–4) in the squares at the intersections of functional limitations and environmental barriers. The total of the points is a measure of the degree of accessibility problems.

A. OUTDOOR ENVIRONMENT	A	B1	B2	X	X	E	F	G	H	X	J	K	X	M	N
General (pp. 37–42, 183–96)															
1. Narrow paths (less than 1.3 m).				3	3								3	3	1
X Irregular walking surface (includes irregular joins, sloping sections, etc.).		2	3	(1)	1		3						(3)	3	
3. Unstable walking surface (loose gravel, sand, clay, etc.).		2	3		3	3	2						3	4	

FIGURE 4.3 Principles for housing accessibility assessment by means of the Housing Enabler instrument (Iwarsson & Slaug, 2001).

tion of the personal component is based on epidemiological data instead of assessments of specific persons, the items are marked as present or not present based on epidemiological knowledge of the user group at target.

The result of this step is expressed in terms of profiles of functional limitations; that is, the significant characteristic of this assessment is that it takes simultaneous occurrence of several different functional limitations into account. In this kind of profile, the presence as well as the absence of any of the functional limitations is crucial, the result of the quantitative analysis (see III below) takes both aspects into account (Carlsson et al., 2002).

2. Assessment of physical environmental barriers: A detailed, on-site observation of physical environmental barriers in the home and the immediate outdoor environment (188 items). Thus, the environmental component of accessibility is operationalized in terms of the presence of physical environmental barriers. The housing environment is divided into four sections: outdoor environment (33 items), entrances (49 items), indoor environment (100 items), and communication features (6 items). A few examples of item definitions are given in Figure 4.3. Approximately 70 percent of the items are defined according to official Swedish norms or guidelines. The remaining items are defined and assessed based on professional experience, primarily occupational therapy expertise. The 188 items constitute a valid source of information, and they are subsequently entered into the quantitative analysis (see 3 below; Figure 4.3). If the objective of the assessment is to serve as the basis for planning of practical intervention, such as individual housing adaptation or planning for rebuilding in order to meet the needs of a specific user group, collection of additional qualitative information is recommended. During the on-site observation the rater is recommended to take additional notes, make sketches, et cetera, that might be useful in the planning process. Even if this section of the instrument is very complex and comprises many items, it fulfills high inter-rater reliability requirements, kappa$=0.68$ (Iwarsson & Isacsson, 1996).

3. Calculation of accessibility score: This step is a quantitative analysis of accessibility. It is a calculation of a total score predicting the demand caused by a particular combination of functional limitations in an individual or a group and physical environmental barriers (environmental design features), i.e., the degree of objective, norm-based accessibility problems in housing. For each environmental barrier item, the instrument comprises predefined points (1 to 4), adopted from the original Enabler Concept (Steinfeld et al., 1979), quantifying the severity of the problems predicted to arise in the specific case. Based on the rater's dichotomous assessments in steps 1 and 2 of the administration procedure, the predefined points 1 to 4 already fixed in the instrument format (Figure 4.3) yield a score summing up the degree of accessibility problems anticipated, i.e., predictive physical environmental demand. In cases where no functional limitations or dependence on mobility devices are present in the person, the score

always is zero. In cases where the person has functional limitations and/or is dependent on mobility devices, higher scores mean more accessibility problems and higher environmental demand. A computerized tool for more efficient data analyses, on individual as well as group level, is available (Slaug & Iwarsson, 2001).

In 1994/95, the Housing Enabler was applied in empirical studies carried out in Sweden (Iwarsson, 1997). On home visits to 133 elderly people living in ordinary housing, data were collected with the Housing Enabler, in combination with an ADL instrument and a self-assessment instrument for subjective well-being. Most of the subjects lived in high-standard homes but, nevertheless, there were environmental barriers in all of them (Iwarsson & Isacsson, 1996). The Housing Enabler made it possible to predict at group level which environmental details caused the greatest accessibility problems. Dependence in ADL co-varied with accessibility problems, and the results supported Lawton and Nahemow's docility hypothesis (1973; Iwarsson, Isacsson, & Lanke, 1998). Furthermore, accessibility problems co-varied with subjective well-being (Iwarsson & Isacsson, 1997b).

In 2002, a *Conseil d'Europe* (EC) funded project involving use of the Housing Enabler in an international research project saw its start, namely, the ENABLE-AGE Project (Iwarsson et al., 2001). Within this project, the instrument has been adapted for use in five different European countries. The adaptation process was based on reviews of legislation and norms concerning housing accessibility in Sweden, Germany, the United Kingdom, Hungary, and Latvia, ending up with a project-specific version of the instrument (Iwarsson & Nygren, 2002). In each country, national teams of raters have been established, and all raters have undergone project-specific training in order to optimize data quality. Preliminary results indicate that all five teams have reached sufficient inter-rater reliability. The first wave of data collection was completed in May 2003, and the results will demonstrate the instrument's basic qualities as regards to validity, reliability, and usefulness in an international context.

"USABILITY IN MY HOME," UIMH

The conceptual differences between accessibility and usability that have been pointed out (Iwarsson & Ståhl, 2003) need to be further validated by empirical findings. In other words, we need knowledge on the relationship between objective and subjective housing assessments as well as on how such relationships may differ between different groups of users (Fänge & Iwarsson, 2003).

In order to capture user opinions of physical housing usability, a self-administered instrument entitled *"Usability in My Home"* (UIMH) was developed (Fänge & Iwarsson, 1999). The instrument consists of 23 items, addressing the degree to which the physical housing environment supports personal ADL (e.g., hygiene, dressing, grooming, and going to the toilet) and instrumental ADL (e.g., cooking, washing, doing the dishes, and cleaning), as well as hobby and leisure activities, as assessed by the user. Further questions reflect safety/security, privacy, and ability to maintain social contacts as well as housing accessibility. The questions on accessibility are divided into sections congruent with the Housing Enabler instrument, that is, outdoor environment, entrances, indoor environment, and communication (Iwarsson & Slaug, 2001). By the use of a seven-point rating scale, the user is asked to give his or her opinion on 16 items. The rating scale is graded from 1 to 7, with 1 indicating the most negative and 7 indicating the most positive response alternative. Another seven questions are open-ended; six for definition of the type of accessibility problems experienced in the home environment, and one question for expression of any additional opinions on housing conditions. The instrument is designed to be applicable in various housing conditions, such as one-family houses or blocks of flats, in urban as well as rural areas, and with users experiencing different problems in their daily life. Consequently, (at the most) five questions (three regarding personal or instrumental ADL and two regarding accessibility) are "non-applicable" to some users and should not be responded to. The instrument is a valid and reliable tool for use in research and practice (Fänge & Iwarsson, 1999, 2003).

The UIMH (Fänge & Iwarsson, 1999) and the Housing Enabler (Iwarsson & Slaug, 2001) have been used in an explorative study investigating the relationship between objective, norm-based assessment of housing accessibility and subjective, self-rated housing usability among 131 users receiving housing adaptation grants (Fänge & Iwarsson, 2003). On an overarching level, the results demonstrated that among housing adaptation cases, objective accessibility and subjective usability assessments do correlate. However, according to the results of sub-sample analyses of different age groups, between genders, according to civil status, between subjects with high dependence versus low dependence in ADL, et cetera, in sub-samples with more current experience of performing daily activities in the part of environment in question, stronger correlation between accessibility and usability was identified. The results indicate that different user groups seem to have different preconditions to assess housing usability, most likely primarily depending on whether the user has current experience of performing daily activities in the part of environment in question or not. Thus, the pattern of correlation between accessibility and usability is complex and requires careful consideration. Most important, the study indicated the conceptual differentiation between accessibility and usability, supporting Golant (2003) in highlighting the value of acknowledging activity as a component deserving more attention in future P-E fit research.

METHODOLOGICAL CHALLENGES: ASSESSMENT OF HOUSING ACCESSIBILITY

The major challenge in regards to the personal component of the concept of accessibility is to outline a set of profiles of functional limitations representing different user groups, that is, profiles that could be utilized in more efficient analyses prior to physical planning decisions at the societal level. In an explorative study applying hierarchical cluster analysis, a first step toward increased knowledge about the frequencies of profiles of functional limitations in different population groups has been taken (Carlsson et al., 2002). As expected, the results show that the complexity of profiles of functional limitations increases with age, highlighting the need to develop methods allowing for valid descriptions, such as in relation to different age groups. Most methodological efforts in this respect lie ahead of us, and knowledge about profiles of functional limitations is scarce. In order to arrive at a valid assessment of the personal component, substantial data on the prevalence of functional limitations in different population groups have to be gathered and analyzed.

In regard to the environmental component, in order to achieve an even more valid and reliable assessment of environmental barriers, some specific methodological challenges have to be dealt with. New challenges have gradually become evident as our research activities have been expanded to the public outdoor environment and public transportation (Carlsson, 2002). The spans of variation in dynamic phenomena identified in this research (Jensen et al., 2002) most likely have implications for assessment of environmental barriers in housing as well, and have to be further investigated, even if the problems in housing (given the more limited spaces to be assessed) are expected to be less extensive. When assessing larger areas, predominantly outdoors, the rater easily risks missing an environmental detail, such as a crack in the pavement, jeopardizing reliability as well as validity. In order to achieve reliability and feasibility with preserved validity, it is a substantial challenge to make the environmental assessment not too demanding (Carlsson, 2002). Another crucial question needing to be further explored is how to assess the repetition of environmental demands in an area. An environmental detail occurring once may have identical consequences as repeated environmental demands, but repetition may also increase the demands and result in more accessibility problems. Our knowledge in this respect is still insufficient (Iwarsson, Jensen, & Ståhl, 2000; Jensen et al., 2002). Finally, because norms and guidelines are still lacking for 30 percent of the environmental items of the Housing Enabler and the validity of existing norms is largely unknown (Steinfeld & Danford, 1999), the validity of the Housing Enabler assessment should be further tested and developed. Given the international variation and lack of consensus as regards norms and legislation, this issue poses specific challenges to the use of the Housing Enabler in different countries.

During the work with the third step of the Housing Enabler, the question of the validity of the predefined demand points has been raised. According to Steinfeld et al. (1979; E. Steinfeld, personal communication, June, 1994), points one to four were established on the basis of many years' practical experience of work with accessibility issues. Experience acquired from intensive practical collaboration among experienced architects, occupational therapists, and persons with disabilities was subsequently gathered and systematized. An iterative process of discussions led to the definition of the predefined scores, successively improving content validity. Detailed validation on empirical grounds would appear to be an almost unreasonable task, above all in view of the infinite number of possible combinations of functional limitations and details in the physical environment (E. Steinfeld, personal communication, June, 1994). Studies so far have shown that the instrument has sufficient content and construct validity (Fänge & Iwarsson, 2003; Iwarsson, 1997; Iwarsson & Slaug, 2001). Moreover, it has external validity both in relation to the Swedish National Board of Housing's surveys of implemented adaptation measures (see Boverket, 1996), and in relation to the results of internationally published studies in the field (see Gitlin, 1998; Iwarsson & Isacsson, 1993). It is important to note, however, that a Housing Enabler assessment, despite the degree of detail gives only crude predictive results. In the course of the work it has been found in detailed analyses that there are some inconsistencies in the scoring, but, as it stands, most of the grading in the original instrument (Steinfeld et al., 1979) has been retained. In the present version of the instrument the inconsistencies that have become obvious during several years' work have been changed in accordance with basic reliability and validity principles (Iwarsson & Slaug, 2001). In relation to the extent and richness of detail of the assessment and the often high scores it generates, a discrepancy of a few points because of possible inconsistencies is considered to be of marginal significance.

To sum up, in order to develop the methodology described further, substantial methodological challenges are involved, concerning all three steps of an accessibility assessment.

ASSESSMENT OF USABILITY IN HOUSING

When it comes to usability assessment, research experiences are scarce, and most of the challenges in this respect must be dealt with in forthcoming studies. Given the greater complexity of the concept of usability, it is obvious that more aspects of its components have to be taken into consideration. The delimitation of the personal component made for accessibility assessments by means of the Housing Enabler, that is, to physical capacity, represents one specific methodological deficit. Because usability embraces more of the individual's subjective perceptions of the environment, aspects such as motivation, personality, personal values, and roles must be taken into account. Further, considering the activity component of usability and the transactional P-E-A relationships, usability research implies more of a contextualization in terms of research approaches and methodology. In research targeting elderly people's ability to travel by means of public transport (Carlsson, 2002), participant observation, including the critical incident technique as described by Flanagan (1954), has been successfully applied, demonstrating that it is possible to study usability in its context. It remains to be investigated whether this methodological approach could be useful for further research into usability in housing as well.

ASSESSMENT OF ACTIVITIES OF DAILY LIVING (ADL)

In geriatrics, gerontology, rehabilitation, and occupational therapy, et cetera, ADL assessments are frequently used in research, as well as practice (see Wade, 1994). Considering the CMOP (CAOT, 1997; Law et al., 1996), the definition of usability (Iwarsson & Ståhl, 2003), and the new model presented (Carlsson, 2002), it is obvious that functional performance in terms of ADL should be further reflected upon. In accepting the definition of usability as presented in this chapter, that is, adding the activity component, the concept of usability seems to be related to ADL capacity.

Substantial bodies of ADL assessment instruments as well as ADL research literature are available, representing different instrument administration procedures, measurement levels, and scaling approaches (Wade, 1994). For example, as demonstrated by Jette (1994), different administration procedures yield different results in the same study sample, implying that it is important to reflect upon subjective and objective dimensions of ADL capacity. Furthermore, different measurement levels, such as dependence on personal assistance or assistive devices, or degree of difficulty, affect the prevalence of ADL disability as well (Jette, 1994). Another aspect worth commenting on is the fact that environmental factors affect the prevalence of ADL disability (Iwarsson, 1997). Several studies have demonstrated that environmental factors, such as availability of public transportation, affect the hierarchical structure of ADL dependence (Iwarsson, 1998; Iwarsson & Isacsson, 1997a), and there are also gender differences in patterns of ADL dependence (Avlund & Schultz-Larsen, 1991; Iwarsson, 1998; Iwarsson & Isacsson, 1997a). Even if no results targeting the relationship between ADL capacity and usability are available yet, it seems reasonable that different aspects of ADL affect perceptions of usability, presumably involving coping mechanisms as well.

Having said this, it is of interest to reflect upon the role ADL assessments play in research targeting accessibility and usability, and the kinds of ADL instruments that would be most valuable and valid to include in future research on P-E-A transactions in old age. Even if ADL assessments hitherto have often been used in empirical studies within environmental gerontology, as well as within occupational therapy and geriatric rehabilitation, as regards to the transactional relationships between accessibility, usability, and ADL capacity, much remains yet to be explored.

IMPLICATIONS OF ASSESSING PERSON-ENVIRONMENT FIT IN LATER LIFE

The fact that problems of housing accessibility co-vary with the prevalence of ADL disability in older people (Iwarsson et al., 1998) means that health-promotive and preventive efforts ought to be initiated because reduced everyday activity is health-threatening. The problem is frequent, and it will increase with the growing proportion of older people in the population (Iwarsson, 1997). Among the strategies recommended for efficient public health work are promotion of healthy behavior and creation of healthy and supportive environments (WHO, 1992), shifting the focus from thinking in terms of diseases to thinking in terms of health. Thus, preventive efforts based on risk factors are changed into efforts promoting health in everyday life. Quantitative data are useful for finding broad patterns, which is important in prevention surveys (Steinfeld & Shea, 1993). As stated by Morfitt in 1983, reducing physical environmental demand in the healthy segment of the elderly population is an important preventive strategy, but in practice as well as research such approaches are still rare.

As early as the 1960s, gerontologists displayed an increasing interest in the role of the physical environment (e.g., Lawton & Simon, 1968; Carp & Kahana as cited in Stokols & Altman, 1987), for example, in housing. The home environment is often acknowledged as being a critical determinant for autonomy, participation, and well-being in elderly people, but housing issues have not yet been adequately and sufficiently addressed in research, policy, and practice (Gitlin, 2003; Iwarsson et al., 2001). In order to strengthen the knowledge base required for future policy recommendations and guidelines in housing issues targeting senior citizens, instruments on accessibility and usability represent an important contribution to existing instrument arsenals for environmental gerontology research. Subsequently, different assessment devices have been suggested to assess the physical environment (see Gitlin, 1998; Gitlin, 2003), but, to the best of my knowledge, the methodology presented in this chapter constitutes the only set of rigorously tested instruments explicitly targeting accessibility and usability currently available. An important contribution to existing research is that the instruments presented allow for examinations of relationships between objective housing circumstances and subjective evaluations of the home environment. Such studies would contribute to the provision of evidence-based policy recommendations and guidelines in housing issues targeting the elderly population (Iwarsson et al., 2001) and the creation of healthy and supportive environments (WHO, 1992). Given the problematization presented in this chapter, research needs on relationships between accessibility, usability, and aspects of functional performance in terms of ADL ability represent a challenge for forthcoming studies. More research along these lines will contribute to conceptual and theoretical development within the field of environmental gerontology as well as occupational therapy.

In order to increase housing accessibility and usability, ultimately to promote everyday activity and health among old people, several practice-oriented strategies are suggested:

• By means of valid and reliable assessment methods such as the Housing Enabler and the UIMH, the complex constructs of accessibility and usability can be made concrete. The instruments can be used for individual interventions, such as in geriatric rehabilitation, but because they cover many aspects of architectural design, they could be of general use within the public planning process as well (Iwarsson, 1997). They are useful with persons of different ages and with a wide range of diagnoses.

• With reliable survey data on housing accessibility and usability at hand, public building and planning processes in general could most likely be positively influenced in order to create healthy and supportive environments.

• Based on local environmental surveys, educational programs for senior citizens concerning accessible and safe housing could be developed (Iwarsson, 1997). There is a difficulty in striking a balance between the relative importance of objective assessments and sensitivity to the subjective opinions of people. An attractive approach in health-promotive activities is to teach elderly people how to observe potential risks in their surroundings by themselves, thus encouraging active assumption of personal responsibility (Cwikel & Fried, 1992). It is often difficult to make frail elderly people undertake coping behaviors related to housing consumption (Reschovsky & Newman, 1990), at least until impairments and disabilities increase (Devor, Wang, Renvall, Feigal, & Ramsdell, 1994). To date, little information has been obtained on what could be done by means of active health-promotive efforts in this respect (Trickey, Maltais, Gosselin, & Robitaille, 1993).

CONCLUDING REMARKS

The methodology presented in this chapter represents a means to perform surveys focusing on the prevalence of functional limitations in older people, and on physical environmental barriers and problems of accessibility and usability in their homes. The Housing Enabler and the UIMH instruments have potentials for complementing current methodological approaches used in environmental gerontology. In explicitly introducing accessibility and usability to this field of research focusing on P-E-A transactions, the theoretical reflections outlined deliver novel input to environmental gerontology. Furthermore, in order to collect data underfeeding implementation of practical health-promotive and rehabilitative strategies, the methodology can be applied in practice contexts in health care and social services as well as in health-promotive work at the community level, such as, in public planning.

ACKNOLWEDGMENTS

Acknowledgments are extended to Professor Agneta Ståhl, PhD, Reg. OT Gunilla Carlsson and MSc, Reg. OT Agneta Fänge for outstanding contributions to the knowledge development underlying this book chapter.

REFERENCES

Avlund, K., & Schultz-Larsen, K. (1991). What do 70-year-old men and women do? And what are they able to do? From the Glostrup Survey in 1994. *Aging Clinical and Experimental Research, 3*, 39-49.

Baum, C., & Law, M. (1997). Occupational therapy: Focusing on occupational performance. *American Journal of Occupational Therapy, 51*, (4), 277-288.

Boverket. (1996). *Bostadsanpassningsbidragen 1994-95—Omfattning, kostnadsutveckling och tillämpning.* [Housing adaptation grants 1994-95. Scope, cost development, and application.] Karlskrona, Sweden: Boverket.

Boverket. (2001). *Bostadsanpassningsbidragen 2000. Rapport.* [Housing adaptation grants 2000. Report.] Karlskrona, Sweden: Boverket.

Bränholm, I. B., & Fugl-Meyer, A. R. (1994). On non-work activity preferences: Relationship with occupational roles. *Disability and Rehabilitation, 16*, 205-216.

Campbell, A. J., Busby, W. J., Robertson, M. C., Lum, C. L., Langlois, J. A., & Morgan, F. C. (1994). Disease, impairment, disability and social handicap: a community based study of people aged 70 years and over. *Disability and Rehabilitation, 16*, 72-79.

Canadian Association of Occupational Therapists, CAOT. (1997). *Enabling occupation: An occupational therapy perspective.* Ottawa, Canada: CAOT.

Carlsson, G. (2002). Catching the bus in old age. Methodological aspects of physical accessibility assessments in public transport. Doctoral dissertation. Department of Clinical Neuroscience, Lund University. Lund, Sweden: Studentlitteratur.

Carlsson, G., Iwarsson, S., & Ståhl, A. (2002). The personal component of accessibility at group level: Exploring the complexity of functional capacity. *Scandinavian Journal of Occupational Therapy, 9*, 100-108.

Christophersen, J. (Ed.). (2002). *Universal Design. 17 ways of thinking and teaching.* Oslo, Norway: Husbanken.

Clark, F. (2002). Actions for Activity and Occupation. Address for Core Theme III. The WFOT 13th World Congress, June 23-28, Stockholm, Sweden.

Cwikel, J., & Fried, A. V. (1992). The social epidemiology of falls among the community-dwelling elderly: Guidelines for prevention. *Disability and Rehabilitation, 14*, 113-121.

Devor, M., Wang, A., Renvall, M., Feigal, D., & Ramsdell, J. (1994). Compliance with social and safety recommendations in an outpatient comprehensive geriatric assessment program. *Journals of Gerontology, 49*, M168-M173.

Didón, L. U., Magnusson, L., Millgård, O., & Molander, S. (1987). *Plan- och byg-glagen, en kommentar.* [The Planning and Building Act. A commentary.] Stockholm, Sweden: Norstedts.

El-Faizy, M., & Reinsch, S. (1994). Home safety intervention for the prevention of falls. *Physical and Occupational Therapy in Geriatrics, 12*, 33-49.

Fänge, A., & Iwarsson, S. (1999). Physical housing environment—development of a self-assessment instrument. *Canadian Journal of Occupational Therapy, 66*, 250-260.

Fänge, A., & Iwarsson, S. (in press). Accessibility and usability in housing— Construct validity and implications for research and practice. *Disability and Rehabilitation.*

Feinstein, A. R., Josephy, B.R., & Wells, C. K. (1986). Scientific and clinical problems in indexes of functional disability. *Annals of Internal Medicine, 105*, 413-420.

Flanagan, J. C. (1954). The critical incident technique. *Psychological Bulletin, 51*, 327-358.

Gitlin, L. N. (1998). Testing home modification interventions: Issues of theory, measurement, design, and implementation. In R. Schulz, G. Maddox, & M. P. Lawton, (Eds.), *Annual Review of Gerontology and Geriatrics, 18*, 190-245. New York: Springer.

Gitlin, L. N. (in press). Conducting research on home environments: Lessons learned and new directions. *Gerontologist.*

Golant, S. (in press). Conceptualizing time and behavior in environmental gerontology: A pair of old issues deserving new thought. *Gerontologist.*

Handikappombudsmannen. (1997). Rapport till regeringen 1996. [Report to the government 1996.] Stockholm, Sweden: Handikappombudsmannen.

Iwarsson, S. (1997). Functional capacity and physical environmental demand. Exploration of factors influencing everyday activity and health in the elderly population. Doctoral dissertation. Department of Community Health Sciences, Lund University. Lund, Sweden: Studentlitteratur.

Iwarsson, S. (1998). Environmental influences on the cumulative structure of instrumental ADL: An example in osteoporosis patients in a Swedish rural district. *Clinical Rehabilitation, 12*(3), 221-227.

Iwarsson, S. (1999). The Housing Enabler: An objective tool for assessing accessibility. *British Journal of Occupational Therapy, 62*(11), 491-497.

Iwarsson, S., & Isacsson, Å. (1993). Basic accessibility in modern housing —a key to the problems of care in the domestic setting. *Scandinavian Journal of Caring Sciences, 7*, 155-159.

Iwarsson, S., & Isacsson, Å. (1996). Development of a novel instrument for occupational therapy assessment of the physical environment in the home— A methodologic study on "The Enabler." *Occupational Therapy Journal of Research, 16*(4), 227-244.

Iwarsson, S., & Isacsson, Å. (1997a). On scaling methodology and environmental influences in disability assessments: The cumulative structure of personal and instrumental ADL among older adults in a Swedish rural district. *Canadian Journal of Occupational Therapy, 64*, 240-251.

Iwarsson, S., & Isacsson, Å. (1997b). Quality of life in the elderly population: An example exploring interrelationships among subjective well-being. ADL dependence, and housing accessibility. *Archives of Gerontology and Geriatrics, 26*, 71-83.

Iwarsson, S., Isacsson, Å., & Lanke, J. (1998). ADL dependence in the elderly population living in the community: The influence of functional limitations and physical environmental demand. *Occupational Therapy International, 5*, 173-193.

Iwarsson, S., Jensen, G., & Ståhl, A. (2000). Travel Chain Enabler: Development of a pilot instrument for assessment of urban public bus transportation accessibility. *Technology and Disability, 12*, 3-12.

Iwarsson, S., & Nygren, C. (2002). The Housing Enabler: International research version. Project-specific assessment format within "Enabling autonomy, participation, and well-being in old age: The home environment as a determinant for healthy ageing. ENABLE-AGE." Project funded by the European Commission; QLRT-2001-00334. Department of Clinical Neuroscience, Lund University, Sweden.

Iwarsson, S., Oswald, F., Wahl, H. W., Sixsmith, A., Sixsmith, J., Széman, Z., et al. (2001). Enabling autonomy, participation, and well-being in old age: The home environment as a determinant for healthy ageing. ENABLE-AGE. Proposal to the European Commission; QLRT-2001-00334. Lund University, Sweden.

Iwarsson, S., & Slaug, B. (2001). *The housing enabler. An instrument for assessing and analysing accessibility problems in housing.* Nävlinge and Staffanstorp, Sweden: Veten & Skapen HB & Slaug Data Management.

Iwarsson, S., & Ståhl, A. (1999). Traffic engineering and occupational therapy: A collaborative approach for future directions. *Scandinavian Journal of Occupational Therapy, 6*, 21-28.

Iwarsson, S., & Ståhl, A. (2003). Accessibility, usability and universal design—positioning and definition of concepts describing person-environment relationships. *Disability and Rehabilitation, 25*, 57-66.

Jensen, G., Iwarsson, S., & Ståhl, A. (2002). Theoretical understanding and methodological challenges in accessibility assessments focusing the environmental component: An example from travel chains in urban public bus transport. *Disability and Rehabilitation, 24*, 231-242.

Jette, A. M. (1994). How measurement techniques influences estimates of disability in older populations. *Social Science and Medicine, 38*, 937-942.

Law, M., Cooper, B., Strong, S., Stewart, D., Rigby, P., & Letts, L. (1996). The person-environment-occupation model: A transactive approach to occupational performance. *Canadian Journal of Occupational Therapy, 63*, 9-23.

Lawton, M. P. (1986). *Environment and aging.* 2nd ed. Albany, NY: Center for the Study of Aging.

Lawton, M. P. (1989a). Three functions of the residential environment. *Journal of housing for the elderly, 5*, 35-50.

Lawton, M. P. (1989b). Environmental proactivity in older people. In V. L. Bengtson, & K. W. Schaie (Eds.), *The course of later life. Research and reflections.* New York: Springer.

Lawton, M. P. (1989c). Environmental proactivity and affect in older people. In S. Spaceapan, & S. Oskamp, *The social psychology of aging.* Newbury Park, CA: Sage.

Lawton, M. P., & Nahemow, L. (1973). Ecology and the aging process. In C. Eisdorfer, & M.P. Lawton (Eds.), *The psychologist of adult development and aging.* Washington, DC: American Psychological Association.

Lawton, M. P., & Simon, B. (1968). The ecology of social relationships in housing for the elderly. *Gerontologist, 8*, 108-115.

Lewin, K. (1951). *Field theory in social science.* New York: Harper & Brothers.

Lundh, U. (1992). Vård och omsorg i eget boende på äldre dar. [Care and nursing in the home setting of the elderly.] Doctoral dissertation. Linköping, Sweden: Linköping University.

Miller, B. R., Sieg, K. W., Ludwig, F. M., Shortridge, S. D., & Van Deusen, J. (1988). *Six perspectives on theory for the practice of occupational therapy.* Rockville, MD: Aspen.

Morfitt, J. M. (1983). Falls in old people at home: Intrinsic versus environmental factors in causation. *Public Health, 97*, 115-120.

Oxford Popular Dictionary and Thesaurus. (1998). 3rd ed. Oxford, UK: Oxford University Press.

Pollock, N. (1993). Client-centered assessment. *American Journal of Occupational Therapy, 47*, 298-301.

Preiser, W. F. E., & Ostroff, E. (Eds.). (2001). *Universal design handbook.* New York: McGraw-Hill.

Regeringens proposition 1999/2000: 79. (2000). Från patient till medborgare—en nationell handlingsplan för handikappolitiken. 1999/2000: 79. [Governmental proposition. From patient to citizen—A national agenda for disability policies.] Stockholm, Sweden.

Reschovsky, J. D., & Newman, S. (1990). Adaptations for independent living by older frail households. *Gerontologist, 30*, 543-552.

Schmitt, E., Kruse, A., & Olbrich, E. (1994). Formen der Selbständigkeit und Wohnumwelt—ein empirischer Beitrag aus der Studie "Möglichkeiten und grenzen der selbständigen Lebensführung im Alter." [Independence and the living environment—An empirical contribution from the study "Potential and limits of independent living in old age."] *Zeitschrift für Gerontologie, 27*, 390-398.

Slaug, B., & Iwarsson, S. (2001). Housing Enabler 1.0—A Tool for Housing Accessibility Analysis. Software for PC; demo version available at www.enabler.nu. Staffanstorp & Nävlinge, Sweden: Slaug Data Management AB & Veten & Skapen HB.

Steinfeld, E., & Danford, G. S. (1999). Theory as a basis for research on enabling environments. In E. Steinfeld, & G. S. Danford (Eds.), *Enabling environments: Measuring the impact of environment on disability and rehabilitation* (pp. 11-33). New York: Kluwer Academic/Plenum.

Steinfeld, E., Schroeder, S., Duncan, J., Faste, R., Chollet, D., Bishop, M., et al. (1979). *Access to the built environments: A review of the literature.* Washington, DC: U.S. Government Printing Office.

Steinfeld, E., & Shea, S. (1993). Enabling home environments. Identifying barriers to independence. *Technology and Disability, 2,* 69-79.

Steinfeld, E., & Tauke, B. (2002). Universal designing. In J. Christophersen (Ed.), *Universal Design. 17 ways of thinking and teaching.* Oslo, Norway: Husbanken.

Stokols, D., & Altman, I. (1987). *Handbook of environmental psychology.* New York: John Wiley & Sons.

Svensson, T. (1996). Competence and quality of life: Theoretical views of biography. In J. E. Birren, G. M. Kenyon, J. E. Ruth, J. J. F. Schroots, & T. Svensson (Eds.), *Aging and biography: Exploration in adult development* (pp. 100-116). New York: Springer.

Trickey, F., Maltais, D., Gosselin, C., & Robitaille, Y. (1993). Adapting older persons' homes to promote independence. *Physical and Occupational Therapy in Geriatrics, 12*(1), 1-14.

United Nations (UN). (1993). Standard rules on the equalization of opportunities for persons with disabilities. New York: United Nations.

Wade, D. T. (1994). *Measurement in neurological rehabilitation.* Oxford, UK: Oxford University Press.

Wahl, H. W. (in press). Environmental gerontology at the beginning of the new millennium: Reflections on its historical, empirical and theoretical development. *Gerontologist.*

Wahl, H. W., Oswald, F., & Zimprich, D. (1999). Everyday competence in visually impaired older adults: A case for person-environment perspectives. *Gerontologist, 39,* 140-149.

World Health Organization (WHO). (1991). Action for public health. Sundsvall statement on supportive environments. June 9-15, Sundsvall, Sweden. Geneva, Switzerland: WHO.

World Health Organization (WHO). (1992). ICD-10: The international statistical classification of diseases and related health problems. 10th revision. Geneva, Switzerland: WHO.

World Health Organization (WHO). (2001). ICF: The international classification of functioning, disability and health. Geneva, Switzerland: WHO.

CHAPTER 5

Socio-physical Environments at the Macro Level: The Impact of Population Migration

CHARLES F. LONGINO, JR.
DEPARTMENT OF SOCIOLOGY, WAKE FOREST UNIVERSITY

M igration is the population process that has the greatest impact on small geographical environments. Professors understand this point as they watch the annual comings-and-goings of the student population, and the impact of its ebb and flow on the economic, social, and intellectual micro-environment of the college town. The same can be said in Phoenix, Arizona, or West Palm Beach, Florida, regarding the seasonal migration of retirees. Likewise, the economic, political, and social impacts of retirees can be discerned at the state level in a few heavily impacted states. In the pages of this chapter, the major socio-environmental patterns, types, motivations, and impacts of migrating retirees will be explored, primarily in the context of the United States, summarizing research published nearly entirely in the past decade. These studies are largely demographic, and as such, tend to emphasize macro-level socio-physical environments and perspectives.

PATTERNS OF MIGRATION

The Evolution of State Destinations

The first way of describing migration destinations in the USA is to compare the numbers who moved to different states or counties, ranking the states or counties that received the largest proportions. The top 100 counties or county groups (called *public use microdata areas*, or PUMAs) were ranked in terms of net interstate migration for the 1985-1990 census migration period. Florida contains one-third of these PUMAs. This fact is not surprising considering Florida's seigniorial status as a retirement destination state.

110

Perhaps more interesting, however, the substate destinations are located in counties featuring coastal, mountain, and desert physical environments across the United States from seaside New Hampshire to the Puget Sound in Washington state. Maricopa County, Arizona (Phoenix), and Clark County, Nevada (Las Vegas), rank second and fourth, respectively, and are the leading destinations in the West. Riverside County, California (Palm Springs), ranks 29th and is California's only entry on the list.

Although the Sunbelt pattern generally holds, there are a greater variety of substate destinations than is commonly assumed. Some strong regional destinations, such as Cape Cod, do not show up in interstate migration patterns simply because so many of its migrants come from within state (Cuba, 1992). The state of New Jersey, on the other hand, has consistently received enough retirees from New York and Pennsylvania to keep it among the top 10 interstate destination states since 1960. Most regional retirement locations, especially those outside the Sunbelt, only show up when county-level data are used (Longino, 1995).

Channelization is a nautical term denoting a very busy port; deep channels are dug to accommodate ship traffic. Over half (54 percent in 2000) of older interstate migrants arrive in just 10 of the 50 states. Florida dominates the scene, attracting from a fifth to a quarter of all interstate migrants over 60 in all four census decades (Longino & Bradley, in press). These are national destination states, and over time the list has become dominated by Sunbelt states.

Regional destinations primarily attract migrants from adjacent states and do not necessarily show up in the states listed in Table 5.1. Examples are Cape Cod, Massachusetts, the New Jersey shore, the Pocono Mountains of northeastern Pennsylvania, the Wisconsin Dells, and the Upper Peninsula of Michigan, all located outside the Sunbelt. Other locations in the Appalachian mountain chain, the Ozark region of Missouri and Arkansas, are in the non-coastal Sunbelt (Rowles & Watkins, 1993; Watkins, 1990). Southern and western Nevada and areas in the Pacific Northwest are all retirement areas of strong regional attraction (Cuba & Longino, 1991), and areas frequently cited in retirement guides as good places to retire (Savageau, 2000). Having mentioned the diversity of regional locations, however, it remains true that older migrants, by count, still prefer locations in Sunbelt states.

Census data are helpful in defining the temporal patterns of state inflows and outflows of older migrants. In the matrices, however, the connection between individual migrants and their old and new environments is barely visible.

The changes that do occur, however, point to some long-term trends and processes that should be considered. Humans, and human populations, are not boundless; they are finite and relatively easy to track over time and space. Discerning the long-term patterns in those traces is one of the most

TABLE 5.1 Ten States Receiving Most In-Migrants Age 60+ in Five-Year Periods Ending in 1960, 1970, 1980, and 1990

Rank	State	1960 #	%	State	1970 #	%	State	1980 #	%	State	1990 #	%
1	FL	208,072	22.3	FL	263,200	24.4	FL	437,040	26.3	FL	451,709	23.8
2	CA	126,883	13.6	CA	107,000	9.9	CA	144,880	8.7	CA	131,514	6.9
3	NJ	36,019	3.9	AZ	47,600	4.4	AZ	94,600	5.7	AZ	98,756	5.2
4	NY	33,794	3.6	NJ	46,000	4.3	TX	78,480	4.7	TX	78,117	4.1
5	IL	30,355	3.3	TX	39,800	3.7	NJ	49,400	3.0	NC	64,530	3.4
6	AZ	29,571	3.2	NY	32,800	3.0	PA	39,520	2.4	PA	57,538	3.0
7	OH	27,759	3.0	OH	32,300	3.0	NC	39,400	2.4	NJ	49,176	2.6
8	TX	26,770	2.9	IL	28,800	2.7	WA	35,760	2.2	WA	47,484	2.5
9	PA	25,738	2.8	PA	28,600	2.7	IL	35,720	2.1	VA	46,554	2.4
10	MI	20,308	2.2	MO	25,300	2.3	NY	34,920	2.1	GA	44,475	2.3
Total												
Interstate Migrants		931,012			1,079,200			1,622,120			1,901,105	
% of Total in Top 10 States			**60.7**			**60.4**			**59.5**			**56.3**

interesting speculative aspects of social science. Migration patterns do hint at a long-term macro process. Quality of life, or at least the perception thereof, is at the heart of this process.

A geographical definition of quality of life incorporates the concept of individual well-being but focuses more on environments than on individuals. Quality of life, however, like a coin, has two sides, goals and appraisals (Cutter, 1985). The goal side is subjective and attempts to specify what a good place "ought to be." The appraisal side assesses the actual environment, usually with a variety of measures. It is the subjective nature of the *ideal*, however, that creates the problem in rating places. The "ideal" environment differs from one rater to another, so the reliability of ratings is not always high. The person-environment (P-E) fit, in this case, is largely anticipatory and perceptual.

Some of the subjective goals of older migrants can be discerned from the observed population data. We know, for example, that climatic conditions favor Sunbelt locations. We also know there is a movement out of the most populous states. Moving to a place with less congestion and fewer of the problems that big cities tend to have must be attractive to many retirees. The fact that people often move to the rim states (from New England through Florida and California to the state of Washington), most of which are on the water, must imply that more than a warm climate is involved. An attractive physical environment is also important. Water and mountains, and scenic beauty in general are traditional pulls.

States from which retirees move to the Sunbelt tend overwhelmingly to contain large metropolitan populations. Substate analyses show the leading origin counties to be in these large cities (Longino, 1995). Economic opportunities are greater in metropolitan environments than elsewhere. Cities are places where resources can be accumulated more easily to support such a move in retirement. People who work in large cities also confront higher levels of environmental challenges (pollution, crime, traffic, and noise) than those who live and work in smaller cities and small towns. In addition to climate, therefore, there are quality of life issues, derived from city living, that drive retirement migration. Ordinarily, these are considered "push factors" in traditional push-pull models.

So long as there is a perceived quality of life difference in the environments at origin and destination, the better quality of life will always attract new residents who are retired. The passage of time, however, sometimes alters perceptions. Retired migrants who have lived in a Sunbelt community for 10 or 15 years will often complain that the quality of life has declined since they arrived, and they often blame the decline on the retirees who followed them, and those who keep coming. The reason that they keep coming is that even in its decline, as viewed by migrant old-timers, there is still a quality of life advantage as compared with where the new migrants originated. The quality of life of the environment of origin may also have declined over the past 15 years, at least perceptually, holding the relative advantage of the destination about constant.

When the difference narrows, however, in-migration is gradually choked off, generating pressure for retirement out-migration from the old destination. People who retire in Sunbelt cities sometimes subsequently move to less crowded places with greater scenic beauty and feel that they have traded up on their quality of life.

This is the long-term pattern seen in California. Once a powerful magnet to retirees, California may be better known in the future as an origin than as a destination. In recent years, residents have faced water and electricity shortages, earthquakes, rising crime and riots, skyrocketing housing costs (recently moderated but still much higher than national averages), and generally bad news in the national news media. An increasing rate of out-migration is not surprising in this context. The same principle appears to be at work in certain regions of Florida. Dade County certainly has its share of crowding, crime, and natural disasters, not to mention its negative image in the news media. An exodus of retirees from Dade County as the quality of life has declined in Greater Miami over recent decades has been evident (Longino & Perricone, 1991).

The strategic planner should not forget the long-term as well as the short-term prospects for the quality of life when considering retirement migration. For a future generation that values personal space, convenience, and quality more highly than earlier generations did, unplanned and uncontrolled retirement development may carry within itself the seeds of its own destruction by hastening the decline in the quality of life as it is understood by retirees.

A CYCLICAL PATTERN: SEASONAL MIGRATION

Seasonal migration is a very interesting cyclical pattern, which stands midway between vacationing and permanent change of residence. Seasonal migrants are variously called dual-community residents, winter (or summer) visitors, and snowbirds.

No one knows how many there are. The Census Bureau does not attempt to directly measure seasonal migration. Although it does keep track of the number of persons who completed their census forms away from home at the time of the census, the data from this set of records are not easy to interpret because they have not been broken down by age. However, there have been several local surveys—in Texas, Arizona, and Florida—that provide snapshots of seasonal migrants and their destinations (Longino & Marshall, 1990). Survey results (McHugh & Mings, 1991) have offered a reasonably consistent profile of seasonal migrants, describing them as overwhelmingly white, retired, healthy, married persons mostly in their sixties. These are characteristics associated, in other studies, with lifestyle-driven amenity migration. Another study (Martin, Hoppe, Marshall, & Duciuk, 1992) compared samples of older Canadians who wintered in Florida with U.S. citizens who spent their winters in the Rio Grande Valley of Texas. The aggregate characteristics of the migrants are similar to those studied by McHugh and Mings in Arizona.

Nevertheless, Hogan and Steinnes (1993) argue that seasonal and permanent migrants cannot be estimated well by the same statistical model. And, indeed, the Canadian seasonal migrants in Florida are diverse as well (Tucker, Mullins, Beland, Longino, & Marshall, 1992). English-speaking and French-speaking Canadians tend to settle in different parts of the state. The demographic profiles of the residents in these two settlements of seasonal migrants are very similar in many ways. However, the Francophone Canadians are more youthful, have lower levels of education and monthly income, and have larger families, contributing, by their visits, to larger social support networks in Florida.

McHugh and Mings (1991) were the first to emphasize environmental issues when they considered climate as a motive for seasonal moves. They found that the colder the climate, the more likely retirees are to migrate seasonally. U.S. retirees in states along the Canadian border have a greater propensity to migrate seasonally than those in states located farther south.

A good deal of research has been devoted to the question of whether seasonal migration is only a stage, a precursor to a permanent move (Longino et al., 1991; McHugh, 1990). Whether seasonal migrants settle down at their destination and become permanent residents depends upon the balance between ties to place and persons at origin and destination and the shift in these ties over time. Ties to the environment are important. Furthermore, seasonal migrants are also encouraged to remain year round by their relatives and friends who have already moved permanently to seasonal destinations. The vast majority of seasonal migrants, perhaps 80 percent, apparently do not relocate permanently. They extend or shorten their visits, and they finally end their extended series of visits when their health forces them to do so.

There is an additional environmental issue for seasonal migrants. The fit between environment and the person can become problematic in the face of declining or fluctuating health. McHugh and Mings (1994) examined the health care of seasonal residents in Arizona and found that they tend to adjust to health decrements over time. Their major adjustment strategies include reducing the number of side trips during their winter residence and giving up their recreational vehicles in favor of renting lodging while in Arizona.

Health issues also affect seasonal migration on a policy level. Canadians wintering in Florida tend to limit the length of their stay in response to their nation's national health insurance rules that require them to spend more than half a year in Canada to keep their benefits. These international seasonal migrants understand a strategic orientation toward the Canadian and U.S. health care systems. One study (Marshall et al., 1989) found that most seasonal migrants visited a Canadian doctor for a checkup and stocked up on prescription drugs prior to leaving Canada. One-third left specific instructions with relatives or friends in case of a medical emergency and four-fifths enrolled in a private health insurance plan to supplement their provincial health plan.

Mings (1997) compared seasonal migration in the United States, Canada, and Australia, and found many similarities. He studied winter visitors in a caravan [recreational vehicle] park in tropical northern Queensland. The demographic profiles of persons in the three national categories were very similar, and all maintained high levels of recreational activities. However, the Australians had traveled longer distances to get to their destination, and had a somewhat lower level of social interaction than Canadian and U.S. seasonal migrants. The result was a lower level of social integration among the Australian seasonal migrants. There are apparently macro-environmental differences among seasonal migrants.

McHugh, Hogan, and Happel (1995), argue that temporary residence is much more frequent than we realize. They found that cyclical migration often occurs in stages, beginning with vacationing in midlife and leading to longer stays in the retirement years. Many migrants who had moved permanently to Arizona tended to make extended visits back to their origins when temperatures rose to uncomfortable levels, placing them in the category of cyclical movers as well. In fact, if you combine older persons visiting in the winter with residents leaving in the summer, and add those who move within state seasonally (to higher and cooler places in the summer), the number is substantial. They estimated that, in the winter, one-fourth of older people in Arizona fall into one of these three categories.

Apparently seasonal migration generates its own lifestyle and culture, different from that of permanent migrants but equally valuable in its own right. Once having adopted the lifestyle, seasonal migration is likely to last for several years, finally interrupted and reluctantly terminated.

MOTIVATIONS FOR MIGRATION

The 1990s saw a steady advancement of conceptual models in the study of retirement migration addressed to the "why" and "so what" questions. They do not compete directly with one another, but have different types of starting points: the life course, the migration decision process, housing disequilibrium, and place identity.

THE LIFE COURSE MODELS

One line of theoretical development has tended to make the life course of migrants during the retirement years its central focus, emphasizing those triggering mechanisms associated with life events and probabilities. This conceptualization draws from demographic and human-development perspectives and is congenial with other concerns of gerontological research. Warnes (1992), for example, developed a long list of life course events that occur, on average, at different ages. He sequenced them and discussed the housing needs and mobility patterns associated with them. In later life, the list includes retirement, bereavement, and frailty.

Litwak and Longino (1987) presented a developmental context for the patterns of elderly interstate migration commonly reported from demographic studies. They argue that the nature of modern technology puts the kinship structures of older people under pressures to make three basic types of moves. The first type involves persons who are recently retired, a second type includes persons who are experiencing moderate forms of disability, and a third type is an institutional move when health problems overwhelm the capability of the family to care for older relatives at home. The moves are not necessarily sequenced. The pressure may be slight for the first type of move, but it may increase for the second type and again for the third. It is easy to see, in this model, that the P-E fit is critical, and when it becomes imbalanced, the imbalance creates pressure for a move.

De Jong et al. (1995) and Choi (1996) argue effectively that poor health, reduced social affiliation, economic insecurity, having functional limitations, and getting on with life after a family crisis, all micro-environmental issues, are adequate reasons for moving. The life course model merely arranges some of these motivations around a type of move.

THE MIGRATION DECISION MODELS

A second line of theoretical advancement in the 1990s built upon migration decision-making theory (Wiseman, 1980) to delineate P-E adjustment processes by which the elderly decide whether or not and where to move. Following Ravenstein's (1885) framework, Wiseman (1980) had argued that moves were triggered by push and pull factors, such as climate, environmental hassle level, or cost of living, and facilitated or hampered by indigenous filters such as personal resources or the housing market. Once the decision to move is made, the selection of a destination follows. Only then can the migration outcome be considered. There are feedback loops in Wiseman's model. People who decide not to move, or cannot successfully choose a destination, may adjust their present environment through various mechanisms in order to avoid feeling trapped there. Furthermore, over time, migration outcomes that initially may be improvements generate new pushes and pulls that may eventually trigger another move.

Cuba (1991), studying migrants to Cape Cod, challenged Wiseman's assertion that the decision to move preceded the selection of a destination. Most had not considered other places and knew they wanted to live on the Cape before they had worked out the final decision to move.

Haas and Serow (1993) elaborate on the Wiseman model, fitting it to the circumstance of the recently or nearly retired amenity migrant. They add to the model "remote thoughts" or daydreams about moving (Longino, 1992) that precede the formal process, and the information sources that make the actor aware of push/pull factors. Another important addition to the original decision model, following the move, is developing ties within the community. Community adjustment has been understudied (Serow, 1992). Kallan (1993) suggests that although individual level variables are stronger predictors of the migration of older adults, contextual variables and multilevel interactions improve the explanatory power of the models. The influence of some contextual variables, such as climate, crime rates, and cost of living, varies among elderly subgroups.

The Health and Retirement Survey, a 10-year, 5-panel, national study of persons crossing the retirement threshold, offers the best opportunity for building models that would prospectively predict retirement migration based on social and environmental factors. To this point, the relative weight of the pushes and pulls, especially those rooted in the environments of origin and destination, has not been studied.

THE HOUSING DISEQUILIBRIUM MODEL

Economic incentives due to housing assets may be assessed within the context of the migration decision model. When they are the focus, however, the resulting model is better described as a housing disequilibrium model

(Fournier, Rasmussen, & Serow, 1988). This model, as applied to older migrants (Clark & White, 1990), received much attention from researchers very early in the decade of the 1990s. The push to move from less affordable rental housing tends to motivate central city moves, whereas the pull to more appropriate, owned housing tends to motivate suburban moves.

A study conducted by Steinnes and Hogan (1992) supported the hypothesis that elderly migration to Arizona, both seasonal and permanent, results, in part, from the economic gains made in the housing markets from which migrants move. Americans experience relatively little geographic mobility in the 15 years or so leading up to retirement. As a consequence, they tend to gain through the appreciation of their residential property. Selling a house in California, for example, can net a surplus that can be "spent" on seasonal migration or a move to a more affordable housing market. Of course, the housing disequilibrium model could be easily adapted to an environmental perspective, because the functional match between persons and their housing is always a factor in housing satisfaction. And, as in the Wiseman model, if moving is not an option due to scarce resources or other factors, housing environments can be adapted.

THE PLACE IDENTITY MODELS

A final conceptual framework that is relevant to environmental considerations emerged during the 1990s and may be called the place identity model. Cuba (1989) argues that "selves" as well as "bodies" can be mobile. Moving oneself physically to another community environment does not necessarily mean that one also moves emotionally. There are some migrants who never put down roots but remain emotionally tied to their former communities. Some of them have problems changing from being a vacationer to being a permanent resident after they arrive in their destination communities. Identity can be tied to geographic environment for a number of reasons. Homes and neighborhood settings carry emotional and social significance; they are places in which memories are embedded. Staying in the familiar pre-retirement social and geographic environment promises an environment where retirees understand the rhythms and routines of life (Longino, Perzynski, & Stoller, 2002).

Cuba and Hummon (1993a) argue that identification with one's dwelling, one's community, and one's region, is arrived at differently. Personal possessions and the dwelling itself foster identification with the dwelling as "home," especially for older women; social participation and the size of one's friendship network are essential for strong identification with the community. And, finally, younger migrants more often base their identity on affiliations of friendship, family, and emotional self-attributions, whereas older migrants do so in terms of dwelling and prior experience with place (Cuba & Hummond, 1993b). Weak community identity could hinder adjustment and thereby contribute to a second migration decision cycle.

Finally, we confront shifts in place identity throughout our lives, and the experience that accrues serves to inform future decisions (Watkins, 1999). Place identity, therefore, must be seen as part of a long-term process of adjustments.

IMPACT OF MIGRATION

Economic Impact

The migrant decides to move to a new community environment. However, the migrant's relative value to that community is also being assessed simultaneously. The assumed value of the potential migrant has risen over the past decade in many communities. The decade of the 1990s began with a spate of articles considering the economic impact of retirees at their destination. Longino and Crown (1990) and Crown and Longino (1991) documented the sizable amount of income that was transferred to and from states due to retirement migration. A census item asks for income data in the last year before the census. The 1979 income of all migrants who had moved into Florida between 1975 and 1980 amounted to over $4 billion dollars. In the same year, New York State lost over $2.2 billion from outmigration between 1975 and 1980. Ten years later, the income from 1985-1990 in-migrants had doubled to $8.3 billion for Florida. Considering the fact that older migrants are pumping most of their income into the economy through consumption, but not competing for jobs, this was a sizeable economic boost to Florida's economy. In the same year, New York lost nearly $4 billion (Longino, 1995). The income figures for other states fell in between Florida and New York.

Serow (1990) analyzed the percent of their incomes that older migrants paid in state and local taxes in Florida and concluded that their economic contribution to the state was substantial. And Sastry (1992), using a regional input-output modeling system and data from the Consumer Expenditure Survey, agreed that retirement migration had large, positive, total impacts on the Florida economy. Finally, using data from an expenditure survey of older migrants around Asheville, North Carolina, Serow and Haas (1992) demonstrated the economic dynamics that produce specific benefits for the local and state economies.

Simultaneously, Glasgow and her colleagues were examining rural retirement counties across the country and speculating about the positive economic contribution that retirees could make. They showed that these 515 rural counties, where the older population was growing through migration, outperformed nonmetropolitan area averages for job growth (Reeder & Glasgow, 1990). Retirees were said to establish a "mailbox economy" of social security and pensions (Glasgow, 1991). These studies argued that older migrants had not been an excessive burden on local public service expenditures, which tended to be low in any case (Glasgow & Reeder, 1990; Glasgow, 1995), a point echoed by Joseph and Cloutier (1991) concerning rural Canadians. Voss and Fuguitt (1991) showed that in rural low-income counties in the South, new income from migrants only replaced that taken out by out-migrants. These were not the same set of counties, however, that Glasgow called "retirement counties." Hodge (1991), in his study of smaller communities in the province of British Columbia, Canada, reported data supportive of Glasgow's analysis. Bennett (1992, 1993), in studying high amenity retirement counties on the Atlantic seaboard, offered strong support to Glasgow's observations. Schneider and Green (1992), however, noted that the economic success of the retirement counties should not be attributed simply to retirement migration. Rural counties, when accessible to heavily traveled transportation corridors and abundant with amenities, are attractive to young people as well.

Schneider and Green (1992), along with Glasgow (1990), and Cook (1990), were early contributors to the discussion of the utility of community policies to attract retirees. Fagan and Longino (1993) demonstrated the benefits to rural retirement counties of diversifying their economic development strategy by adding tourism and active retiree recruitment. Deller (1995) used a regional economic model to simulate the impact of a policy of retirement recruitment on the state of Maine. He argued that the short-run beneficial economic impact of retiree recruitment is significant and warrants serious consideration. Finally, the economic benefits of elderly winter residents to Phoenix (Happel, Hogan, & Pflanz, 1988) and, generally, to Arizona (Hogan & Happel, 1994) are also now documented. Finally, Frey and his colleagues (2000) remind us that only in those states with a positive net migration can there be much economic impact from retirement migration.

However, despite the preponderance of evidence, concerns continued to be voiced on the subject of retiree recruitment. The majority of retiring migrants does not have a high income as compared to working people. Nationally, over one-third (35.6 percent) of older interstate migrants have incomes under $20,000 (in 1989 dollars), as compared with the 28.2 percent with incomes over $50,000 (Longino, 1995). Stallmann and Siegel (1995) warned that the long-term effects of aging in place, if retiree recruitment were to fall off, could be negative for rural communities in terms of increased public expenditures for health and long-term care services. This is a concern also shared by Mullins and Rosentraub (1992). Indeed, this anxiety may grow in the years immediately ahead. Due to the long-term effects of fertility decline during and following the Great Depression, the growth of entrants into the retirement years will level off during the early 2000s just before baby boomers retire. This factor alone is likely to produce a greater aging in place effect in retirement communities that are fed by migration but do not *actively* recruit new younger retirees (Longino & Perricone, 1991).

LOCAL POLITICAL ACTIVISM AND SUPPORT FOR PUBLIC SERVICES

As the 1990s dawned, there was a tentative consensus among students of retirement migration that the political impact of migrants was small to nonexistent. Rosenbaum and Button (1989) studied the political impact of the expanding older population on city and county governments in Florida. Their findings suggested that older Floridians are politically active at the local level but seldom get involved in organized advocacy for the elderly, and they are not against local policies largely beneficial to other groups. They did find a private anxiety among many municipal and county officials, however, that the elderly might someday have a negative political impact on their communities.

This picture seems quite naïve a decade later. Political research of the past decade tells a more complex story. Local voting studies have tended to examine the results of local school budget referenda. Using the results of school district bond elections in Florida, Button (1992), and especially MacManus (1997), both found that a higher percent of elderly residents and voters in a school district are associated with lower support for schools. This finding is consistent with recent research by Simonsen and Robbins (1996), who found that citizens, and senior citizens, in particular, were much less supportive of public services that they do not expect to use. This would include schools.

IMPACT ON COMMUNITY SOCIAL STRUCTURE AND VALUES

Longino (1990) argued that retirement enclaves in rural counties tend to be worlds unto themselves, relatively unattached to local social structure. Cuba (1992) even asserted that, on Cape Cod, the distinguishing characteristics of older migrants make them susceptible to scapegoating by non-migrants and younger migrants.

Later studies have seen migrants as more proactive and as change agents in their communities. Rowles and Watkins (1993), for example, provide case studies of three contrasting Appalachian communities at different stages of development as retirement destinations. They draw from their analysis a temporal model of community development involving overlapping phases of emergence, recognition, restructuring, and saturation. This study is refreshingly insightful because it analyzes retirement migration in a broader social context. *Place identity* theory is also useful as it focuses on adaptive dynamics in retirement communities. For example, middle-class retirees, moving to a small town in the mountains or on the seashore, are likely to band together to protect the environmental ambiance of the community. They may, for instance, oppose the local chamber of commerce as it attempts to develop land for housing or to invite in light industry. Local opinion may see the migrants as selfishly obstructing attempts to create economic opportunities that would raise the standard of living for the next generation of local residents. The lure of economic development through retiree recruitment, in some small towns, could have disappointing consequences for local boosters as the size and power of the older population increases.

COHORT CHANGE IN MIGRATION

The Baby Boom Arrives Soon

Will the retirees of the baby boom generation be different from those of earlier generations? The leading edge of that cohort of persons born between 1946 and 1964 is approaching retirement. The fact that the number of new retirees will increase rapidly between 2008 and 2026 will mean that there will also be a rapid increase in persons making retirement moves in the United States. The rate at which persons over age 60 make interstate moves has changed little since 1960. The great increase in mobility both among the retired and the general population between 1975 and 1980 is considered an aberration of the general trend before and since due to the social turmoil the United States was experiencing during that period. There is no reason to suspect that it will change radically when the baby boomers begin retiring. If that is the case, then the number of migrants will no doubt also increase as a function of population aging.

Will the patterns of migration destination change radically when the baby boomers retire? Even if the leading destination states continue to lose their attractiveness to older migrants, their lost market share would have to be radical to actually reduce the number of retirees moving into those states between 2010 and 2020. The increasing numbers will offset moderate proportional changes.

On the other hand, those states that have been developing strategies for courting retirees, because they expect them to have a beneficial economic impact on their destination communities, will interpret the rising tide of retired migrants as a validation of their recruitment efforts. Further, the states in which regional retiree destinations have existed for decades will experience a burgeoning of their older in-migrants, making them much more visible than before. Attention will be paid to the allure of Cape Cod, the Ozarks, and even Michigan's Upper Peninsula, Montana, and Idaho, as the baby boomers crowd in, drawing some attention away from the traditional Sunbelt locations.

THE BABY BOOMERS DEPART

After the baby boomers have retired, those who moved will age in place, although a few will make additional moves. The reduction in the numbers of newly retired migrants will no longer make retirees seem younger in communities where they have tended to move in large numbers. They will age, as a part of the U.S. population, from 2020 to 2050, by which time they are expected to have largely died out, finally removing the generational bulge from the age-sex structure. During this 30-year period, the concentrations of older persons created by the out-migration of the young, and the in-migration of the old, will receive increasing attention as concentrations of age-related needs of all kinds. Because the nonmobile majority of the baby boom will be aging in place also, retirement destinations will only seem to be special examples of a general phenomenon, thus eroding their uniqueness.

CONCLUSION

The former British colonies on the continents of North America and Australia have high mobility rates. This may be true of retirees in those countries as well. The European Union has reduced or eliminated barriers between formerly independent states, and population movement between those states are expected to increase as a result (Convey & Kupiszewski, 1995; Penninx, 1986). The seasonal and permanent migration between

Northern and Southern Europe that was recently documented by Warnes and Patterson (1998), Williams, King, and Warnes (1997), and Williams and Patterson (1998) provides a baseline against which future European studies may be compared.

This chapter has not attempted to thoroughly summarize the research on the migration of retirees throughout the world. Space limitations prohibited such a far-ranging discussion. Instead, it has focused primarily, and more narrowly, on research in the United States, primarily in the past decade, and drawing heavily from other integrative and summarizing works of the author (Longino, 2001). It has focused largely on the macro level of analysis. The gerontology journals are the ones most thoroughly reviewed. This strategy always runs the risk of ignoring pockets of important research beyond the view of the writer that are developing in other disciplines, locations, or from other theoretical perspectives. Nonetheless, the basic patterns of retirement migration, particularly in the United States, have now been explored.

REFERENCES

Bennett, D. G. (1992). The impact of retirement migration on Carteret and Brunswick counties, N.C. *North Carolina Geographer, 1*, 25-38.
Bennett, D. G. (1993). Retirement migration and economic development in high-amenity, nonmetropolitan areas. *The Journal of Applied Gerontology, 12*(4), 466-481.
Button, J. W. (1992). A sign of generational conflict: The impact of Florida's aging voters on local school and tax referenda. *Social Science Quarterly, 73*(4), 786-797.
Chevan, A. (1995). Holding on and letting go. *Research on Aging, 17*(3), 278-302.
Choi, N. G. (1996). Older persons who move: Reasons and health consequences. *The Journal of Applied Gerontology, 15*(3), 325-344.
Clark, W. A. V., & White, K. (1990). Modeling elderly mobility. *Environment and Planning A, 22*, 909-924.
Convey, A., & Kupiszewski, M. (1995). Keeping up with Schengen: Migration and Policy in the European Union. *International Migration Review, 29*(4), pp. 939-963.
Cook, A. K. (1990). Retirement migration as a community development option. *Journal of the Community Development Society, 21*(1), 83-101.
Crown, W. H., & Longino, C. F., Jr. (1991). State and regional policy implications of elderly migration. *Journal of Aging and Social Policy, 3*, 185-207.
Cuba, L. J. (1989). Retiring from vacationland: From visitor to resident. *Generations, 13*(2), 63-67.
Cuba, L. J. (1991). Models of migration decisions making reexamined: The destination search of older migrants to Cape Cod. *The Gerontologist, 31*(2), 204-209.

Cuba, L. J. (1992). *The Cape Cod retirement migration study: A final report to the National Institute of Aging*. Wellesley, MA: Wellesley College.

Cuba, L. J., & Hummon, D. M. (1993a). A place to call home: Identification with dwelling, community and religion. *The Sociological Quarterly, 34*, 111-131.

Cuba, L. J., & Hummon, D. M. (1993b). Constructing a sense of home: Place affiliation and migration across the life-cycle. *Sociological Forum, 8*(4), 547-572.

Cuba, L. J., & Longino, C. F., Jr. (1991). Regional retirement migration: The case of Cape Cod. *Journal of Gerontology: Social Sciences, 46*, S33-S42.

DeJong, G. F., Wilmoth, J. M., Angel, J. L., & Cornwell, G. T. (1995). Motives and the geographic mobility of very old Americans. *Journal of Gerontology: Social Sciences, 50B*(6), S395-S404.

Deller, S. C. (1995). Economic impact of retirement migration. *Economic Development Quarterly, 9*(1), 25-38.

Fagan, M., & Longino, C. F., Jr. (1993). Migrating retirees: A source for economic development. *Economic Development Quarterly, 7*(1), 98-106.

Fournier, G. M., Rasmussen, D. W., & Serow, W. J. (1988). Elderly migration as a response to economic incentives. *Social Science Quarterly, 69*, 245–260.

Frey, W. H., Kao- Lee, L., & Lin, G. (2000). State magnets for different elderly migrant types in the United States. *International Journal of Population Geography, 6*, 21-44.

Glasgow, N. L. (1990). Attracting retirees as a community development option. *Journal of the Community Development Society, 21*(1), 102-114.

Glasgow, N. L. (1991). A place in the country. *American Demographics, 13*(3), 24-30.

Glasgow, N. L. (1995). Retirement migration and the use of services in nonmetropolitan counties. *Rural Sociology, 60*(2), 224-243.

Glasgow, N. L., & Reeder, R. J. (1990). Economic and fiscal implications of nonmetropolitan retirement migration. *The Journal of Applied Gerontology, 9*(4), 433-451.

Haas, W. H., III, & Serow, W. J. (1993). Amenity retirement migration process: A model and preliminary evidence. *The Gerontologist, 33*(2), 212-220.

Happel, S. K., Hogan, T. D., & Pflanz, E. (1988). The economic impact of elderly winter residents in the Phoenix area. *Research on Aging, 10*(1), 199-133.

Hodge, G. (1991). The economic impact of retirees on smaller communities. *Research on Aging, 13*(1), 39-54.

Hogan, T. D., & Happel, S. K. (1994). 1993-94 winter residents important to AZ economy. *Arizona Business, 41*(7), 1-4.

Hogan, T. D., & Steinnes, D. N. (1993). Elderly migration to the Sun belt: Seasonal versus permanent. *Journal of Applied Gerontology, 12*, 246-260.

Joseph, A. E., & Cloutier, D. S. (1991). Elderly migration and its implications for service provision in rural communities: An Ontario perspective. *Journal of Rural Studies, 7*(4), 433-444.

Kallan, J. E. (1993). A multilevel analysis of elderly migration. *Social Science Quarterly, 74*, 403-416.

Litwak, E., & Longino, C. F., Jr. (1987). Migration patterns among the elderly: A developmental perspective. *The Gerontologist, 27*(3), 266-272.

Longino, C. F., Jr. (1990). Geographical distribution and migration. In R.H. Binstock & L. K. George (Eds.), *Handbook of aging and the social sciences* (3rd ed., pp.

45-63). San Diego, CA: Academic Press.

Longino, C. F., Jr. (1992). The forest and the trees: Micro-level considerations in the study of geographic mobility in old age. In A. Rogers (Ed.), *Elderly migration and population redistribution* (pp. 23-24). London: Belhaven Press.

Longino, C. F., Jr. (1995). *Retirement migration in America*. Houston, TX: Vacation Publications.

Longino, C. F., Jr. (2001). Geographic distribution and migration. In R. H. Binstock and L. K. George (Eds.), *Handbook of Aging and The Social Sciences* (5th ed., pp. 103-124). San Diego, CA: Academic Press.

Longino, C. F., Jr., & Bradley, D. E. (in press). A first look at retirement migration trends through 2000. *The Gerontologist, 44*, in press.

Longino, C. F., Jr., & Crown, W. H. (1990). Retirement migration and interstate income transfers. *The Gerontologist, 30*, 784-789.

Longino, C. F., Jr., & Marshall, V. W. (1990). North American research on seasonal migration. *Ageing and Society, 10*, 229-235.

Longino, C. F., Jr., Marshall, V. W., Mullins, L. C., & Tucker, R. D. (1991). On the nesting of snowbirds. *Journal of Applied Gerontology, 10*, 157-168.

Longino, C. F., Jr., & Perricone, P. J. (1991). The elderly population of south Florida, 1950-1990. *The Florida Geographer, 25*, 2-19.

Longino, C. F., Jr., Perzynski, A. T., & Stoller, E. P. (2002). Pandora's briefcase: Unpacking the retirement migration decision. *Research on Aging, 24*, 29-49.

MacManus, S. (1997). Selling school taxes and bond issues to a generationally diverse electorate: Lessons from Florida referenda. *Government Finance Review, April*, 17-22.

Marshall, V. W., Longino, C. F., Jr., Tucker, R. D., & Mullins, L. G. (1989). Health care utilization of Canadian snowbirds: An example of strategic planning. *Journal of Aging and Health, 1*, 150-168.

Martin, H. W., Hoppe, S. K., Marshall, V. W., & Daciuk, J. F. (1992). Socio-demographic and health characteristics of Anglophone Canadian and U.S. Snowbirds. *Journal of Aging and Health, 4*, 500-513.

McHugh, K. E. (1990). Seasonal migration as a substitute for, or precursor to, permanent migration. *Research on Aging, 12*, 229-245.

McHugh, K. E., Hogan, T. D., & Happel, S. K. (1995). Multiple residence and cyclical migration: A life course perspective. *Professional Geographer, 47*(3), 251-267.

McHugh, K. E., & Mings, R. C. (1991). On the road again: Seasonal migration to a Sunbelt metropolis. *Urban Geography, 12*, 1-18.

McHugh, K. E., & Mings, R. C. (1994). Seasonal migration and health care. *Journal of Aging and Health, 6*, 111-122.

Mings, R. C. (1997). Tracking "snowbirds" in Australia: Winter sun seekers in far north Queensland. *Australian Geographical Studies, 35*, 168-182.

Mullins, D. R., & Rosenstraub, M. S. (1992). Fiscal pressure?: The impact of elder recruitment on local expenditures. *Urban Affairs Quarterly, December*, 337-354.

Penninx, R. (1986). International migration in Western Europe since 1973: Developments, mechanisms, and controls. *International Migration Review, 20*, 951-972.

Ravenstein, E. G. (1885). Law of migration. *Journal of the Statistical Society of London,* *48*, 167-235.

Reeder, R. J., & Glasgow, N. L. (1990). Nonmetro retirement counties' strengths and weaknesses. *Rural Development Perspectives, 6*(2), 12-17.

Rosenbaum, W. A., & Buton, J. W. (1989). Is there a gray peril?: Retirement politics in Florida. *The Gerontologist, 29,* 300-306.

Rowles, G. D., & Watkins, J. F. (1993). Elderly migration and development in small communities. *Growth and Change, 24,* 509-538.

Sastry, M. L. (1992). Estimating the economic impacts of elderly migration: An input-output analysis. *Growth and Change, 23*(1), 54-79.

Savageau, D. (2000). *Retirement places rated.* New York: Macmillan.

Schneider, M. J., & Green, B. L. (1992). A demographic and economic comparison of nonmetropolitan retirement and nonretirement counties in the U.S. *Journal of Applied Sociology, 9,* 63-84.

Serow, W. J. (1990). Economic implications of retirement migration. *The Journal of Applied Gerontology, 9*(4), 452-463.

Serow, W. J. (1992). Unanswered questions and new directions in research on elderly migration: Economic and demographic perspectives. *Journal of Aging Social Policy, 4*(3/4), 7389.

Serow, W. J., & Haas W. H. (1992). Measuring the economic impact of retirement migration: The case of western North Carolina. *The Journal of Applied Gerontology, 47*(1), 538-543.

Simonsen, W., & Robbins, M. (1996). Does it make any difference anymore? Competitive versus negotiated municipal bond issuance. *Public Administration Review, 56*(1), 57-64.

Stallmann, J. I., & Siegel, P. B. (1995). Attracting retirees as an economic development strategy: Looking into the future. *Economic Development Quarterly, 9*(4), 372-382.

Steinnes, D. N., & Hogan, T. D. (1992). Take the money and the sun: Elderly migration as a consequence of gains in unaffordable housing markets. *Journal of Gerontology: Social Sciences, 47*(4), S197-S203.

Tucker, R. D., Mullins, L. C., Beland, F., Longino, C. F., Jr., & Marshall, V. W. (1992). Older Canadians in Florida: A comparison of Anglophone and Francophone seasonal migrants. *Canadian Journal on Aging, 11,* 281-297.

Voss, P. R., & Fuguitt, G. V. (1991). The impact of migration on southern rural areas of chronic depression. *Rural Sociology, 56*(4), 660-679.

Warnes, A. M. (1992). Migration and the life course. In T. Champion & T. Fielding (Eds.), *Migration processes and patterns* (pp. 175-187). London: Belhaven Press.

Warnes, A.M., & Patterson G. (1998). British retirees in Malta: components of the cross-national relationship. *International Journal of Population Geography, 4,* 113-33.

Watkins, J. F. (1990). Appalachian elderly migration. *Research on Aging, 12,* 409-429.

Watkins, J.F. (1999). Life course and spatial experience: A personal narrative approach in migration studies. In K. Pandit & S. Davies-Wiothers (Eds.), *Migration and Restructuring in the United States* (pp. 294-312). Boulder, CO: Rowman and Littlefield.

Williams, A. M., King, R., & Warnes, A. M. (1997). A place in the sun: International retirement migration from northern to southern Europe. *European Urban and Regional Studies, 4,* 115-134.

Williams, A., and Patterson, G. 1998. An empire lost but a province gained: A cohort analysis of British international retirement in the Algarve. *International Journal of Population Geography, 4*(2), 135-56.

Wiseman, R. F. (1980). Why older people move. *Research on Aging, 2*(2), 141-154.

CHAPTER 6

Everyday Competence and Everyday Problem Solving in Aging Adults: The Role of Physical and Social Context

MANFRED DIEHL
UNIVERSITY OF FLORIDA

SHERRY L. WILLIS
THE PENNSYLVANIA STATE UNIVERSITY

Although the concept of everyday competence has theoretical roots in different traditions in psychology and gerontology, in its broadest sense it refers to individuals' capacity to interact effectively with their environment (Bandura, 1997; White, 1959). This definition emphasizes that competence is shown in persons' transactions with their *physical-spatial* and *social-interpersonal* surroundings and that an examination of competent behavior needs to focus on at least two major factors. The first factor is the *person* with his or her skills, abilities, beliefs, developmental history, and other personal resources. The second factor is the *environment*, which can facilitate or impede the application of the person's skills, abilities, and resources. Thus, competent behavior in everyday life always reflects the confluence, or interaction, of personal and environmental factors and focuses on individuals' abilities to adapt to the challenges of different environmental conditions (Diehl, 1998; Lawton, 1989a; Lewin, 1935; Willis, 1991, 2000).

This chapter has several objectives:

1. We will define the conceptual space associated with the construct of everyday competence. In doing so, we will advocate for a transactional view of everyday competence and a conceptualization of person and environment as being multidimensional and dynamic.

2. We will discuss the physical-spatial and social-interpersonal features of the environment that facilitate or impede competent behavior in older adults.

3. We will review the literature on predictors of everyday competence. In this section, we will draw as much as possible on available research to show how personal and environmental variables interact to facilitate or impede the expression of competence in everyday life.

4. We will discuss some emerging trends and future directions in this area of aging research, including a focus on driving competence and associated aspects of person-environment (P-E) fit.

It needs to be noted that this chapter focuses on everyday competence and everyday problem solving in relatively healthy, community-residing, older adults. Thus, we will not discuss everyday competence in institutionalized older adults, although we may refer to this specific environmental context for illustration purposes (see M. Baltes & Horgas, 1997; Regnier & Pynoos, 1992).

DEFINING THE CONCEPTUAL SPACE

Several authors have presented models describing the conceptual components of everyday competence (e.g., M. Baltes, Maas, Wilms, & Borchelt, 1999; Willis, 1991). Building on this earlier work, Figure 6.1 displays the conceptual space that we consider of relevance in our discussion of everyday competence and everyday problem solving in adulthood and old age.

As can be seen in Figure 6.1, a person's everyday competence with regard to several domains of performance, ranging from basic, obligatory, self-care activities to expanded discretionary activities, emerges out of the confluence of characteristics of the person and the environment. On the person side, we distinguish biological/functional, social (see Section V, "Effects of the Social-Interpersonal Environment on Older Adults' Everyday Competence"), and psychological resources (see Section VI, "Predictors of Everyday Competence and Everyday Problem Solving in Late Adulthood"). These resources interact in complex ways with each other and the environment to produce a person's actual behavior in a given situation. For example, a person with some visual or motor impairment may apply his or her cognitive abilities, coping strategies, and social resources in a somewhat different way than a person without such limitations. At the same time, such a person may also consider features of the physical-spatial and social-interpersonal environment in different ways (e.g., avoiding nighttime driving or relying on public transportation or another person) than a person without limitations. Thus, competent behavior in everyday life does not exist in a vacuum, but is expressed and

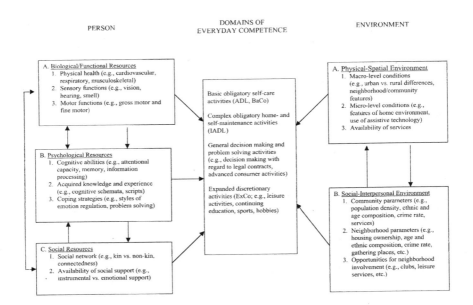

PERSON   DOMAINS OF   ENVIRONMENT
                     EVERYDAY COMPETENCE

FIGURE 6.1   The conceptual space of everyday competence as a function of person and environment.

receives its validation in transactions with the actual physical and social environment. To say it differently, we propose that competent behavior resides neither within the person nor within the environment, but in the interaction between person and environment. Both person and environment have to be conceptualized as dynamic entities (see Willis, 2000).

Taking into account this conceptual space, we define everyday competence as a person's potential to perform a broad array of activities considered essential for independent living, even though the individual may not perform all of these activities on a regular basis (M. Baltes et al., 1999; Lawton, 1982; Willis, 1991, 1996a). Several aspects of this definition warrant further discussion:

1. Everyday competence refers to a person's potential, or capability, to perform certain tasks, not the actual daily behavior of the person (Salthouse, 1990). The distinction between potential and actual performance is consistent with the notions of intra-individual reserve capacity and behavioral plasticity and has received attention from lifespan developmental (P. Baltes, 1987; P. Baltes & M. Baltes, 1990) and cognitive researchers alike (Park, 1992; Salthouse, 1990, 1996). Furthermore, the distinction between performance potential and actual performance has become of interest to legal scholars in the context of competency assessment and guardianship decisions (Grisso, 1986; Sabatino, 1996; Smyer,

Schaie, & Kapp, 1996). It needs to be noted, however, that the emphasis on performance potential should not distract from the fact that adults' *actual* performance on tasks of daily living provides valuable baseline information from which the examination of their performance potential can be launched (P. Baltes, 1987).

2. Although most of the literature on everyday competence and everyday problem solving has focused on older adults' capacity to perform *activities of daily living* (ADLs) (Katz, Ford, Moskowitz, Jackson, & Jaffe, 1963; Katz & Stroud, 1989) and *instrumental activities of daily living* (IADLs) (Fillenbaum, 1985, 1988; Lawton & Brody, 1969), more recent conceptualizations have argued for the inclusion of discretionary activities as part of the competence construct. For example, M. Baltes et al. (1999) have presented a two-component model that distinguishes between a *basic* (BaCo) and an *expanded level of competence* (ExCo). The latter encompasses expanded discretionary activities such as leisure time and out-of-house activities (e.g., participation in continuing education, sports, travel, etc.) that are often indicative of successful aging (P. Baltes & M. Baltes, 1990; Horgas, Wilms, & M. Baltes, 1998). Indeed, some authors have argued that the role of the physical-spatial environment may play a more crucial role with regard to discretionary and out-of-house activities (Wahl, Oswald, & Zimprich, 1999).

3. Several authors have argued that everyday competence is a *multidimensional* and *dynamic* construct (Sansone & Berg, 1993; Willis, 1991). For example, Willis (1991) presented a model that distinguishes between antecedents, components, mechanisms, and outcomes of everyday competence. Two aspects of this model are of particular importance. First, Willis's (1991) conceptualization implies that everyday competence serves as a moderator between outcomes and age-related, health-related, and psychosocial losses (see also M. Baltes et al., 1999). Second, Willis's (1991) model also suggests that older adults' competencies and their application in different domains are best conceptualized as a dynamic and recursive process. That is, physical and psychological outcomes at one point in time are likely to affect a person's future competency beliefs, thus becoming the antecedents for future functioning. Moreover, a dynamic element is also introduced when environmental conditions change because a person may perform at a high level of competence in a familiar environmental condition (e.g., using public transportation in one's home town), but may behave at a lower level of competence in a less familiar environment (e.g., using public transportation in an unfamiliar city).

In summary, a transactional view of everyday competence emphasizes the mutual and reciprocal relations between person and environment (Lawton, 1982). The person side encompasses physical, psychological, and social resources, which interact with each other and the environmental conditions (i.e., physical-spatial and social-interpersonal) and determine a person's potential to meet the diverse challenges of everyday life. Consistent with the focus of this volume, we will first discuss environmental and then personal factors that influence adults' everyday competence. Throughout the chapter, we will highlight interactions between personal and environmental factors as they affect adults' everyday competence and everyday problem solving.

ENVIRONMENTAL INFLUENCES ON EVERYDAY COMPETENCE: GENERAL FRAMEWORK

Environmental perspectives have a long-standing tradition in gerontology (Kleemeier, 1959; Lawton, 1977, 1983; Parmelee & Lawton, 1990; Wahl, 2001). Kleemeier (1959) already emphasized that the aging process is modified by the relations between person and external environment. He also coined the term *prosthetic environments* to indicate that environmental conditions can serve as "prosthetics" that compensate for aging-related impairments or losses, either naturally or by design. Similarly, Scheidt and Windley (1985) pointed out that research on the effects of the environment on the aging process has always been intervention oriented and has sought to improve the fit between person and environment, with the ultimate goal of enhancing older adults' quality of life.

A great deal of theorizing has focused on the *person-environment* (P-E) relations and the role of environmental conditions in the aging process, resulting in several elaborate theoretical models (see Wahl, 2001, Table 9.1, p. 227). One of the most widely recognized models is the *competence-press model* of Lawton and Nahemow (1973). In this model, an older person's level of adaptive behavior is seen as the result of environmental demands that are commensurate with the bio-behavioral competence of the person. Although the different models emphasize different aspects of the P-E relationship, they basically all focus on two main functions of the physical and psychosocial environment. Specifically, the physical and psychosocial environment is conceptualized either as serving a *supporting* or an *impeding* role as individuals deal with the challenges of later adulthood (Scheidt & Windley, 1985; Wahl, 2001). Conceptualizing the physical and social environment either as a source of stress or a source of support builds on the notion that stress challenges individuals' adaptive capacity, whereas support tends to stabilize adaptive behaviors (see Lazarus & Folkman, 1984).

How the planned design of the environment can facilitate desirable and reduce undesirable behavior has been specifically studied in the context of nursing homes and special care units (Parmelee & Lawton, 1990; Regnier & Pynoos, 1992; Wahl, 2001). Far less research has focused on the P-E relations in natural and unplanned surroundings. In the following, we will examine which ways the environment can either facilitate or impede older adults' everyday competence in natural settings. For clarity of presentation, we will review the literature separately for the physical-spatial and the social-interpersonal environment, although these two components of the environment often interact with each other.

EFFECTS OF THE PHYSICAL-SPATIAL ENVIRONMENT ON OLDER ADULTS' EVERYDAY COMPETENCE

The Physical-Spatial Environment as a Source of Stress
Physical-spatial features can become sources of stress in the immediate home environment (i.e., the microenvironment) or the extended environment, such as the neighborhood or community (i.e., the macroenvironment), in which older adults reside. With regard to features of the macroenvironment, extensive research by Lawton and his colleagues showed that attributes of neighborhoods, such as community size, accessibility of buildings, neighborhood resources, crime risk, and degree of age segregation, were significantly associated with older adults' activity level, motility, and well being (Lawton, Nahemow, & Yeh, 1980). Moreover, environmental features of neighborhoods, in more than half of the studies, accounted for more variance in well-being than did personal characteristics of the older adults (Lawton, 1983; Scheidt & Windley, 1985). Similarly, Regnier (1983) found that the cognitive representations of neighborhoods were significantly related to the percentage and frequency of trips taken by older adult residents. Specifically, environmental factors such as street traffic, topography, bus routes, accessibility of buildings, and number of services in the neighborhood, together with social factors such as population density, crime rates, and ethnic mix, were factors that affected older adults' motility and their activity radius (Regnier, 1976). More recent research has shown that these effects are exacerbated in older adults with vision and mobility impairments (Wahl, Schilling, Oswald, & Heyl, 1999). Moreover, research that focuses on the incorporation of human factors considerations into the design of more age-appropriate environments has shown that taking into account basic performance parameters, such as older adults' average walking speed, can be used to design more elderly-friendly environments (e.g., implementing more age-appropriate intersection crossing times; for a review see Charness & Bosman, 1990; Fisk & Rogers, 1997).

In summary, it is well documented that physical-spatial features of the macro-environment affect older adults' motility and consequently their radius of activities. Although research is limited, it can also be concluded that the activities that are most affected by impeding conditions of the macro-environment are those that belong to an *expanded definition of everyday competence* (ExCo), such as leisure time activities, traveling, and outdoor activities (Wahl, 2001). Older adults often respond to unfavorable physical neighborhood conditions by voluntarily limiting their activities outside of their home, which also tends to reduce their personal contact with social interaction partners. Such self-chosen restrictions of the activity radius contain the risk of starting a slow but progressive erosion process due to the disuse of physical, social, and cognitive functions. Such a downward spiraling effect, resulting in progressive disuse and increased risk of injury, has been documented in the literature on falls in older adults (Friedman, Munoz, West, Rubin, & Fried, 2002; Tinetti, Speechley, & Ginter, 1988).

With regard to the micro-environment, many older adults seem to respond proactively to changes in their functional abilities with modifications to their home environment (Lawton, 1989b; Wahl, 2001). Despite such proactive and adaptive modifications, the home environment can nevertheless present certain risks. For example, for elderly adults for whom it becomes increasingly difficult to climb stairs due to arthritis in knees and hips, the presence of any stairs in their home environment is likely to increase the risk for falls and subsequent disability (Campbell, Borrie, & Spears, 1989; Tinetti et al., 1988). The height and depth of cupboards and countertops in the kitchen area (Charness & Bosman, 1990) may affect an older adult's ability and willingness to prepare meals and the lack of grab bars in bathtub and shower areas may affect a person's willingness to engage in activities related to personal hygiene (Pynoos, Cohen, Davis, & Bernhardt, 1987; Regnier & Pynoos, 1987). Similarly, inadequately lit spaces in entryways and hallways, slippery floor conditions, or the use of decorative items in the home, such as throw rugs, may increase visually or mobility-impaired elders' risk for falls and other injuries (Charness & Bosman, 1990; Gill, Williams, Robison, & Tinetti, 1999).

In a population-based study, Gill, Williams, Robison, and Tinetti (1999) found that the prevalence of environmental hazards in the homes of older adults was high. These researchers used a room-to-room assessment protocol to examine hazards related to transfers, balance, and gait in older adults' home environment. Findings showed that grab bars in the tub/shower were absent in 61 percent of homes; loose throw rugs and obstructed pathways were present in nearly 80 percent and 50 percent of homes, respectively. Similarly, dim lighting, shadows, or glare were identified in 44 percent of the rooms and nightlights were not present or not near 67.6 percent of the examined staircases. Overall, two or more hazards were identified in 59 percent of bathrooms and in 23 to 42 percent of the other rooms. Subsequently, Gill, Robison, Williams, and Tinetti (1999) showed that these environmental hazards did not only exist in the home environment of vigorous older adults but that they were equally, and in some instances even more, prevalent in the home environment of physically impaired elders. The authors comment on these findings by stating that environmental hazards are highly prevalent in the homes of frail older adults and that the need for environment-focused interventions is vastly underestimated.

These assessments of the physical-spatial home environment of active and impaired older adults are consistent with findings from other studies. For example, Tinetti et al. (1988) reported findings from a one-year prospective study showing that the majority of reported falls (77 percent) occurred at home. A likely contribution of environmental factors was reported for 44 percent of the falls. The most frequently mentioned environmental factors were objects tripped over and stairs (Tinetti et al., 1988). From this and other studies, it can be concluded that conditions in the home environment that require an elderly person to displace their center of gravity, to bend over or reach up, or step up and step down will increase the risk for falls and the likelihood for subsequent declines in everyday competence (see also Charness & Bosman, 1990; Sterns, Barrett, & Alexander, 1985). In addition, inadequately lit spaces such as staircases and hallways in combination pose a risk to older adults with regard to falls or unintended injury (Gill et al., 1999).

In summary, certain aspects of the home environment can represent challenges or threats to older adults' everyday competence. Although many older adults proactively modify their home environment to adjust to diminishing functional abilities (Lawton, 1989b, 1990), current surveys suggest that a larger number of older adults could benefit from a systematic evaluation of the interior and exterior conditions of their environment with regard to the maintenance of their independent functioning (Charness & Bosman, 1990; Gill et al., 1999).

The Physical-Spatial Environment as a Source of Support

The physical environment, however, should not only be seen as a source of constraints and barriers to older adults' everyday competence. The physical environment can also facilitate older adults' day-to-day functioning and, especially in the home environment, can assume an important prosthetic function over an extended period of time (Gitlin, 1998; Regnier & Pynoos, 1992; Reschovsky & Newman, 1990; Wahl, 2001). In the following, we will elaborate on the supportive functions of older adults' physical-spatial environment. In particular, we will focus on older adults' proactive modifications of their environment (Lawton, 1989b, 1990) to optimize their P-E fit and to maximize their potential for living independently as long as possible.

Numerous authors have pointed out that the physical environment serves not only supportive functions in terms of its objective features, but also in terms of cognitive representations and feelings of belonging and attachment (Golant, 1984; Wahl, 2001). Rubinstein and Parmelee (1992), for example, defined the construct of *place attachment* as "a set of feelings about a geographic location that emotionally binds a person to that place as a function of its role as a setting for experience" (p. 139). These authors consider place attachment as important as objective housing conditions in explaining older adults' P-E fit and view it as a central construct in explaining well-being in later life. Moreover, the concept of place attachment exemplifies that the physical and social environment are often inseparably connected because older adults' emotional bond to their place of living may not only be a function of the familiarity with the physical setting, but also a function of the social relations and the social support that exist in that setting.

From a macro-environmental perspective, place attachment relates to older adults' familiarity with and emotional bond to their community and neighborhood in which they may have lived for many years. As a consequence, they may have established a P-E fit that allows them to live independently even when physical and cognitive impairments begin to challenge their everyday competence (Oswald, Schilling, Wahl, & Gäng, 2002; Wahl, 2001). For example, having lived in a neighborhood for a long time may afford older adults with a number of formal community-based services (e.g., visits from a home health care nurse, meals at a senior center, transportation services) and informal services from family members, long-time neighbors, and other highly familiar individuals who watch out for them. Informal services from neighbors and long-time friends (e.g., weekly delivery from the neighborhood grocery store, transportation to doctor appointments, etc.) in the community may be particularly important for older adults with low income and for individuals who lack kin in close proximity. Thus, it is not surprising that older adults' sense of place attachment influences their decision to age in place and to not consider relocation until objective housing and neighborhood conditions change to their disadvantage (Krause, 1993; Speare, Avery, & Lawton, 1991; Thompson & Krause, 1998). In contrast, proactive home-to-home relocations, with the objective to maximize the supportive function of the home and the community environment, are more frequently considered by older adults with a higher socioeconomic status and higher educational level, and tend to occur early in the post-retirement years (Oswald et al., 2002; Wahl, 2001).

From a micro-environmental perspective, place attachment and the feeling of belonging refer to elderly adults' sense that their home is a "save haven" and a protective environment. Moreover, there is growing evidence that the protective role of the home environment becomes more important as physical and cognitive impairments become more severe (Gitlin, 1998; Lawton, 1990; Oswald et al., 2002; Wahl et al., 1999). Because the home environment takes on such a crucial role for the everyday competence of older adults, it is important to understand to what extent older adults engage in proactive modifications of their environment in order to maintain their independent life style (Gitlin, 1998; Lawton, 1989b, 1990). Although Gitlin (1998) points out that home safety inspections and environmental modifications have long been an integral part of occupational therapy practice, home care, geriatric rehabilitation, and, more recently, fall-prevention programs, similar systematic approaches have been lacking in the domain of everyday competence assessment.

With regard to everyday competence, home modifications are most often made with a focus on maintaining a person's ability to perform basic *self-care activities* (e.g., bathing, toileting, eating) and to move safely around the home (Gitlin, 1998). For example, data from several national surveys (see Table 7.1 in Gitlin, 1998) have shown that a large number of older adults use mobility aids and other assistive devices in order to be able to live in their own home. Gitlin (1998) also points out that environmental strategies are usually "adapted in a progressive, stepwise fashion, with behavioral change used as the primary coping mechanism, followed by the use of an adaptive device and possibly minor physical environmental adjustments" (p. 196). The progression of environmental modifications tends to be dictated by the experienced impairments or anticipated disabilities and ranges from the use of slip-resistant footwear to the installation of grab bars in tubs and showers, the reconstruction of kitchen countertops, and the installation of special stovetops and other aging-friendly appliances. Gitlin (1998) points out that modifications that involve alterations to the physical structure of the home (e.g., widening doors to accommodate a wheel chair, removal of walls, etc.) and/or the installation of special equipment (e.g., stair lift, alarm system) are less likely and tend to be the last or to be considered by older adults. In addition, frail older adults usually report the need for more home modifications to support their everyday activities (Gitlin, Schemm, Landsberg, & Burgh, 1996; Mann, Karuza, Hurren, & Tomita, 1993; Reschovsky & Newman, 1990). Thus, it does not come as a surprise that the best predictor of whether an individual will pursue an environmental modification is disability level, as manifested by the number of limitations in ADLs and IADLs (Gitlin, 1998).

Evidence that older adults actively restructure their living space to optimize its supportive features has been provided by intensive observational studies. For example, Rowles (1981) showed that older adults often intentionally restrict their physical-spatial environment to a residential *surveillance zone*, which includes the residence and the immediate spaces surrounding the residential unit. This surveillance zone serves as the primary source for social interactions but also provides the space in which the older adult can function safely. Within the home environment, older adults, especially when mobility or vision impaired, often tend to arrange special *functional spaces* as sort of command centers that allow them to perform certain tasks of daily living while providing them with a maximum amount of security and comfort (Oswald et al., 2002). Such functional spaces seem to be of particular importance with regard to the performance of IADLs such as taking medications or using the telephone. For example, older adults may keep their medications in a prominent spot in the kitchen or the dining area as a reminder that they will take them with meals. In addition, elders may optimize the supportive nature of their environment through the use of external memory aids such as timers or other environmental cues (e.g., reminder notes posted in prominent places) to remind them to perform certain activities of daily living. Because researchers have recognized the importance of aging in place, there have been increased efforts to provide assistive devices to older adults helping them to maintain their functional independence (Fernie, 1997; Mann, Hurren, Tomita, & Charvat, 1995).

In summary, there is a good amount of evidence showing that older adults actively structure their home environment with the objective to maximize their everyday functioning. These efforts range from small modifications to the setting up of specific functional spaces and to the use of specific assistive devices. Although the use of assistive devices is a particularly promising approach to extending older adults' functional independence, currently little is known about the psychosocial factors that influence the acceptance and long-term use of such devices. Some studies, however, have shown that older adults with moderate to severe disabilities who used assistive devices in their homes reported greater self-efficacy in comparison to older adults who relied on personal assistance (Verbrugge, Rennert, & Madans, 1997). This suggests that the use of assistive devices may have positive psychological side effects.

EFFECTS OF THE SOCIAL-INTERPERSONAL ENVIRONMENT ON OLDER ADULTS' EVERYDAY COMPETENCE

We already pointed out that the physical-spatial and the social-interpersonal environment are often interrelated. For example, older adults' place attachment is not only a function of the familiarity with their physical-spatial surrounding, but also a function of the social relations that exist in that surrounding. Thus, it is also important to understand the contributions of the social-interpersonal environment to older adults' everyday competence and well-being (Antonucci & Akiyama, 1997). These contributions can be conceived in terms of stress and burden or in terms of resources and support.

The Social-Interpersonal Environment as a Source of Stress
Close interpersonal relationships involve a combination of positive and negative features (Rook, 1984; Rowe & Kahn, 1998). Although most of the research on social relations in old age has focused on their beneficial fea-

tures, researchers have increasingly recognized that the social-interpersonal environment can also be a source of stress and negative experiences (Lakey, Tardiff, & Drew, 1994; Manne & Zautra, 1989; Okun, Melichar, & Hill, 1990; Rook, 1984; Stephens, Kinney, Norris, & Ritchie, 1987). Negative social exchanges, for example, can take the form of criticizing, demanding, misunderstanding, or overprotecting and can undermine a person's sense of mastery and autonomy. Moreover, negative social relationships may add additional burden to older adults' lives by letting them know that their social support resources may not be available when bad things will happen (Ingersoll-Dayton, Morgan, & Antonucci, 1997; Okun et al., 1990). For example, Ingersoll-Dayton et al. (1997) found, in a national probability sample of adults aged 50 to 95, that negative social exchanges were associated with negative affect and that this relationship was significantly stronger in the subgroup that had experienced more negative life events. Okun et al. (1990) reported similar findings for a sample of community-residing older adults. Stephens et al. (1987) showed for a sample of elderly adults recovering from stroke that their social networks not only provided resources, but also created liabilities. These researchers showed that negative and positive social exchanges differentially accounted for variance in morale, psychiatric symptoms, and cognitive functioning in older adults recovering from stroke. In particular, negative social interactions were associated with poorer morale and more psychiatric symptoms. Interestingly, older adults who reported and those who did not report negative interactions did not differ significantly from each other on a variety of social and demographic variables previously shown to predict social interactions and well-being.

Several authors have suggested that unwanted social support may increase distress by inducing feelings of dependence and that negative social exchanges may erode older adults' sense of autonomy and mastery (Kuypers & Bengtson, 1973; Lawton, 1982; Silverstein, 1997). Smith and Goodnow (1999) conducted a study that addressed this general hypothesis with regard to *unasked-for support* and *unsolicited advice*. Findings from this study showed that at all ages, unasked-for support was experienced as more unpleasant than pleasant. Among the reasons why they perceived unsolicited support as unpleasant, study participants indicated most frequently that it implied incompetence. Moreover, the implication of incompetence ("it indicated that the other person saw me as incompetent or incapable") was most pronounced in life situations related to financial matters, cognitive performance, and general competence (Smith & Goodnow, 1999), areas in which older adults may be particularly vulnerable to declines in performance.

In summary, it is important to be mindful about the potential negative effects that unwanted support and unsolicited advice may have on older adults' everyday competence (Rowe & Kahn, 1998; Smith & Goodnow,

1999). Individuals who assist older adults with tasks of daily living should provide their assistance in a well-dosed manner and in a way that does not undermine older adults' sense of self-efficacy and autonomy. On the other hand, research by M. Baltes (1996) has shown that older adults' dependent behavior represents an effective way by which they seek social stimulation and attention from individuals in their environment.

The Social-Interpersonal Environment as a Source of Support

In contrast to the physical-spatial environment, the social-interpersonal environment is often automatically viewed as a source of support and assistance for older adults (Antonucci, 2001; Lang, 2001). Indeed, there is a large amount of sociological and epidemiological literature showing that the availability of social relations reliably predicts morbidity and mortality across the adult lifespan (Antonucci & Akiyama, 1997; Berkman & Syme, 1979; Blazer, 1982; House, Robbins, & Metzner, 1982). Although the positive effects of social relations on adults' physical and mental well-being is well established (Antonucci, 2001; Baumeister & Leary, 1995; Lang, 2001), similar data regarding the effects of social relations on elderly adults' everyday competence as a behavioral outcome are less sound.

Two theoretical models suggest that the provision of social support may be relevant for older adults' everyday competence. These two models are the *convoy model of social relations* by Kahn and Antonucci (1980) and the *socioemotional selectivity theory* by Carstensen (1993). The convoy model proposes that from childhood to old age individuals are surrounded by a number of persons with whom they interact and socialize on a regular basis (Kahn & Antonucci, 1980). This "social convoy" accompanies the person over time and across different life contexts and serves a number of functions. Among these functions is the provision of instrumental and emotional support in times of need (Antonucci, 2001; Antonucci & Akiyama, 1997). It is well known that social convoys are organized in a hierarchical fashion with family members and close friends being the ones that are most often drawn upon for support and assistance (Antonucci & Akiyama, 1997). Neighbors, acquaintances, and other individuals with whom the person interacts on a regular basis (e.g., church members) follow family members and close friends in importance.

A good deal of evidence suggests that individuals' social relationships are highly specialized (Antonucci, 1985; Carstensen, 1993). That is, older adults are not indiscriminant with regard to whom, when, and for what kind of support they ask. In addition, there is evidence suggesting that older adults monitor the provision and receipt of support from others to assure that their "support account" remains balanced (Antonucci, 1985; Silverstein, 1997). We suggest that the functions of the social-interpersonal environment with regard to older adults' everyday competence have to be studied within this context of hierarchical organization and specialization (Heller & Thompson, 1991; Messeri, Silverstein, & Litwak, 1993).

With regard to the tasks of daily living that are essential for independent living (i.e., instrumental support), the majority of support is provided by family members, such as spouses, adult children, or siblings (Antonucci, 1985; Gatz, Bengtson, & Blum, 1990; Hobfoll & Freedy, 1990). Thus, following a hierarchy of filial responsibility, spouses and adult children are most likely to help with the performance of ADLs and IADLs, such as self-care activities, preparing meals, managing finances, or providing transportation (Gatz et al., 1990; Horowitz, 1985). However, if family members do not live close by, these types of assistance may be provided by neighbors or acquaintances. The latter may be particularly the case if an older adult has lived for a long time in the same neighborhood and is well-known by his or her neighbors so that a non-family-based support network has emerged and is available to the elderly person as a social compensation mechanism. Antonucci and Akiyama (1997) emphasized that although supportive relationships tend to have a generalized positive effect on well-being (see also Pinquart & Sörensen, 2000), in the case of deficits in specific domains of competenc,e it is more reasonable to assume that supportive behaviors that directly address these specific deficits will be most beneficial (see also Carstensen & Lang, 1997; Silverstein, 1997).

The second theory that has focused on the role of social relations in old age and their effect on older adults' well-being is the *socioemotional selectivity theory* (SST) (Carstensen, 1993). Although SST emphasizes the instrumental purposes of social relationships during the early lifespan (i.e., the acquisition of knowledge), with regard to old age SST focuses primarily on the emotional functions of social relations (Carstensen & Lang, 1997). Specifically, Carstensen and her colleagues (Carstensen, Isaacowitz, & Charles, 1999; Lang & Carstensen, 1994) have shown in a series of studies that in late life social relationships are selected based on their degree of emotional closeness and in terms of the emotional gratification that they provide. Thus, from this perspective the influence of the social-interpersonal environment on older adults' everyday competence is conceptualized as being indirect via its effects on their psychological competence (Carstensen & Lang, 1997).

Consistent with Antonucci and Jackson's (1987) support-efficacy model, Carstensen and Lang (1997) have proposed that social relations can exert effects on older adults' everyday competence by enhancing their self-efficacy beliefs in three possible ways. First, the availability of social support provides older adults with the opportunity to decide when and from whom to accept assistance. This, in turn, may strengthen their sense of control and may allow them "to receive support without experiencing it as threatening to their self-competence" (Carstensen & Lang, 1997, p. 217). Second, if an elderly person has lost the capability to competently perform in a particular domain, a social proxy may be able to perform on his or her behalf, thus providing the older adult with a form of secondary control

(Heckhausen & Schulz, 1995). Third, older adults' experience with managing the positive and the negative aspects of their social ties over long periods of time provides them with a "database" on which they can draw to regulate the giving and receiving of social support. It is reasonable to assume that older adults draw on this database in order to avoid unwanted feelings of dependency or unwanted intrusions on their autonomy (Bandura, 1997).

In conclusion, the social-interpersonal environment can enhance older adults' everyday competence in multiple ways (Rowe & Kahn, 1998). First, family, close friends, and neighbors provide a great deal of support for daily functioning in the form of instrumental assistance (Antonucci, 1985, 2001). This instrumental assistance helps to compensate for declines in elderly adults' functioning and provides the social prosthetic that is necessary for independent living. Second, older adults tend to draw on their social relationships in ways that emphasize selection and reciprocity, thereby avoiding one-sidedness and dependency in their social relations (Lang, 2001). Third, social relationships also affect older adults' everyday competence indirectly by providing them with a sense of control and mastery over their interpersonal matters and thus giving them an opportunity to compensate for possible declines in other areas of functioning (Lang, 2001).

PREDICTORS OF EVERYDAY COMPETENCE AND EVERYDAY PROBLEM SOLVING IN LATE ADULTHOOD

A transactional conceptualization of everyday competence rests on the premise that a person's exchanges with the physical and social environment contribute to the development and maintenance of competence in different life domains. Although a person's level of performance may not be equally high in every life domain, it is important to understand the interactions that result in high levels of performance and to isolate the predictors that contribute to the maintenance of competent behavior into old age. Adopting Willis's (1991) model of everyday competence, we review findings on long-term antecedents of older adults' everyday competence. Whenever possible, our review will emphasize how these antecedents interact with environmental conditions.

Physical Health
Significant yet moderate associations between clinician ratings or self-ratings of physical health and self-reported everyday competence have been found in numerous studies (see Idler & Kasl, 1995). Fillenbaum (1985, 1988) reported the relationships between ratings of physical health and ratings of everyday competence to be on the order of .54. In a summary of sev-

eral studies, Lawton (1986) reported associations between self-reports of everyday competence and physical health in the range of .30 to .40. More recent studies have focused on specific medical conditions and their impact on older adults' everyday competence. Using data from a multi-stage probability sample of all non-institutionalized U.S. civilians age 70 or older, Boult, Kane, Louis, Boult, and McCaffrey (1994) reported that the best predictors of the development of functional limitations in ADLs and IADLs were cerebrovascular disease, arthritis, and coronary artery disease (see also Furner, Rudberg, & Cassel, 1995).

Several studies have focused on sensory impairments and their effect on elderly adults' everyday competence. Branch, Horowitz, and Carr (1989) compared changes in self-reports of everyday competence over a five-year period for a group of elderly adults with good vision and a group of elderly adults who reported a decline in vision. Older adults with vision problems were twice as likely to report needing assistance with shopping and paying bills. They also were less likely than the nonimpaired elders to leave their residence and travel by car. Rudberg, Furner, Dunn, and Cassel (1993) used data from the Longitudinal Study of Aging to examine the relationship of visual and hearing impairments with ADL disability in adults aged 70 and older. They found that persons with visual impairment were at an increased risk to develop functional disability in ADLs compared to individuals without visual impairment. In contrast, hearing impairment was not independently related to increased ADL disability. Wahl et al. (1999) found in a German sample that the majority of the visually impaired older adults showed low P-E fit with regard to their home environment. Moreover, under conditions of low P-E fit, older adults were more likely to show lower IADL performance. Thus, this research illustrates how person and environment interact to produce a certain level of everyday competence. That is, in individuals with visual impairment, a poorly structured physical environment will exacerbate the effects of vision loss, whereas a well-designed environment is more likely to assume a compensatory role, resulting in a higher level of everyday competence (Wahl et al., 1999).

Willis and Marsiske (1991) found a significant but modest negative relationship between the number of cardiac drugs along with the total number of drugs taken and performance on a paper-and-pencil test of everyday competence (i.e., the Basic Skills Assessment Test). Diehl, Willis, and Schaie (1995) showed significant relationships between general health, cardiovascular health, and hearing impairment and older adults' performance on a set of *Observed Tasks of Daily Living* (OTDL). Interestingly, health factors affected older adults' performance on the OTDL indirectly via basic cognitive abilities such as speed of processing and memory.

In summary, older adults' everyday competence and everyday problem solving are positively related to their general physical health and sensory functioning. Moreover, several studies have shown that different medical conditions (e.g., stroke, arthritis, heart disease) affect the development of IADL impairment differentially (Furner et al., 1995; Rudberg et al., 1993). To the extent that older adults' declining health is related to lifestyle factors, such as poor nutrition or lack of physical exercise, targeting these lifestyle factors for interventions may be a viable route to prevent functional decline and increase the likelihood for maintaining a high level of everyday competence (Chernoff, 2001; DiPietro, 2001; King, 2001; McAuley & Katula, 1998).

Cognitive Abilities and Factors Related to their Maintenance
Despite the ongoing debate about the relationship between basic cognitive abilities and everyday competence (Sternberg & Wagner, 1986), there is increasing evidence showing that cognitive abilities are important predictors of practical intelligence and everyday competence (Allaire & Marsiske, 1999; Diehl et al., 1995; Willis & Marsiske, 1991; Willis & Schaie, 1986, 1993). Willis and Marsiske (1991), for example, showed that over 50 percent of the variance in older adults' performance on a test of everyday problem solving was accounted for by basic cognitive abilities. Both fluid and crystallized abilities accounted for everyday task performance, although a somewhat greater portion of the variance was accounted for by fluid abilities. Diehl et al. (1995) showed that fluid intelligence was the strongest correlate of older adults' performance on a set of behavioral tasks of daily living. Smaller yet significant associations between everyday problem solving and basic mental abilities have been reported by Camp, Doherty, Moody-Thomas, and Denney (1989) and by Cornelius and Caspi (1987). Cockburn and Smith (1991) showed that older adults' performance on a test of everyday memory was significantly related to fluid intelligence as well as to age and participation in social and domestic activities.

Willis and Schaie (1986, 1993) proposed a hierarchical relationship between basic cognitive abilities and everyday cognition, suggesting that basic cognitive abilities and processes are necessary but not sufficient antecedents for competence in everyday problem solving. Support for this proposition comes from a study by Willis, Jay, Diehl, and Marsiske (1992) and from longitudinal data from the Seattle Longitudinal Study (Schaie, 1996). Specifically, Willis et al. (1992) examined the directionality of the relationship between basic cognitive abilities and everyday cognitive competence over a seven-year period. Structural equation models showed that fluid ability at the first time of assessment predicted everyday task performance seven years later; however, everyday cognitive competence predicted basic abilities at the second occasion of assessment less well. Similarly, Schaie (1996) documented for the relatively healthy community-residing participants of the Seattle Longitudinal Study that mean-level changes in everyday cognitive competence were small in the '60s, but that the rate of decline increased in the '70s and in the '80s, mimicking the rate of decline that has been observed for traditional measures of psychometric intelligence. Schaie (1996) also found that older adults with a lower level of education functioned at a lower level of everyday cognitive competence at all ages. However, the rate of decline became particularly steep for less educated older adults in the '80s (see Figure 1 in Willis, 1996a).

From an environmental perspective, these findings are relevant because individuals performing at different levels of cognitive functioning are likely to interact differently with their physical and social environment, resulting in different patterns of P-E fit. For example, an older adult who is still able to process information fast and accurately is more likely to show competent driving behavior under a variety of traffic conditions, whereas the driving competency of a person with lower cognitive functioning is more likely to be limited (see Willis, 2000). Similar principles may also apply to exchanges with the social-interpersonal environment.

To the extent that cognitive abilities are the foundation for older adults' everyday cognitive competence, it is reasonable to assume that the same long-term antecedents that contribute to the maintenance of basic intellectual abilities also contribute to the maintenance of everyday competence. Besides physical health, Schaie (1994, 1996) identified a number of individual difference variables that predicted the maintenance of high levels of intellectual functioning into old age. A first group of variables was described as "living in favorable environmental circumstances" (Schaie, 1994, p. 310), as would be the case for persons with high socio-economic status. Such circumstances included "above-average education, histories of occupational pursuits that involve high complexity and low routine, above-average income, and the maintenance of intact families" (Schaie, 1994, p. 310). A second group of variables included involvement in activities high in complexity and intellectual stimulation, such as extensive reading, participation in continuing education activities, or participation in clubs and professional organizations (Gribbin, Schaie, & Parham, 1980; Schaie, 1994). A third set of variables involved a flexible personality style at midlife, as assessed by self-report questionnaires and objective measures of motor-cognitive rigidity/flexibility. Being married to a spouse with high cognitive status and being satisfied with one's life's accomplishments in midlife or early old age represented an additional set of predictors, underscoring the importance of a stimulating social-interpersonal environment (Schaie, 1994). Finally, individuals who maintained high levels of perceptual processing speed also tended to maintain high levels of functioning in other cognitive domains.

In summary, a solid database exists suggesting that *multiple cognitive components* (Allaire & Marsiske, 1999; Diehl et al., 1995; Willis, 1996b) and factors of *environmental complexity* are involved in maintaining high levels of everyday competence into late adulthood (Lawton, 1983; Schaie, 1994, 1996; Schooler, 1987). Indeed, there is some evidence that the dimensions of cognitive functioning and environmental complexity distinguish resource-rich from resource-poor older adults (M. Baltes & Lang, 1997). Moreover, the physical and social factors of environmental complexity suggest promising avenues for interventions in older adults' everyday environment.

Personality Characteristics

Findings with regard to the influence of personality characteristics on older adults' everyday competence and everyday problem solving are limited. However, because there is evidence that environmental complexity, both in terms of the physical and social environment, is positively related to the maintenance of everyday cognitive competence (Schaie, 1994; Schooler, 1987), it can be reasoned that personality characteristics that expose individuals to more complex environments should be positively associated with the maintenance of competent behavior. Among the candidates for such personality characteristics are openness to experience (Costa & McCrae, 1992), behavioral and cognitive flexibility (Schaie, 1994), tolerance for ambiguity, and individuals' beliefs of control (Lachman, Ziff, & Spiro, 1994) and self-efficacy (Bandura, 1997).

In general, adults who have a strong belief in their own capabilities display a number of behaviors that should be conducive to the maintenance of high levels of everyday competence (Bandura, 1997). For example, older adults who believe that aging is associated with positive changes have been shown to benefit more from memory training than older adults who engage in negative self-stereotyping (Levy, 1996). Similarly, adults who have a strong belief in their memory capabilities remember things more accurately and effectively than adults with weak self-efficacy beliefs (Berry, West, & Dennehey, 1989; Lachman, Steinberg, & Trotter, 1987).

Several cross-sectional studies have shown significant relationships between self-efficacy and everyday functioning in community-residing older adults (Berkman et al., 1993; Tinetti, Mendes de Leon, Doucete, & Baker, 1994). Using a prospective design, Mendes de Leon, Seeman, Baker, Richardson, and Tinetti (1996) showed, for a large sample of community-residing older adults, that high ADL-related self-efficacy was associated with less functional decline among older individuals who had declined in physical capacity over an 18-month period. In contrast, among older adults who had not declined in physical capacity, self-efficacy was unrelated to changes in functioning. Taken together these findings suggest that instilling beliefs of self-efficacy and control in older adults represents a powerful tool for fostering the maintenance of everyday competence into old age (Langer & Rodin, 1976; Lachman, Weaver, M. Bandura, Elliott, & Lewkowicz, 1992; Tennstedt, Howland, Lachman, Peterson, Kasten, & Jette, 1998).

To the best of our knowledge, there are no studies that have examined the relations between openness to experience, one of the Big Five personality factors (Costa & McCrae, 1992), and maintenance of everyday competence across the adult lifespan. However, some findings exist with regard to other personality characteristics with conceptual similarity to openness of experience. For example, earlier we already discussed that Schaie (1994) reported a positive relationship between a flexible personality style at midlife and maintenance of intellectual functioning into old age. Similarly, research that has focused on the constructs of tolerance for ambiguity and cognitive style has shown that greater tolerance for ambiguity is associated with more detailed processing of consumer information (Cox, 1967; Schaninger & Schiglimpaglia, 1981) and more effective medical decision-making (E. A. Leventhal, H. Leventhal, Schaefer, & Easterling, 1993).

In summary, although the role of personality characteristics with regard to the maintenance of everyday competence is not well researched at this point in time, there is sufficient evidence suggesting that individual difference variables, such as tolerance for ambiguity, cognitive and behavioral flexibility, and beliefs of control are very likely important moderators of the effects of aging on older adults' everyday competence (Lachman et al., 1994; Schaie, 1994; Willis, 1996b).

EMERGING TRENDS AND FUTURE DIRECTIONS

Throughout this chapter we have emphasized that everyday competence is a function of personal and environmental factors. Because environmental conditions are subject to sociocultural and technological changes, we want to focus on some of the emerging trends and future challenges that we see evolving with regard to the definition and assessment of older adults' everyday competence. Specifically, we will focus on the impact of new technologies and the changing social-interpersonal context on older adults' everyday competence. Furthermore, we will discuss some recent developments in the assessment of everyday competence. Finally, we will use the sample case of driving competence to exemplify the importance of P-E fit when talking about everyday competence.

New Technologies and Everyday Competence
Older adults use their skills, abilities, and knowledge to respond to their social and physical environment; in turn, their competence is affected by their social and physical environment. Such a reciprocal relationship implies that the nature and definition of competent behavior may change with changes in the larger environment. Some of the macro-level changes that increasingly affect older adults' everyday competence are related to the advent of new technologies. Among these technologies, the use of personal computers, microelectronic devices, and communication technologies deserve particular attention from aging researchers (Czaja, 1997).

Computer technology can be used in a number of ways to support older adults' quality of life. For example, it is possible to use home computers to

carry out routine errands such as shopping, bill paying, financial management, and obtaining health and medical information (Czaja, 1997).
Similarly, the use of personal computers and other communication technologies (e.g., wireless phones and phone-based networks) can facilitate
social interaction and enhance the intellectual and leisure activities of older
adults (Czaja, Guerrier, Nair, & Landauer, 1993; Eilers, 1989; Garbe,
Stockler, & Wald, 1993). Even if future generations of aging adults will be
well versed in the use of computers and communication devices, current
generations of older adults often show some anxiety and reservations
toward these new technologies (Czaja, 1997), although most studies show
that older adults' attitude toward the use of personal computers becomes
more positive with experience (Jay & Willis, 1992). These positive findings
have encouraged researchers to design and test user-computer interfaces,
taking into account the specific circumstances of aging adults, such as age-
related changes in vision, hearing, and fine motor skills (Charness &
Bosman, 1992; Morrell & Echt, 1997). In general, redesigned user-computer
interfaces facilitate adults' acquisition of computer-related knowledge and
increase the use of computers in everyday life (Charness, Shulmann, &
Boritz, 1992; Garfein, Schaie, & Willis, 1988; Hahm & Bikson, 1989).

Computer and microelectronic technology will also continue to affect
older adults everyday competence through their incorporation into *assistive
devices* (Fernie, 1997), such as mobility devices or medication organizers
(Park & Jones, 1997). For example, research with microelectronic medic-
ation-event-monitoring systems suggests that such systems can be adopted
to improve the accuracy of older adults' medication-taking behavior and,
in turn, reduce unintended side effects due to nonadherence (Park & Jones,
1997). Similarly, microelectronic technology may be used to assist vision-
impaired elderly to navigate their home environment more safely by
designing mobility-enhancing assistive devices (Czaja, 1997; Fernie, 1997).

In summary, the recent advent of computer and communication technologies underscores that societal and technological changes affect not
only the definition, but the very nature of competent behavior in everyday
life. Although new technologies may challenge the everyday competence
of many older adults, overall they hold great promise for facilitating independent living and enhancing older adults' quality of life.

Collaborative Cognition and Older Adults' Everyday Competence
Another emerging trend focuses on the social-interpersonal context of
older adults' everyday competence. Early assessments already acknowledged the social nature and context of the definition and solution of everyday problems (Cornelius & Caspi, 1987; Demming & Pressey, 1957; Denney
& Pearce, 1989). However, the focus on the social-interpersonal nature of
many everyday problems and individuals' attempts to solve these problems has become more prominent with theoretical developments on the
social foundations of cognition (P. Baltes & Staudinger, 1996; Meacham &

Emont, 1989; Rogoff & Lave, 1984) and the social-contextual embedding of human intelligence (Berg & Sternberg, 1985; Sternberg & Wagner, 1994). Thus, recent studies have drawn on the theoretical notions of *collaborative cognition* and *interactive minds* (Goodnow, 1996; Gould & Dixon, 1993) and have examined how adults define their everyday problems (Berg, Calderone, Sansone, Strough, & Weir, 1998) and how they solve them collaboratively (Berg, Johnson, Meegan, & Strough, 2003; Margrett & Marsiske, 2002; Meegan & Berg, 1997; Strough, Berg, & Sansone, 1996; Strough, Cheng, & Swenson, 2002).

In general, findings from this research have shown that a large proportion of adults' self-reported everyday problems was defined as social-interpersonal in nature and required the cooperation of social partners in finding an optimal solution (Berg et al., 1998; Strough et al., 1996). For example, Margrett and Marsiske (2002) showed that older adults solved their everyday problems more effectively when they collaborated on a problem solution than when they worked individually, supporting the notion that "two heads are better than one" (see also Meegan & Berg, 1997; Strough et al., 2002). However, there were interesting qualifications to this notion. First, collaboration tended to be most effective when individuals first had a chance to work alone. This suggests that prior practice had activated individual competence to higher levels, so that individuals could then more fully profit from the collaborative experience. Second, familiarity of collaborator mattered, such that working with a spouse yielded better performance than working with a stranger (see also Gould & Dixon, 1993). Indeed, working in the presence of a spouse even boosted individual, noncollaborative performance—suggesting that familiar partners might also shape the motivational context and aid in anxiety reduction. Third, when dyad members were classified into "better" and "worse" partners, it was the worse partners who seemed to gain disproportionately from the collaboration, suggesting that a compensatory process might have best characterized the collaborative interactions (Margrett & Marsiske, 2002).

The emerging focus on collaborative problem solving holds a great deal of promise not only because it complements laboratory-based research, but it also complements findings from a longitudinal study showing that being affiliated with a social partner (e.g., spouse) with a high cognitive status tends to be associated with maintenance or an increase in intellectual functioning across the adult lifespan (Schaie, 1994). Thus, these findings point at social partners as important players with regard to adults' competence and everyday functioning. They also point to future research that may draw on these social partners as "tools" of planned interventions and agents of change.

Although research on collaborative problem solving underscores the compensatory nature of social relationships (Dixon & Bäckman, 1995), there are also a number of concerns and challenges that result from recent changes in family composition and family relationships (see Himes, 1992). These changes are likely to affect the availability of family members' support for future generations of older adults and potentially will have negative effects on older adults' everyday competence and quality of life. Specifically, changes in past and future levels of fertility, marriage, and divorce patterns will affect the likelihood that older adults of the future have family members who will be available as "social prostheses." For example, patterns of marital stability and divorce will affect the availability of spousal support, the most important form of support for older adults (Antonucci, 2001). Similarly, increased divorce rates are likely to lead to a situation in which the loyalties of children to their divorced parents are unclear and where elderly parents may not have the benefit to rely on their offspring for support (see Himes, 1992). This may be specifically the case for adult children who had little contact with a particular parent because of divorce and therefore may feel little responsibility with regard to providing support to that parent. Thus, sociocultural changes of family composition and the family life course may create new challenges with regard to the social resources that traditionally have been available to older adults in their old age.

New Measurement Approaches: Performance-Based Assessment of Everyday Competence

The last decade or so has seen a number of new approaches with regard to the assessment of everyday competence (see Diehl, 1998). Among these approaches have been single (e.g., Hershey, Walsh, Read, & Chulef, 1990; Park & Jones, 1997) and multi-domain assessments, such as the *Everyday Problem Solving Inventory* (EPSI) (Cornelius & Caspi, 1987), the *Everyday Problems Test* (EPT) (Willis & Marsiske, 1993), or the *Everyday Cognition Battery* (ECB) (Allaire & Marsiske, 1999). The latter instruments are paper-and-pencil measures of everyday problem solving and have shown consistent relations with basic cognitive abilities and with measures of functional status.

Several researchers have suggested that the use of behavioral, performance-based assessments could provide more accurate and objective information with regard to older persons' everyday competence (Diehl et al., 1995; Guralnik, Seeman, Tinetti, Nevitt, & Berkman, 1994; Kuriansky & Gurland, 1976). Although, in principle, this argument may be correct, a major challenge for test developers has been to design assessment procedures that assess a wide range of functioning (see Guralnik et al., 1994). Researchers have responded to this challenge in two ways. On one hand, measures have been developed for older adults who show signs of mild to moderate cognitive impairment and may be at risk for institutionalization (Loewenstein et al., 1989; Mahurin, DeBettignies, & Pirozzolo, 1991; Morris, Sherwood, & Mor, 1984). On the other hand, measures have been developed for healthy community-residing older adults to assess their competencies in a variety of domains (Diehl et al., 1995; Guralnik et al., 1994; Odenheimer et al., 1994; Owsley, Sloane, McGwin, & Ball, 2002).

The performance-based measures that are currently available are the *Performance Test of Activities of Daily Living* (PADL) (Kuriansky & Gurland, 1976), the *Direct Assessment of Functional Skills* (DAFS) (Loewenstein et al., 1989), and the *Structured Assessment of Independent Living Skills* (SAILS) by Mahurin et al. (1991). All of these assessments measure adults' performance on a mixture of ADLs and IADLs using multiple items per functional domain. The psychometric properties of these measures have been established and their predictive validity has been examined in samples of elderly adults showing early symptoms of dementia (Loewenstein et al., 1989; Kuriansky & Gurland, 1976; Mahurin et al., 1991).

Cognitively more demanding tasks of daily living are included in the OTDL (Diehl et al., 1995) and the *Timed Instrumental Activities of Daily Living* (TIADL) (Owsley et al., 2002). Specifically, the OTDL require older adults to perform tasks related to food preparation, telephone use, and medication-taking behavior. The OTDL have shown significant correlations with basic cognitive abilities such as fluid and crystallized intelligence, perceptual speed, and memory (Diehl et al., 1995), and a revised and shortened version has been used in the ACTIVE multisite clinical trial (Jobe et al., 2001). The TIADL (Owsley et al., 2002) assess performance with regard to five IADLs (i.e., communication, finance, cooking, shopping, and taking medications). Adults are required to perform each task as fast and as accurately as they can. The TIADL is used as another everyday competence measure in the ACTIVE clinical trial and preliminary findings support its psychometric properties and its predictive validity (Owsley et al., 2002).

In summary, recent years have seen a number of efforts to assess adults' actual performance on everyday tasks more objectively. Results from this research have shown that the traditionally used self-report assessments have serious limitations and should, whenever possible, be complemented by other methods of assessment. Observational assessments and evaluations from proxies (e.g., spouse and caregiver) who are intimately familiar with the focus person's day-to-day behavior represent valuable complements to older adults' self-reports.

Emphasizing Person-Environment Fit: Driving Competence as a Sample Case
Throughout this chapter, we have emphasized that everyday competence does not reside solely in the person nor in the environment, but in the interaction between the person and environment. Perhaps the best support for this argument comes from research that focuses on older adults' driving competence. Willis (2000), for example, defined driving competence "as the congruence or fit between the driver and the environment" (p. 270) and discussed a number of environmental and personal factors that con-

tribute to driving competence. On the environmental side, researchers have investigated

1. the physical environment, including the weather;
2. the environment within the automobile (including the placement of equipment such as mirrors, turn signals, etc.);
3. structural (e.g., number of lanes and types of signals) and dynamic aspects (e.g., traffic flow and the size of oncoming vehicles) of the roadway;
4. the social aspects of the driving context (e.g., driving alone or with others, and the aggressive behavior of other drivers)

As Willis (2000) has pointed out "these environmental factors are important to the extent that they increase or decrease the mental load required of the driver" (p. 272). That is, these factors become important in interaction with the sensory (i.e., vision and hearing) and cognitive capabilities (e.g., simple and complex reaction time, speed of processing, working memory) of the older driver, resulting in the actual driving competence that is displayed in a particular traffic situation. We suggest that research on older adults' driving competence can serve an important function by providing a more dynamic perspective and research tools that recognize explicitly that everyday competence always exists in the interaction between person and environment.

CONCLUDING REMARKS

Maintaining a high level of functioning in everyday life is one of the most important goals for older adults and a sign of successful aging (M. Baltes & Lang, 1997). Willis (1996c) stated that "what the elderly fear most, often even more than dying, is the loss of independence—the inability to care for oneself, to manage one's affairs, and to live independently in the community" (p. 87). Thus, individuals' ability to interact independently, competently, and meaningfully with their physical and social environment, and to respond to the challenges of everyday life constructively, is a central topic of aging research.

The objective of this chapter was to provide a review of the role of the physical and social environment in the context of everyday competence and everyday problem solving in later life. We conceptualized everyday competence as a transactional construct and emphasized its multidimensional nature. An important implication of such a conceptualization is that assessment procedures do not only need to take into account older adults' actual performance on day-to-day tasks, but also their performance potential, including the reserve capacities that may be activated under favorable environmental conditions. In addition, assessment of an older person's everyday competence needs to take into account the available physical and social resources and the person's motivational and emotional states. We believe that such a conceptualization is most appropriate for capturing the dynamic and reciprocal nature of the competence construct.

Studies that have adopted such a transactional and multidimensional view of everyday competence have shown that complex models and greater differentiation are needed to account for older adults' performance on different tasks of daily living (Allaire & Marsiske, 1999; Diehl et al., 1995; Marsiske, Klumb, & M. Baltes, 1997; Wahl et al., 1999). Most notably, research on the dual-component model of everyday competence by M. Baltes and her colleagues (1999) has shown that in community-residing elderly adults, different components of everyday competence are associated with different physical, social, and psychological correlates. Similarly, research by Wahl et al. (1999) on everyday competence in visually impaired older adults has shown that different combinations of environmental and personal factors are at play depending on whether everyday competence is conceptualized as outcome, process, or predictor variable.

The overwhelming majority of studies on everyday competence conducted to date have been correlational in nature. We believe that a next step in this area of aging research needs to also focus on experimental studies that examine P-E interactions under more controlled conditions. For example, the simulation of different driving conditions in the laboratory is one way in which environmental conditions (e.g., road conditions such as traffic flow, weather, etc.) and person factors (e.g., cognitive load) can be systematically manipulated and actual driving competence can be observed. Other examples are the testing-the-limits approach to examine the performance potential or range of plasticity of older adults' everyday competence under conditions of optimal environmental support (see P. Baltes & M. Baltes, 1990) or research on human factors and aging (Charness & Bosman, 1992). These efforts need to be complemented by research designs that explicitly test for P-E interactions and incorporate both physical and social aspects of older adults' environment.

Finally, we highlighted some of the emerging trends and future challenges in this research area. Recent developments in computer and communication technology challenge established definitions of everyday competence and suggest that different skill repertoires will be necessary in order to be considered competent in daily life in the future. Similarly, sociocultural changes in family composition and family relationships, due to large-scale changes in fertility, marriage, and divorce patterns, represent challenges to the established forms of social support (Antonucci, 2001; Himes, 1992). Aging researchers need to adapt their definitions, assessment instruments, and research methodologies to these changes in order to serve the aging population appropriately in the twenty-first century (Czaja, 1997).

REFERENCES

Allaire, J. C., & Marsiske, M. (1999). Everyday cognition: Age and intellectual ability correlates. *Psychology and Aging, 14,* 627-644.

Antonucci, T. C. (1985). Personal characteristics, social support, and social behavior. In R. H. Binstock & E. Shanas (Eds.), *Handbook of aging and the social sciences* (2nd ed., pp. 94-128). New York: Van Nostrand Reinhold.

Antonucci, T. C. (2001). Social relations: An examination of social networks, social support, and sense of control. In J. E. Birren & K. W. Schaie (Eds.), *Handbook of the psychology of aging* (5th ed., pp. 427-453). San Diego, CA: Academic Press.

Antonucci, T. C., & Akiyama, H. (1997). Social support and the maintenance of competence. In S. L. Willis, K. W. Schaie, & M. Hayward (Eds.), *Societal mechanisms for maintaining competence in old age* (pp. 182-206). New York: Springer.

Antonucci, T. C., & Jackson, J. S. (1987). Social support, interpersonal efficacy, and health: A life course perspective. In L. L. Carstensen & B. A. Edelstein (Eds.), *Handbook of clinical gerontology* (pp. 291-311). New York: Pergamon.

Bandura, A. (1997). *Self-efficacy: The exercise of control.* New York: Freeman.

Baltes, M. M. (1996). *The many faces of dependency in old age.* New York: Cambridge University Press.

Baltes, M. M., & Horgas, A. L. (1997). Long-term care institutions and the maintenance of competence: A dialectic between compensation and overcompensation. In S. L. Willis, K. W. Schaie, & M. Hayward (Eds.), *Societal mechanisms for maintaining competence in old age* (pp. 142-164). New York: Springer.

Baltes, M. M., & Lang, F. R. (1997). Everyday functioning and successful aging: The impact of resources. *Psychology and Aging, 12,* 433-443.

Baltes, M. M., Maas, I., Wilms, H. U., & Borchelt, M. (1999). Everyday competence in old and very old age: Theoretical considerations and empirical findings. In P. B. Baltes & K. U. Mayer (Eds.), *The Berlin aging study: aging from 70 to 100* (pp. 384-402). New York: Cambridge University Press.

Baltes, P. B. (1987). Theoretical propositions of life-span developmental psychology: On the dynamics between growth and decline. *Developmental Psychology, 23,* 611-626.

Baltes, P. B., & Baltes, M. M. (1990). Psychological perspective on successful aging: The model of selective optimization with compensation. In P. B. Baltes & M. M. Baltes (Eds.), *Successful aging: Perspectives from the behavioral sciences* (pp. 1-34). New York: Cambridge University Press.

Baltes, P. B., & Staudinger, U. M. (Eds.). (1996). *Interactive minds: Life-span perspectives on the social foundation of cognition.* New York: Cambridge University Press.

Baumeister, R. F., & Leary, M. R. (1995). The need to belong: Desire for interpersonal attachments as a fundamental human motivation. *Psychological Bulletin, 117,* 497-529.

Berg, C. A., Calderone, K. S., Sansone, C., Strough, J., & Weir, C. (1998). The role of problem definitions in understanding age and context effects on strategies for solving everyday problems. *Psychology and Aging, 13,* 29-44.

Berg, C. A., Johnson, M. M. S., Meegan, S. P., & Strough, J. (2003). Collaborative problem-solving interactions in young and old married couples. *Discourse Processes, 15,* 33-58.

Berg, C. A., & Sternberg, R. J. (1985). A triarchic theory of intellectual development during adulthood. *Developmental Review, 5,* 334-370.

Berkman, L. F., Seeman, T. T., Albert, M., Blazer, D., Kahn, R., Mohs, R., et al. (1993). High, usual, and impaired functioning in community-dwelling older men and women: Findings from the MacArthur Foundation Research Network on Successful Aging. *Journal of Clinical Epidemiology, 46,* 1129-1140.

Berkman, L. F., & Syme, S. L. (1979). Social networks, host resistance and mortality: A nine-year follow-up study of Alameda County residents. *American Journal of Epidemiology, 109,* 186-204.

Berry, J. M., West, R. L., & Dennehey, D. (1989). Reliability and validity of the memory self-efficacy questionnaire. *Developmental Psychology, 25,* 701-713.

Blazer, D. (1982). Social support and mortality in an elderly community population. *American Journal of Epidemiology, 115,* 684-694.

Boult, C., Kane, R. L., Louis, T. A., Boult, L., & McCaffrey, D. (1994). Chronic conditions that lead to functional limitations in the elderly. *Journal of Gerontology: Medical Sciences, 49,* M28-M36.

Branch, L. G., Horowitz, A., & Carr, C. (1989). The implications for everyday life of incident self-reported visual decline among people over age 65 living in the community. *The Gerontologist, 29,* 359-365.

Camp, C. J., Doherty, K., Moody-Thomas, S., & Denney, N. W. (1989). Practical problem solving in adults: A comparison of problem types and scoring methods. In J. D. Sinnott (Ed.), *Everyday problem solving: Theory and applications* (pp. 211-228). New York: Praeger.

Campbell, A. G., Borrie, M. J., & Spears, G. F. (1989). Risk factors for falls in a community-based prospective study of people 70 years and older. *Journal of Gerontology: Medical Sciences, 44,* M112-M117.

Carstensen, L. L. (1993). Motivation for social contact across the life span: A theory of socioemotional selectivity. In J. Jacobs (Ed.), *Nebraska Symposium on Motivation: Vol. 40. Developmental perspectives on motivation* (pp. 209-254). Lincoln: University of Nebraska Press.

Carstensen, L. L., Isaacowitz, D. M., & Charles, S. T. (1999). Taking time seriously: A theory of socioemotional selectivity. *American Psychologist, 54,* 165-181.

Carstensen, L. L., & Lang, F. R. (1997). Commentary: Social relationships in context and as context: Social support and the maintenance of competence in old age. In S. L. Willis, K. W. Schaie, & M. Hayward (Eds.), *Societal mechanisms for maintaining competence in old age* (pp. 207-222). New York: Springer.

Charness, N., & Bosman, E. A. (1990). Human factors and design for older adults. In J. E. Birren & K. W. Schaie (Eds.), *Handbook of the psychology of aging* (3rd ed., pp. 446-463). San Diego, CA: Academic Press.

Charness, N., & Bosman, E. A. (1992). Human factors and aging. In F. I. M. Craik & T. A. Salthouse (Eds.), *The handbook of aging and cognition* (pp. 495-545). Hillsdale, NJ: Erlbaum.

Charness, N., Schulmann, C. E., & Boritz, G. M. (1992). Training older adults in word processing: Effects of age, training technique, and computer anxiety. *International Journal of Technology and Aging, 5,* 79-106.

Chernoff, R. (2001). Nutrition and health promotion in older adults. *Journals of Gerontology: Series A, 56A (Special Issue II),* 47-53.

Cockburn, J., & Smith, P. T. (1991). The relative influence of intelligence and age on everyday memory. *Journal of Gerontology: Psychological Sciences, 46,* P31-P36.

Cornelius, S., & Caspi, A. (1987). Everyday problem solving in adulthood and old age. *Psychology and Aging, 2,* 144-153.

Costa, P. T., Jr., & McCrae, R. R. (1992). *NEO-PI-R: Revised NEO Personality Inventory and NEO Five-Factor Inventory (NEO-FFI).* Odessa, FL: Psychological Assessment Resources.

Cox, D. F. (Ed.). (1967). *Risk taking and information handling in consumer behavior.* Cambridge, MA: Harvard University Press.

Czaja, S. J. (1997). Using technologies to aid the performance of home tasks. In A. D. Fisk & W. A. Rogers (Eds.), *Handbook of human factors and the older adult* (pp. 311-334). San Diego, CA: Academic Press.

Czaja, S. J., Guerrier, J. H., Nair, S. N., & Landauer, T. K. (1993). Computer communication as an aid to independence for older adults. *Behavior and Information Technology, 12,* 197-207.

Demming, J. A., & Pressey, S. L. (1957). Tests "indigenous" to the adult and older years. *Journal of Counseling Psychology, 4,* 144-148.

Denney, N. W., & Pearce, K. A. (1989). A developmental study of practical problem solving in adults. *Psychology and Aging, 4,* 438-442.

Diehl, M. (1998). Everyday competence in later life: Current status and future directions. *The Gerontologist, 38,* 422-433.

Diehl, M., Willis, S. L., & Schaie, K. W. (1995). Everyday problem solving in older adults: Observational assessment and cognitive correlates. *Psychology and Aging, 10,* 478-491.

DiPietro, L. (2001). Physical activity in aging: Changes in patterns and their relationship to health and function. *Journals of Gerontology: Series A, 56A (Special Issue II),* 13-22.

Dixon, R. A., & Bäckman, L. (1995). Concepts of compensation: Integrated, differentiated, and Janus-faced. In R. A. Dixon & L. Bäckman (Eds.), *Compensating for psychological deficits and declines: Managing losses and promoting gains* (pp. 3-19). Mahwah, NJ: Erlbaum.

Eilers, M. L. (1989). Older adults and computer education: "Not to have the world a closed door." *International Journal of Technology and Aging, 2,* 56-76.

Fernie, G. (1997). Assistive devices. In A. D. Fisk & W. A. Rogers (Eds.), *Handbook of human factors and the older adult* (pp. 289-310). San Diego, CA: Academic Press.

Fillenbaum, G. G. (1985). Screening the elderly: A brief instrumental activities of daily living measure. *Journal of the American Geriatrics Society, 33,* 698-706.

Fillenbaum, G. G. (1988). *Multidimensional functional assessment of older adults: The Duke Older Americans Resources and Services Procedures.* Hillsdale, NJ: Erlbaum.

Fisk, A. D., & Rogers, W. A. (Eds.). (1997). *Handbook of human factors and the older adult.* San Diego, CA: Academic Press.

Friedman, S. M., Munoz, B., West, S. K., Rubin, G. S., & Fried, L. P. (2002). Falls and fear of falling: Which comes first? A longitudinal prediction model suggests strategies for primary and secondary prevention. *Journal of the American Geriatrics Society, 50,* 1329-1335.

Furner, S. E., Rudberg, M. A., & Cassel, C. K. (1995). Medical conditions differentially affect the development of IADL disability: Implications for medical care and research. *The Gerontologist, 35,* 444-450.

Garbe, D., Stockler, F., & Wald, R. (1993). The state of the art: Telecommunication and the elderly. In H. Bouma & J. A. M. Graffmans (Eds.), *Gerontechnology* (pp. 283-292). Amsterdam: ISO Press.

Garfein, A. J., Schaie, K. W., & Willis, S. L. (1988). Microcomputer proficiency in later middle-aged and older adults: Teaching old dogs new tricks. *Social Behaviour, 3,* 131-148.

Gatz, M., Bengtson, V. L., & Blum, M. J. (1990). Caregiving families. In J. E. Birren & K. W. Schaie (Eds.), *Handbook of the psychology of aging* (3rd ed., pp. 404-426). San Diego, CA: Academic Press.

Gill, T. M., Robison, J. T., Williams, C. S., & Tinetti, M. E. (1999). Mismatches between home environment and physical capabilities among community-living older adults. *Journal of the American Geriatrics Society, 47,* 88-92.

Gill, T. M., Williams, C. S., Robison, J. T., & Tinetti, M. E. (1999). A population-based study of environmental hazards in the homes of older persons. *American Journal of Public Health, 89,* 553-556.

Gitlin, L. N. (1998). Testing home modification interventions: Issues of theory, measurement, design, and implementation. In R. Schulz, G. Maddox, & M. P. Lawton (Eds.), *Annual Review of Gerontology and Geriatrics* (Vol. 18, pp. 1-16). New York: Springer.

Gitlin, L. N., Schemm, R. L., Landsberg, L., & Burgh, D. Y. (1996). Factors predicting assistive device use in the home by older persons following rehabilitation. *Journal of Aging and Health, 8,* 554-575.

Golant, S. M. (1984). *A place to grow old: The meaning of environment in old age.* New York: Columbia University Press.

Goodnow, J. J. (1996). Collaborative rules: How are people supposed to work with one another? In P. B. Baltes & U. M. Staudinger (Eds.), *Interactive minds: Life-span perspectives on the social foundation of cognition* (pp. 163-197). New York: Cambridge University Press.

Gould, O. N., & Dixon, R. A. (1993). How we spent our vacation: Collaborative storytelling by young and old adults. *Psychology and Aging, 8,* 10-17.

Gribbin, K., Schaie, K. W., & Parham, I. A. (1980). Complexity of life style and maintenance of intellectual abilities. *Journal of Social Issues, 36,* 47–61.

Grisso, T. (1986). *Evaluating competencies: Forensic assessments and instruments.* New York: Plenum.

Guralnik, J. M., Seeman, T. E., Tinetti, M. E., Nevitt, M. C., & Berkman, L. F. (1994). Validation and use of performance measures in a non-disabled older population: MacArthur Studies of Successful Aging. *Aging Clinical Experimental Research, 6,* 410-419.

Hahm, W., & Bickson, T. (1989). Retirees using e-mail and networked computers. *International Journal of Technology and Aging, 2,* 113-124.

Heckhausen, J., & Schulz, R. (1995). A life-span theory of control. *Psychological Review, 102,* 284-302.

Heller, K., & Thompson, M. G. (1991). Support interventions for older adults: Confidante relationships, perceived family support, and meaningful role activity. *American Journal of Community Psychology, 19,* 139–146.

Hershey, D. A., Walsh, D. A., Read, S. J., & Chulef, A. S. (1990). The effects of expertise on financial problem solving: Evidence for goal-directed problem-solving scripts. *Organizational Behavior and Human Decision Processes, 46,* 77-101.

Himes, C. L. (1992). Future caregivers: Projected family structures of older persons. *Journal of Gerontology: Social Sciences, 47*, S17-S26.

Hobfoll, S. E., & Freedy, J. R. (1990). The availability and effective use of social support. *Journal of Social and Clinical Psychology, 9*, 91-103.

Horgas, A. L., Wilms, H. U., & Baltes, M. M. (1998). Daily life in very old age: Everyday activities as expression of successful living. *The Gerontologist, 38*, 556-568.

Horowitz, A. (1985). Family caregiving to the frail elderly. In M. P. Lawton & G. L. Maddox (Eds.), *Annual Review of Gerontology and Geriatrics* (Vol. 5, pp. 194-246). New York: Springer.

House, J. S., Robbins, C., & Metzner, H. M. (1982). The association of social relationships and activities with mortality: Prospective evidence from the Tecumseh Community Health Study. *American Journal of Epidemiology, 116*, 123-140.

Idler, E. L., & Kasl, S. V. (1995). Self-ratings of health: Do they also predict change in functional ability? *Journal of Gerontology: Social Sciences, 50B*, S344-S353.

Ingersoll-Dayton, B., Morgan, D., & Antonucci, T. (1997). The effects of positive and negative social exchanges on aging adults. *Journal of Gerontology: Social Sciences, 52B*, S190-S199.

Jay, G. M., & Willis, S. L. (1992). Influence of direct computer experience on older adults' attitudes toward computers. *Journal of Gerontology: Psychological Sciences, 47*, P250-P257.

Jobe, J. B., Smith, D. M., Ball, K., Tennstedt, S., Marsiske, M., Willis, S. L., Rebok, G., Morris, J. N., Helmers, K., Leveck, M. D., & Kleinman, K. (2001). ACTIVE: A cognitive intervention trial to promote independence in older adults. *Controlled Clinical Trials, 22*, 453-479.

Kahn, R. L., & Antonucci, T. C. (1980). Convoys over the life course: Attachment, roles, and social support. In P. B. Baltes & O. G. Brim, Jr. (Eds.), *Life-span development and behavior* (Vol. 3, pp. 253-286). New York: Academic Press.

Katz, S., Ford, A. B., Moskowitz, R. W., Jackson, B. A., & Jaffee, M. W. (1963). Studies of illness in the aged. The index of ADL: A standardized measure of biological and psychological function. *Journal of the American Medical Association, 185*, 94-101.

Katz, S., & Stroud, M. W. (1989). Functional assessment in geriatrics: A review of progress and directions. *Journal of the American Geriatrics Society, 37*, 267-271.

King, A. C. (2001). Interventions to promote physical activity by older adults. *Journals of Gerontology: Series A, 56A (Special Issue II)*, 36-46.

Kleemeier, R. W. (1959). Behavior and the organization of the bodily and the external environment. In J. E. Birren (Ed.), *Handbook of aging and the individual* (pp. 400-451). Chicago: University of Chicago Press.

Krause, N. (1993). Neighborhood deterioration and social isolation in later life. *International Journal of Aging and Human Development, 36*, 9-38.

Kurianksy, J., & Gurland, B. (1976). The Performance Test of Activities of Daily Living. *International Journal of Aging and Human Development, 7*, 343-352.

Kuypers, J. A., & Bengtson, V. L. (1973). Social breakdown and competence: A model of normal aging. *Human Development, 16*, 181-201.

Lachman, M. E., Steinberg, E. S., & Trotter, S. D. (1987). Effects of control beliefs and attributions on memory self-assessments and performance. *Psychology and Aging, 2*, 266-271.

Lachman, M. E., Weaver, S. L., Bandura, M., Elliott, E., & Lewkowicz, C. J. (1992). Improving memory and control beliefs through cognitive restructuring and self-generated strategies. *Journal of Gerontology: Psychological Sciences, 47,* P293-P299.

Lachman, M. E., Ziff, M. A., & Spiro, A. (1994). Maintaining a sense of control in later life. In R. P. Abeles, H. C. Gift, & M. G. Ory (Eds.), *Aging and quality of life* (pp. 216-232). New York: Springer.

Lakey, B., Tardiff, T. A., & Drew, J. B. (1994). Negative social interaction: Assessment and relations to social support, cognition, and psychological distress. *Journal of Social and Clinical Psychology, 13,* 42-62.

Lang, F. R. (2001). Regulation of social relationships in later adulthood. *Journal of Gerontology: Psychological Sciences, 56B,* P321-P326.

Lang, F. R., & Carstensen, L. L. (1994). Close emotional relationships in late life: Further support for proactive aging in the social domain. *Psychology and Aging, 9,* 315-324.

Langer, E. J., & Rodin, J. (1976). The effects of choice and enhanced personal responsibility for the aged: A field experiment in an institutional setting. *Journal of Personality and Social Psychology, 34,* 191-198.

Lawton, M. P. (1977). The impact of the environment on aging and behavior. In J. E. Birren & K. W. Schaie (Eds.), *Handbook of the psychology of aging* (pp. 276-301). New York: Van Nostrand Reinhold.

Lawton, M. P. (1982). Competence, environmental press, and the adaptation of older people. In M. P. Lawton, P. G. Windley, & T. O. Byerts (Eds.), *Aging and environment: Theoretical approaches* (pp. 33-59). New York: Springer.

Lawton, M. P. (1983). Environment and other determinants of well-being in older people. *The Gerontologist, 23,* 349-357.

Lawton, M. P. (1986). Contextual perspectives: Psychosocial influences. In L. W. Poon (Ed.), *Handbook for clinical memory assessment of older adults* (pp. 32-42). Washington, DC: American Psychological Association.

Lawton, M. P. (1989a). Behavior-relevant ecological factors. In K. W. Schaie & C. Schooler (Eds.), *Social structure and aging: Psychological processes* (pp. 57-78). Hillsdale, NJ: Erlbaum.

Lawton, M. P. (1989b). Environmental proactivity in older people. In V. L. Bengtson & K. W. Schaie (Eds.), *The course of later life* (pp. 15-23). New York: Springer.

Lawton, M. P. (1990). Residential environment and self-directedness among older people. *American Psychologist, 45,* 638-640.

Lawton, M. P., & Brody, E. M. (1969). Assessment of older people: Self-maintaining and instrumental activities of daily living. *The Gerontologist, 9,* 179-185.

Lawton, M. P., & Nahemow, L. E. (1973). Ecology and the aging process. In C. Eisdorfer & M. P. Lawton (Eds.), *The psychology of adult development and aging* (pp. 619-674). Washington, DC: American Psychological Association.

Lawton, M. P., Nahemow, L. E., & Yeh, T. (1980). Neighborhood environment and the well-being of older tenants in planned housing. *International Journal of Aging and Human Development, 11,* 211-227.

Lazarus, R. S., & Folkman, S. (1984). *Stress, appraisal, and coping.* New York: Springer.

Leventhal, E. A., Leventhal, H., Schaefer, P. M., & Easterling, D. (1993). Conservation of energy, uncertainty reduction, and swift utilization of medical care among the elderly. *Journal of Gerontology: Psychological Sciences, 48,* P78-P86.

Levy, B. (1996). Improving memory in old age through implicit self-stereotyping. *Journal of Personality and Social Psychology, 71,* 1092-1107.

Lewin, K. (1935). *A dynamic theory of personality.* New York: McGraw-Hill.

Loewenstein, D. A., Amigo, E., Duara, R., Guterman, A., Hurwitz, D., Berkowitz, N., Wilkie, F., Weinberg, G., Black, B., Gittelman, B., & Eisdorfer, C. (1989). A new scale for the assessment of functional status in Alzheimer's disease and related disorders. *Journal of Gerontology: Psychological Sciences, 44,* P114-P121.

Mahurin, R. K., DeBettignies, B. H., & Pirozzolo, F. J. (1991). Structured assessment of independent living skills: Preliminary report of a performance measure of functional abilities in dementia. *Journal of Gerontology: Psychological Sciences, 46,* P58-P66.

Mann, W. C., Hurren, D., Tomita, M., & Charvat, B. (1995). The relationship of functional independence to assistive device use of elderly persons living at home. *The Journal of Applied Gerontology, 41,* 225-247.

Mann, W. C., Karuza, J., Hurren, M. D., & Tomita, M. (1993). Needs of home-based older persons for assistive devices. *Technology and Disability, 2,* 1-11.

Manne, S. L., & Zautra, A. J. (1989). Spouse criticism and support: Their association with coping and psychological adjustment among women with rheumatoid arthritis. *Journal of Personality and Social Psychology, 56,* 608-617.

Margrett, J. A., & Marsiske, M. (2002). Gender differences in older adults' everyday cognitive collaboration. *International Journal of Behavioral Development, 26,* 45-59.

Marsiske, M., Klumb, P., & Baltes, M. M. (1997). Everyday activity patterns and sensory functioning in old age. *Psychology and Aging, 12,* 444-457.

McAuley, E., & Katula, J. (1998). Physical activity interventions in the elderly: Influence on physical health and psychological function. In R. Schulz, G. Maddox, & M. P. Lawton (Eds.), *Annual Review of Gerontology and Geriatrics* (Vol. 18, pp. 111-153). New York: Springer.

Meacham, J. A., & Emont, N. C. (1989). The interpersonal basis of everyday problem solving. In J. D. Sinnott (Ed.), *Everyday problem solving: Theory and applications* (pp. 7-23). New York: Praeger.

Meegan, S. P., & Berg, C. A. (1997). *The interpersonal context of appraisal and coping with developmental life tasks.* Unpublished manuscript, University of Utah, Salt Lake City.

Mendes de Leon, C. F., Seeman, T. E., Baker, D. I., Richardson, E. D., & Tinetti, M. E. (1996). Self-efficacy, physical decline, and change in functioning in community-living elders: A prospective study. *Journal of Gerontology: Social Sciences, 51B,* S183-S190.

Messeri, P., Silverstein, M., & Litwak, E. (1993). Choice of optimal social supports among the elderly: A meta-analysis of competing theoretical perspectives. *Journal of Health and Social Behavior, 34,* 122-137.

Morrell, R. W., & Echt, K. V. (1997). Designing written instructions for older adults: Learning to use computers. In A. D. Fisk & W. A. Rogers (Eds.), *Handbook of human factors and the older adult* (pp. 335-361). San Diego, CA: Academic Press.

Morris, J. N., Sherwood, S., & Mor, V. (1984). Assessment tool for use in identifying functionally vulnerable persons in the community. *The Gerontologist, 24,* 373-379.

Odenheimer, G. L., Beaudet, M., Jette, A. M., Albert, M. S., Grande, L., & Minaker, K. L. (1994). Performance-based driving evaluation of the elderly driver:

Safety, reliability, and validity. *Journal of Gerontology: Medical Sciences, 49*, M153-M159.

Okun, M. A., Melichar, J. F., & Hill, M. D. (1990). Negative daily events, positive and negative social ties, and psychological distress among older adults. *The Gerontologist, 30*, 193-199.

Oswald, F., Schilling, O., Wahl, H. W., & Gäng, K. (2002). Trouble in paradise? Reasons to relocate and objective environmental changes among well-off older adults. *Journal of Environmental Psychology, 22*, 273-288.

Owsley, C., Sloane, M., McGwin, G., & Ball, K. (2002). Timed instrumental activities of daily living tasks: Relationship to cognitive function and everyday performance assessments in older adults. *Gerontology, 48*, 254-265.

Park, D. C. (1992). Applied cognitive aging research. In F. I. M. Craik & T. A Salthouse (Eds.), *The handbook of aging and cognition* (pp. 449-493). Hillsdale, NJ: Erlbaum.

Park, D. C., & Jones, T. R. (1997). Medication adherence and aging. In A. D. Fisk & W. A. Rogers (Eds.), *Handbook of human factors and the older adult* (pp. 257-287). San Diego, CA: Academic Press.

Parmelee, P. A., & Lawton, M. P. (1990). The design of special environments for the aged. In J. E. Birren & K. W. Schaie (Eds.), *Handbook of the psychology of aging* (3rd ed., pp. 464-488). San Diego, CA: Academic Press.

Pinquart, M., & Sörensen, S. (2000). Influences of socioeconomic status, social network, and competence on subjective well-being in later life: A meta-analysis. *Psychology and Aging, 15*, 187-224.

Pynoos, J., Cohen, E., Davis, L. J., & Bernhardt, S. (1987). Home modifications: Improvements that extend independence. In V. Regnier & J. Pynoos (Eds.), *Housing the aged: Design directives and policy considerations* (pp. 277-303). New York: Elsevier.

Regnier, V. (1976). Neighborhoods as service systems. In M. P. Lawton, R. Newcomer, & T. Byerts (Eds.), *Community planning for an aging society* (pp. 240-257). Stroudsburg, PA: Dowden, Hutchinson and Ross.

Regnier, V. (1983). Urban neighborhood cognition: Relationships between functional and symbolic resources. In G. D. Rowles & R. J. Ohta (Eds.), *Aging and milieu: Environmental perspectives on growing old* (pp. 63-82). New York: Academic Press.

Regnier, V., & Pynoos, J. (Eds.). (1987). *Housing the aged: Design directives and policy considerations.* New York: Elsevier.

Regnier, V., & Pynoos, J. (1992). Environmental intervention for cognitively impaired older persons. In J. E. Birren, R. B. Sloane, & G. D. Cohen (Eds.), *Handbook of mental health and aging* (2nd ed., pp. 763-792). San Diego, CA: Academic Press.

Reschovsky, J. D., & Newman, S. J. (1990). Adaptations for independent living by older frail households. *The Gerontologist, 30*, 543-552.

Rogoff, B., & Lave, J. (Eds.). (1984). *Everyday cognition: Its development in social context.* Cambridge, MA: Harvard University Press.

Rook, K. S. (1984). The negative side of social interaction: Impact on psychological well-being. *Journal of Personality and Social Psychology, 46*, 1097-1108.

Rowe, J. W., & Kahn, R. L. (1998). *Successful aging: The MacArthur Foundation Study.* New York: Pantheon.

Rowles, G. D. (1981). The surveillance zone as meaningful space for the aged. *Gerontology, 3,* 304-311.

Rubinstein, R. L., & Parmelee, P. A. (1992). Attachment to place and representation of life course by the elderly. In I. Altman & S. M. Low (Eds.), *Human behavior and environment: Vol. 12. Place attachment* (pp. 139-163). New York: Plenum.

Rudberg, M. A., Furner, S. E., Dunn, J. E., & Cassel, C. K. (1993). The relationship of visual and hearing impairment to disability: An analysis using the Longitudinal Study of Aging. *Journal of Gerontology: Medical Sciences, 48,* M261-M265.

Sabatino, C. P. (1996). Competency: Refining our legal fictions. In M. A. Smyer, K. W. Schaie, & M. B. Kapp (Eds.), *Older adults' decision making and the law* (pp. 1- 28). New York: Springer.

Salthouse, T. A. (1990). Cognitive competence and expertise in aging. In J. E. Birren & K. W. Schaie (Eds.), *Handbook of the psychology of aging* (3rd ed., pp. 310-319). San Diego, CA: Academic Press.

Salthouse, T. A. (1996). A cognitive psychologist's perspective on the assessment of cognitive competency. In M. A. Smyer, K. W. Schaie, & M. B. Kapp (Eds.), *Older adults' decision making and the law* (pp. 29-39). New York: Springer.

Sansone, C., & Berg, C. A. (1993). Adapting to the environment across the life span: Different processes or different inputs? *International Journal of Behavioral Development, 16,* 215-241.

Schaie, K. W. (1994). The course of adult intellectual development. *American Psychologist, 49,* 304-313.

Schaie, K. W. (1996). *Intellectual development in adulthood: The Seattle Longitudinal Study.* New York: Cambridge University Press.

Schaninger, D. M., & Schiglimpaglia, D. (1981). The influence of cognitive personality traits and demographics on consumer information acquisition. *Journal of Consumer Research, 8,* 208-216.

Scheidt, R. J., & Windley, P. G. (1985). The ecology of aging. In J. E. Birren & K. W. Schaie (Eds.), *Handbook of the psychology of aging* (2nd ed., pp. 245-258). New York: Van Nostrand Reinhold.

Schooler, C. (1987). Psychological effects of complex environments during the life span: A review and theory. In C. Schooler & K. W. Schaie (Eds.), *Cognitive functioning and social structure over the life course* (pp. 24-49). Norwood, NJ: Ablex.

Silverstein, M. (1997). Commentary: Emerging theoretical and empirical issues in the study of social support and competence in later life. In S. L. Willis, K. W. Schaie, & M. Hayward (Eds.), *Societal mechanisms for maintaining competence in old age* (pp. 223-231). New York: Springer.

Smith, J., & Goodnow, J. J. (1999). Unasked-for support and unsolicited advice: Age and the quality of social experience. *Psychology and Aging, 14,* 108-121.

Smyer, M. A., Schaie, K. W., & Kapp, M. B. (Eds.). (1996). *Older adults' decision making and the law.* New York: Springer.

Speare, A., Avery, R., & Lawton, M. P. (1991). Disability, residential mobility, and changes in living arrangements. *Journal of Gerontology: Social Sciences, 46,* S133-S142.

Stephens, M. A. P., Kinney, J., Norris, V., & Ritchie, S. W. (1987). Social networks as assets and liabilities in recovery from stroke by geriatric patients. *Psychology and Aging, 2,* 125-129.

Sternberg, R. J., & Wagner, R. K. (Eds.). (1986). *Practical intelligence: Nature and origins of competence in the everyday world.* New York: Cambridge University Press.

Sternberg, R. J., & Wagner, R. K. (Eds). (1994). *Mind in context: Interactionist perspectives on human intelligence.* New York: Cambridge University Press.

Sterns, H. L., Barrett, G. V., & Alexander, R. A. (1985). Accidents and the aging individual. In J. E. Birren & K. W. Schaie (Eds.), *Handbook of the psychology of aging* (2nd ed., pp. 703-724). New York: Van Nostrand Reinhold.

Strough, J., Berg, C. A., & Sansone, C. (1996). Goals for solving everyday problems across the life span: Age and gender differences in the salience of interpersonal concerns. *Developmental Psychology, 32,* 1106-1115.

Strough, J., Cheng, S., & Swenson, L. M. (2002). Preference for collaborative and individual everyday problem solving in later adulthood. *International Journal of Behavioral Development, 26,* 26-35.

Tennstedt, S., Howland, J., Lachman, M., Peterson, E., Kasten, L., & Jette, A. (1998). A randomized, controlled trial of a group intervention to reduce fear of falling and associated activity restriction in older adults. *Journal of Gerontology: Psychological Sciences, 53B,* P384-P392.

Thompson, E. E., & Krause, N. (1998). Living alone and neighborhood characteristics as predictors of social support in late life. *Journal of Gerontology: Social Sciences, 53B,* S354-S364.

Tinetti, M. E., Mendes de Leon, C. F., Doucete, J. T., & Baker, D. I. (1994). Fear of falling and fall-related efficacy in relationship to functioning among community-living elders. *Journal of Gerontology: Medical Sciences, 49,* M140-M147.

Tinetti, M. E., Speechley, M., & Ginter, S. F. (1988). Risk factors for falls among elderly persons living in the community. *New England Journal of Medicine, 319,* 1701-1707.

Verbrugge, L. M., Rennert, C., & Madans, J. H. (1997). The great efficacy of personal and equipment assistance in reducing disability. *American Journal of Public Health, 87,* 384-392.

Wahl, H. W. (2001). Environmental influences on aging and behavior. In J. E. Birren & K. W. Schaie (Eds.), *Handbook of the psychology of aging* (5th ed., pp. 215-237). San Diego, CA: Academic Press.

Wahl, H. W., Oswald, F., & Zimprich, D. (1999). Everyday competence in visually impaired older adults: A case for person-environment perspectives. *The Gerontologist, 39,* 140-149.

Wahl, H. W., Schilling, O., Oswald, F., & Heyl, V. (1999). Psychosocial consequences of age-related visual impairment: Comparison with mobility-impaired older adults and long-term outcome. *Journal of Gerontology: Psychological Sciences, 54B,* P304-P316.

White, R. W. (1959). Motivation reconsidered: The concept of competence. *Psychological Review, 66,* 297-333.

Willis, S. L. (1991). Cognition and everyday competence. In K. W. Schaie & M. P. Lawton (Eds.), *Annual Review of Gerontology and Geriatrics* (Vol. 11, pp. 80-109). New York: Springer.

Willis, S. L. (1996a). Everyday cognitive competence in elderly persons: Conceptual issues and empirical findings. *The Gerontologist, 36,* 595–601.

Willis, S. L. (1996b). Everyday problem solving. In J. E. Birren & K. W. Schaie (Eds.), *Handbook of the psychology of aging* (4th ed., pp. 287-307). San Diego, CA: Academic Press.

Willis, S. L. (1996c). Assessing everyday competence in the cognitively challenged elderly. In M. A. Smyer, K. W. Schaie, & M. B. Kapp (Eds.), *Older adults' decision making and the law* (pp. 87-127). New York: Springer.

Willis, S. L. (2000). Driving competence: The person x environment fit. In K. W. Schaie & M. Pietrucha (Eds.), *Mobility and aging* (pp. 269-277). New York: Springer.

Willis, S. L., Jay, G. M., Diehl, M., & Marsiske, M. (1992). Longitudinal change and prediction of everyday task competence in the elderly. *Research on Aging, 14,* 68-91.

Willis, S. L., & Marsiske, M. (1991). A life-span perspective on practical intelligence. In D. Tupper & K. Cicerone (Eds.), *The neuropsychology of everyday life* (pp. 183-198). Boston: Kluwer.

Willis, S. L., & Marsiske, M. (1993). *Manual for the everyday problems test.* University Park: The Pennsylvania State University.

Willis, S. L., & Schaie, K. W. (1986). Practical intelligence in later adulthood. In R. J. Sternberg & R. K. Wagner (Eds.), *Practical intelligence: Nature and origins of competence in the everyday world* (pp. 236-268). New York: Cambridge University Press.

Willis, S. L., & Schaie, K. W. (1993). Everyday cognition: Taxonomic and methodological considerations. In J. M. Puckett & H. W. Reese (Eds.), *Life-span developmental psychology: Mechanisms of everyday cognition* (pp. 33-53). Hillsdale, NJ: Erlbaum.

CHAPTER 7

Interior Living Environments in Old Age

GRAHAM D. ROWLES
PROFESSOR OF GEOGRAPHY, BEHAVIORAL SCIENCE AND NURSING
DIRECTOR, PHD PROGRAM IN GERONTOLOGY
ASSOCIATE DIRECTOR, SANDERS-BROWN CENTER ON AGING
UNIVERSITY OF KENTUCKY

FRANK OSWALD
GERMAN CENTER FOR RESEARCH ON AGING AT THE UNIVERSITY OF HEIDELBERG

ELIZABETH G. HUNTER
GHEENS FELLOW
PHD PROGRAM IN GERONTOLOGY
UNIVERSITY OF KENTUCKY

With advancing years and increasing length of residence in a single setting, many elders spend a greater proportion of their time at home amidst a lifetime of accumulated possessions. They inhabit a dwelling that becomes both a locus of control and self-preservation and a source of identity and meaning. Discussions of such interior environments are often limited to consideration of physical design and other objective contextual characteristics. The primary concern is with ways in which the environment might be modified to facilitate *activities of daily living* (ADLs) or *instrumental activities of daily living* (IADLs). In this chapter, moving beyond this perspective and adopting an experiential perspective that emphasizes the phenomenology of place, we focus on the role of residential interior environments including houses, apartments, mobile homes, long-term care facilities, and other permanent living quarters in determining the quality of life and well-being of elders. In what ways is an elder's quality of life, viewed in the context of changing circumstances (health, mobility, etc.), influenced and shaped by evolving transactions with such "inside" environments? Our approach is to consider this trajectory as the outcome of a complex interweaving of individual aging and environmental change.

First, we focus on *experiential dimensions of elders' "dwelling" in interior space*, and explore the manner in which these dimensions are interwoven in creating the meanings of interior spaces. Within this rubric, we report what is known about the sociocultural context of interior spaces in old age. To what extent are the uses and meanings of interior residential spaces influenced by others—peers, family members, or friends with whom elders may cohabitate—and by the cultural mores and values of the society in which they reside (Lawrence, 1987)? Emphasis is also placed on gender differences in the use and meaning of interior spaces to elders. To what extent does an elderly female homemaker's experience, often resulting from decades of inhabiting and raising children in a single interior space, contrast with that of her male spouse who may have spent the majority of those years working at other locations? Does home space evoke different meanings for men and women following retirement?

A second theme permeating the chapter is *adaptation to change*. Initially, the focus is on the immediate creation of relationships with interior spaces as elders occupy an interior space for the first time or on a short-term or temporary basis. We are also concerned with long-term adaptive processes as, over the life course, elders come to imbue interior environments with more permanent meanings and develop characteristic strategies in adapting to each new setting. Third, we consider *developmental aspects* of the manner in which elders appear to evolve a qualitatively different gestalt in the experience of interior settings as they grow older. Finally, we consider the *loss of control* and disruption of long-term relationships with interior spaces that may accompany the changing life circumstances of elders.

A final motif is a focus on *well-being*. As a result of exponential growth in the number of older adults living independently in the community, relationships between immediate interior environmental settings and outcomes such as physical health, psychological well-being, and life quality become especially deserving of attention (Evans, Kantrowitz, & Eshelman, 2002). Discussion of well-being considers objective physical and mental health outcomes as well as subjective indicators, including residential satisfaction and a sense of being in place. We contend that an elder's relationship with his or her interior residential environment and the manner in which he or she accommodates to changes in this relationship (either resulting from increasing personal frailty or the increased press of environmental changes) is closely tied to well-being. Our exploration begins by providing background information on the interior residential environments that elders inhabit.

INTERIOR LIVING ENVIRONMENTS: PHYSICAL CONTEXTS AND THEIR USES

What are the basic characteristics of elders' interior environments? Although it is widely assumed that interior spaces become increasingly important as a result of universal physical and health-related limitations associated with growing older, data to underscore such assumptions are primarily drawn from Western societies. In this chapter our focus remains exclusively on such societies with a primary focus on the two nations with which we are most familiar: the United States and Germany.

LIVING ARRANGEMENTS IN OLD AGE

The large majority of older adults live independently in their communities, most of them in single-person or couple households, and not in institutional settings. In the United States, about 95 percent of persons 65 and older live in community settings (U.S. Bureau of the Census, 1996). In Germany, the equivalent figure is 93 percent (Bundesministerium für Familie, Senioren, Frauen und Jugend [Federal Ministry for Family Affairs, Senior Citizens, Women and Youth], 2001). Although the likelihood of living in a nursing facility increases with age, and the number of elders residing in an array of alternative purpose-built homes is increasing in modern Western societies (Regnier, in press), the vast majority of older adults live in ordinary dwellings. Elders have a high degree of residential stability. For instance, German data from a national survey of about 4,000 persons showed that participants aged 70 to 85 years had lived an average of 31.6 years in the same apartment and 50.3 years in the same town (Motel, Künemund, & Bode, 2000). Finally, it is important to note that an increasing proportion of elders in most Western societies are living alone and that this propensity increases with age, especially for women (Treas, 1995).

Contemporary architects and design professionals are becoming increasingly sensitive to the special housing needs of elders, including the need to provide for independent negotiation of interior spaces and improved access to outdoor spaces (Regnier, 1994). This is likely to become increasingly important for the rapidly growing population of community dwelling elders beyond 80 years of age. Although older adults, more often than young adults, have a tendency to live in older and often less well-equipped residences as a consequence of lengthy residence, virtually all of the housing occupied by elders in the United States is equipped with basic facilities, and most units have modern appliances that enhance quality of life. Complete plumbing facilities (hot piped water, a bathtub or shower, and a flush toilet) are available in 97 percent of residential units (U.S. Bureau of the Census, 1996). Similarly, in Germany, the percentage of persons over 65 years of age who live in modern apartments (with hot piped water, a bathtub or shower, a flush toilet, and central heating) is 94 percent in the western and 85 percent in the eastern part of the country (Statistisches Bundesamt [Federal Bureau of Census], 2000).

HOW DO ELDERS USE INTERIOR SPACES?

Considering the dynamics of elders' everyday life, there is evidence to support a progressive reduction of the spatial range of activities, especially in very old age (Moss & Lawton, 1982; Rowles, 1978). As a result, elders tend to spend more time at home in interior environments than do younger people. Recent data show that elders (65 years of age and older) in Germany spend, on average, 80 percent of each day at home (Küster, 1998). About 80 percent of elders' daily activities take place at home and include a considerable amount of leisure activity (38 percent; Baltes, Maas, Wilms, & Borchelt, 1999; Baltes, Wahl, & Schmid-Furstoss, 1990). Thus, interior space is key living space in old age; both in terms of time spent at home and the creation of place as a setting for activities.

The majority of elders wish to live independently for as long as possible (Kendig & Pynoos, 1996). This preference has resulted in growing emphasis on aging-in-place as a policy priority in Western societies, including the United States and Germany (BMFSFJ, 2001; Callahan, 1992; Rowles, 1993; Tilson, 1990). However, physiological changes associated with aging and a growing risk of chronic illness tend to result in lifestyle changes as a consequence of reduced environmental competence and increasing environmental vulnerability. Indeed, consistent with the "environmental docility" hypothesis (Lawton & Simon, 1968; Lawton & Nahemow, 1973; Lawton, 1987, 1998), research has shown a strong correlation between loss of competence and both environmental changes and behavioral adaptations in old age, especially in very old age.

Elders are by no means passively reduced to life at home. Rather, they are able to actively modify their environment, even when suffering from a loss of environmental competence. Considering this insight on a conceptual level, Lawton introduced the notion of "environmental proactivity" (1989). He argued that being at home could be seen as an expression of maintaining independence and autonomy consistent with a lifestyle developed over the years to facilitate successful coping with environment-relevant impairments such as mobility limitation or vision loss (Wahl, Oswald, & Zimprich, 1999; Wahl, Schilling, Oswald, & Heyl, 1999).

Home modification becomes " . . . an increasingly recognized component of services intended to keep frail older persons in their own homes and communities" (Pynoos, 1995, p. 467; see also, Gitlin, 1998; Lanspery & Hyde, 1997; Regnier, 2003; Reschovsky & Newman, 1990; Sit, 1992; Watzke

& Kemp, 1992). The *American Association of Retired Persons* (AARP) "Fixing to Stay" study in the United States, which included 2,000 persons 45 years of age and older, showed that many Americans modify their homes and make simple changes to make them easier to live in (AARP, 2000). Although systematic analysis of home modifications for older adults has revealed somewhat mixed results (Gitlin, 1998), there is evidence for positive outcomes with respect to maintaining daily activities and enhancing ability to perform ADLs and IADLs (Mann, 2001; Niepel, 1999; Thomas, 1996). In addition, the emergence of universal design and growing recognition of the value of smart home technologies is transforming the potential for elders to remain in and function effectively in familiar settings (Fisk, 2001; Frain & Carr, 1996; Kose, 1998; Mace, 1998; Peterson, 1998; Story, 1998).

Moving beyond environmental modification, there is evidence of behavioral adaptation in the use of interior spaces. Observational data have shown a recurring tendency for environmental centralization, especially around the most favored places at home. The adaptive potential of this lies in maintaining and enhancing competence in the immediate environment and thus, through a process of miniaturization, establishing "control centers" or "living centers" (Lawton, 1985; Oswald & Wahl, in press a; Rubinstein & Parmelee, 1992).

Studies of the *person-environment* (P-E) relationship characteristically focus on external, easily monitored dimensions, such as the availability of resources and barriers to mobility. But such research, emphasizing environmental accessibility, usability, and the reduction of risk through the creation of physically enabling environments, sometimes neglects equally important internal, psychologically-based ties between person and place that enhance quality of life (Oswald, in press; Steinfeld & Danford, 1999). For example, the most comfortable and favored places in the home may not only allow for the manipulation of necessary and preferred items close at hand, but also may be selected to afford a good view out of the window —thus creating a surveillance zone facilitating vicarious participation in the world outside as well (Rowles, 1981).

BEING IN PLACE: DWELLING IN AN INTERIOR ENVIRONMENT

Personal Dimensions of Being in Place in Interior Spaces

Interior living environments are far more than merely the physical spaces we inhabit. For most people, these environments nurture a sense of "being in place." Being in place has multiple overlapping and complexly interwoven dimensions. Frequently occupied interior spaces become physiologically familiar as repeated daily routines of use generate a "body awareness" of the setting through a process of habituation (Gallimore & Lopez, 2002; Rowles, 2000, 2003; Seamon, 2002). Routines and habits are embedded in all aspects of life. They order our days around personal and social expectations and provide a stability and predictability within the personal narrative of daily life (Rubinstein, 1986). Generally operating below the level of consciousness, habitual routines allow individuals to live life without having to constantly reinvent themselves with every physical action they undertake. Routines allow for increased efficiency, decreased decision making, and the conservation of energy. Over time, through repeated use, we come to wear interior settings like a glove as the rhythms, routines, and rituals of daily use become taken-for-granted, and as our bodies develop a comfortable and comforting familiarity with the architectural configuration of these spaces. As one of the subjects in O'Bryant's (1982) study of the value of home to elderly widows commented, "I can walk around my place in the dark because I know where everything is" (p. 352). Such a physical affinity serves to sharply differentiate the visceral intimacy of "inside" space from the uncertainty of less well known "outside" space beyond the threshold.

The differentiation of interior residential spaces from spaces beyond the threshold means that interior spaces tend to become the fulcrum around which we organize our lives. Such spaces become our territory (Altman, 1970; Porteous, 1970). It has been argued that humans have an inherent need for territory and that the possession and ownership of interior spaces satisfies a primal need we share with most mammals (Ardrey, 1966). The interior space of home, in particular, may become a place of territorial centering, the locus from which we venture forth and to which we return (Buttimer, 1980; Rubinstein, 1989). Home may be a place in which the individual may experience a sense of ownership and control (Rutman & Freedman, 1988). The interior space of home may become a place of safety and security. Indeed, a person's residence may become sacred; a locale in which he or she feels protected and shielded from a profane world beyond (Bachelard, 1969; Buttimer, 1980; Eliade, 1959).

In part, the security and safety of home stems from detailed *cognitive awareness* of the architectural configuration of its interior spaces. This is manifest in mental schema that provide knowledge of the contents of interior spaces, and their arrangement—our knowledge of where things are. Such "mental maps" are useful not only for finding our way around interior spaces, but also are invaluable in recalling where various possessions are located and providing a sense of structure and stability in our lives (Rowles, 1978).

Over time, a sense of "dwelling" or "being in place" tends to develop as an expression not only of the routines of use and cognitive awareness of the interior spaces of our residence, but also as a result of a psychological fusion of person and place in the evolving meaning of such spaces

(Heidegger, 1962; Oswald & Wahl, 2001, in press a; Rowles, 1993, 2003). This, in itself, may involve multiple dimensions. Interior spaces evoke emotions as a result of events that transpired within them—the sudden death of a spouse from a heart attack in the living room, the fond memories of the way the upstairs room was redecorated and refurnished for the arrival of a newborn son who now has children of his own, recollections of the flickering log fire on a cold winter's night before the central heating was installed—all become part of the emotional aura of familiar interior space. For many people, the interior of their residence may assume deep meaning as a mirror of the self (Marcus, 1995). It may reflect not only personal preferences but also personality traits, such as extraversion or introversion, that are manifest in the decoration of individual rooms or areas of the dwelling (Gosling, Ko, Mannarelli, & Morris, 2002).

Emotions that contribute to a sense of being in place in an interior space may be reinforced and nurtured by the stimulus to more active processes of selective reminiscence and vicarious reimmersion in places of the elder's past that are provided by objects and personal possessions contained in the space. Each artifact may serve as a cue to reminiscence, to the resurrection in consciousness of events that convey a continuing sense of identity (Boschetti, 1995; Csikszentmihalyi & Rochberg-Halton, 1981; Marcus, 1995; Rowles, 1978; Rubinstein, 1989).

Our sense of identity may be established, modified, and maintained through the possessions with which we fill interior spaces and the manner in which we display these possessions to project our persona (Rowles & Watkins, 2003). The memorabilia in the cabinets or on the shelves, the pictures on the walls, and the choice and arrangement of furniture provide an expression of the self; they reflect not only our personal style, preferences, temperament, and aesthetic values, but also our historical and cultural persona. They tell the story of our life. There is a growing literature on the meanings of possessions that eloquently expresses this theme (Boschetti, 1995; Csikszentmihalyi & Rochberg-Halton, 1981; Marcus, 1995; Paton & Cram, 1992; Rubinstein, 1987; Sherman & Newman, 1977; Whitmore, 2001). As Redfoot & Back (1988, p. 168) note, possession-filled interior spaces may transform elders' rooms into "museums of their lives."

Shared Dimensions of Being in Place in Interior Spaces

For many people, interior spaces are shared with a roommate, spouse, or family members. Being in place is rarely a completely personal process. It is something that, over time, is socially negotiated (Pruchno, Dempsey, Carder, & Koropeckyj-Cox, 1993). For example, the interior spaces of a home may be differentiated into primarily individual locations, such as the separate rooms where individual children sleep, shared territories such as the bedroom of their parents, as well as communal spaces such as the living room and kitchen that are fully shared among all inhabitants (Csikszentmihalyi & Rochberg-Halton, 1981, pp. 135-139; Marcus, 1995, pp. 159-184).

Each space evokes a different sense of being in place for each resident. Each locale in the interior space is characterized by routines of uses, reflected, for example, in a communally accepted and taken-for-granted sequence in which we use the bathroom each morning, "ownership" of the chair where we customarily sit to watch the television, and "our place" at the dining room table. Each resident develops his or her own cognitive map of the dwelling, generally one centered on the room where he or she sleeps. And each inhabitant develops his or her own unique feelings about various locations in the interior space that reflect uniquely significant elements of his or her own personal history of use of the space, preferences, and aesthetic sensibilities. Finally, for each resident a different set of images and reminiscences may be evoked by the setting and by the artifacts it contains. As Csikszentmihalyi & Rochberg-Halton explain:

> When certain artifacts, rooms and activities are preferentially selected by various family members to embody different patterns of meaning, then different family members can be seen as inhabiting different symbolic environments even though in the same household. So every physical house might contain different "homes," and the character of these homes might change over time as the goals and patterns of attention that make up the selves of its members change. (1981, p.138)

On occasion, the juxtaposition of diverse senses of being in place in a shared space may generate tensions—for example, tension over the appropriate placement of furniture or artifacts to be displayed in shared spaces, or tensions over noise or daily routines between elders and young people living in multigenerational settings (Marcus, 1995; Pruchno, Dempsey, Carder, & Koropeckyj-Cox, 1993; Rowles, 1983). However, those who share interior spaces characteristically are able to reconcile their different modes of being in place and to develop and maintain a harmonious social order in the use of the space. Such an ordering of interior space, a shared sense of being in a communal place, may be reflected in accepted rituals of use and in the arrangement and use of furniture in a manner conducive to the well-being of the group. For example, it may be deemed inappropriate for an individual to leave items of clothing on the living room floor or in other shared spaces. Such rules and norms of conduct may not apply in the individual's room. Our room may be furnished with a plethora of personal items of significance only to ourselves—it may become a home within a home—the place to which we retreat for privacy and to be alone and where we may strew our clothes all over the floor if we so choose.

Although there is some work on the theme of the familial use of interior spaces (Lawrence, 1987; Marcus, 1995; Pruchno et al., 1993), to our knowledge, limited research has been undertaken on the manner in which more complex aspects of being in place are negotiated and reconciled among elders. Nor is there sufficient work on the manner in which sociocultural norms and expectations condition elders' uses and meanings of interior spaces. What is the role of cultural heritage and socialization in determining the manner in which interior spaces are utilized (Boesch, 1991; Miller, 2001)?

Gender Dimensions of Being in Place in Interior Spaces

Bonds between women and the places where they live can be complex and quite different from those of men (Howell, 1994; Marcus, 1995; Saegert & McCarthy, 1998). The house is a place of work as much as family life for many women (Ahrentzen, 1992). Research on women and home uncovers differences of interpretation of the house between men and women. Women interpret the house as a symbol of family life, whereas men tend to interpret their attachment in terms of recreation and retreat (Ahrentzen 1992; Ciskszentmihalyi & Rochberg-Halton, 1981). Ahrentzen points out that the idea of creating "family life" is historically part of "women's work." Swenson (1998) found that for the women she interviewed, home was the center of caring for themselves, their families, and for the home itself. It was a nurturing place in which they were the primary caregivers. In fact, home was the place where all of the women in her study had cared for their dying husbands.

Research in Great Britain found that women expressed more complex and contradictory attitudes toward the meaning of home than men did. For example, housework was seen as both a source of pride and a source or resentment (Gurney, 1997). Historically, women's work took place in the home, whether paid or unpaid. In more recent times, home, for many women, has become the locus of a "second shift" after an eight-hour day at the office or factory. Women's attachment to home reflects socially constructed beliefs, options, roles, values, and cultural expectations associated with being female (Ahrentzen, 1992; Saegert & McCarthy, 1998).

With advancing age, the meaning of the interior space of home for both women and men may change (Csikszentmihalyi & Rochberg-Halton, 1981). The most important meaning, from the perspective of elders themselves, may become an increasingly significant association between this interior space and continuing independence (Russell, 1999). Indeed, the symbolic meaning of home as a seat of identity and continuing independence is a critical underpinning of the aging-in-place imperative.

There is also some evidence of life course and role-related gender differences in the use and meaning of the interior space of home to elders (Lawrence, 1982). As Russell (1999, p. 38) notes:

One image that consistently emerges from the gerontological literature is that of the home as the domain of the older woman. "Men are constructed . . . as newcomers to the home" (Hearn, 1995, p.101) who, if still married, may represent nuisance value for their wives; if widowed, they are depicted as somewhat pathetic, powerless figures. It is often suggested, for instance that widowed men find household tasks "unfamiliar and daunting." (Davison et al., 1993, p. 103)

Empirical data on the meaning of home in old age revealed stronger behavioral and somewhat weaker emotional bonding among women compared to men in a group of community dwelling healthy and impaired elders, aged 62 to 92 years old (Oswald & Wahl, in press a). These patterns may reflect historically based gender roles in the assessed cohorts of older adults where women, for the most part, stayed at home and men went out to work. Consequently, old women became familiar with the territory via everyday behavior and not via feelings of privacy and retreat, in contrast to their spouses. However, there is still a need for more research on the manner in which the uses and meanings of interior spaces differ between elderly men and women (Saegert & McCarthy, 1998). Such research would facilitate the development of housing design options more suited to the lifestyles and preferences of single elderly men and women living alone (Saegert & McCarthy, 1998, p. 81). More work is also needed on the processes involved as elderly couples accommodate, or fail to accommodate, to the changing uses and meanings of shared interior home space that occur following retirement. To what extent does the kitchen remain the domain of the older woman? (Lawrence, 1987) Particularly needed in this context are studies exploring gender differences in the uses and meanings of interior spaces among different cohorts. In the future, will older men and women view the interior spaces of home in the same way as current generations? Or will a trend toward more diverse lifetime experiences and gender equity lead toward androgyny in the experience of home? (Saegert & McCarthy, 1998)

ADAPTATION TO CHANGE

Adaptation to change is often considered solely in terms of the effects of home modification or the physical consequences of relocation. We suggest that the meanings of interior places may also be considered as important resources in the individual's adaptation to change, and particularly so for elders, who, over their life course, have accumulated a wealth of such meanings. The uses and meanings of interior spaces are dynamic on several levels.

First is the immediate process of taking possession of unfamiliar interior space—a process that occurs repeatedly in our daily lives as we occupy new spaces—often on a temporary basis. Second is the more long-term process of inhabiting and making a new residence our own, of transferring an inherent style of being in place from one location to another as we move through the life course inhabiting a series of residences and, with each move, becoming more proficient in accommodating to new interior spaces. A third dynamic component of being in place in interior spaces involves developmental changes that occur as a direct result of our aging and the need to accommodate to changing personal capabilities. Finally, it is important to consider enforced and unanticipated disruptions of relationships with interior spaces. Such disruptions may result from either environmental disasters (exogenous influences) or sudden unforeseeable personal health crises (endogenous influences) that make a rapid move to a more physically and socially supportive but nonetheless alien environment inevitable. Often, such moves occur at a time of great environmental vulnerability. Each will be considered in turn.

CREATION OF IMMEDIATE SHORT-TERM RELATIONSHIPS WITH INTERIOR SPACES

Moving to a new environment requires immediate accommodation to the setting—a process of "setting up" in the interior space. This may involve something as ephemeral as setting up our space when we check into a motel room. We develop a ritual use of the space: unpacking our bag and placing items in the drawers, setting out our toiletries, adjusting the thermostat, selecting a familiar side of the bed, and perhaps even setting up the pillow we have brought from "home" to facilitate a restful night's sleep. Essentially, we transform the space of the room into a temporary home that enables us to nurture an immediate sense of being in place. Recognition that habitation of such space is temporary means that although we seek to develop a sense of comfortable and immediate affinity, there is no anticipation of establishing a rooted sense of being in place. It is notable that the similarity and uniformity of motel room design is intended to facilitate this sense of familiarity, of instant being in place, for the guest in a home away from home (Relph, 1976). An awareness of the elements of this process of immediate occupancy may well be adaptive, especially for frail elders. It may provide an effective initial transitional phase in the often stressful first hours and days following an enforced relocation such as a hospital stay or a short-term residential care situation, and an important precursor to the more complex long-term process of putting down roots in the new environment for a person who is environmentally vulnerable.

CREATION OF LONG-TERM RELATIONSHIPS WITH INTERIOR SPACES

If a person relocates relatively frequently, there may develop a learned process of "place making" that involves the transference of elements of previous experience in creating a comfortable interior space consonant with an evolving sense of personal identity (Rowles & Watkins, 2003; Wheeler, 1995). Place making has a number of components. It involves reconciling elements of previously established patterns of inhabiting interior spaces (the places of our past) with the constraints and opportunities provided by the size, architecture, and spatial configuration of each new interior setting (the places of our present). This entails the selective transference of possessions such as furniture, photographs, and other treasured artifacts (Belk, 1992; Boschetti, 1995; Paton & Cram, 1992). There may be a conscious attempt to arrange furniture in a configuration similar to that of our former environment (Hartwigsen, 1987; Toyama, 1988). There may also be a process of recreating or transferring elements of the socio-cultural ambience and patterns of use of the previous environment, particularly if we relocate with family members or others with whom we shared the previous residence. Over a succession of moves, there is a tendency to establish a distinctive style of place making as each new environment is transformed from a space to a place and endowed with meanings that blend the old and familiar with the new and novel (Reed, Payton, & Bond, 1998; Rowles & Watkins, 2003; Wheeler, 1995).

We hypothesize that for some older people, particularly those with a history of frequent relocations, recreating a sense of being in place in a new interior environment is relatively rapid and easy. Emotional identification and bonding may be achieved without difficulty. For others, particularly those with a history of few previous moves, the process may be highly stressful and take much longer. For yet others, we suspect that it may prove impossible to adapt to the new setting even over a lengthy period of occupancy. Finally, for a growing number of contemporary elders both in the United States and in Europe, there is evidence that the process of place making involves an annual sequence of temporary place attachments to two or more meaningful interior spaces as they alternate between winter and summer residences (McHugh & Mings, 1996). Such "snowbirds," in a proactive and creative use of their environments extending far beyond mere adaptation to environmental press, may develop a distinctive style of being in place within each residence and decorate each interior space accordingly (McHugh & Mings, 1996).

INTERIOR SPACES AND DEVELOPMENTAL CHANGE IN OLD AGE

Transforming new spaces into places may become more difficult as people grow older as a result of normative developmentally-related changes associated with aging that make them more environmentally vulnerable (Lawton & Nahemow, 1973). On a physiological level, reduced capabilities can make it more difficult to climb stairs or get into the shower in a new residence. An elder may not be able to compensate for the loss of body awareness of familiar interior space that enabled him or her to function effectively in a former residence—at a level where the familiarity of routine facilitated transcendence of increasing physical limitations. Indeed, the process of hyperhabituation (an overdependence on familiar patterns of behavior) may actually become maladaptive with respect to place making when a relocation is necessitated because the individual is unable to transcend the limitations of long-established routine behavior as he or she tries to accommodate to a new environment (Kastenbaum, 1981; Norris-Baker & Scheidt, 1989).

From a sociocultural perspective, it may also be difficult to develop comfortable relationships with new people who share our interior space. A new roommate might have a different style of using the nursing facility room we share (Everard, Rowles, & High, 1994). She may have a different daily routine, an incompatible preference for the arrangement of furniture and "control" of her own part of the room, and irritating habits in the use and placement of personal artifacts. These may contrast with the rules and norms of behavior we negotiated with cohabitants of our former space. Similar potential for tension may also explain why independent community-dwelling elders who develop a close relationship with a new partner after years of widowhood elect to maintain separate residences and are reluctant to move in with each other. Beyond the desire to remain independent "just in case" the relationship does not work out, there may be a fear of inability to accommodate to their partner's style of inhabiting their interior space. In addition, bonding with a lifelong home may effectively override the power of a new and close personal relationship to result in abandonment of this familiar place.

Normative developmental and life course transitions associated with growing old may be accompanied by concomitant changes in the use and meaning of space (Bronfenbrenner, 1979, 1999; Oswald & Wahl, in press b). Framed in terms of an ongoing person-context dynamic, the transaction between the person and the social/physical environment characteristically becomes increasingly multifaceted from childhood through adult life and into old age as a result of the accumulation of layer upon layer of life experiences and place meanings. Interior spaces are especially important during certain phases of this lifelong dynamic. For instance, home space is generally the fulcrum of life space during childhood when the child's world may be limited to the dwelling and its immediate surroundings. With the transition into adolescence, the challenge for each developing child is to find a balance between basic needs for a secure, safe, and stable base (i.e. the interior living environment of home) on the one hand and higher-order needs encouraging exploration, stimulation, and environmental mastery on the other (Balint, 1955).

Increasing complexity in the individual's life arises from an ever-extending spatial range and diversity of activity (e.g., the individual's progressive ability to crawl, walk, leave home, ride a bus alone, and later, to drive or even fly to different parts of the globe). During adulthood, life experience tends to remain complex and spatially extensive.

As old age approaches, the spatial extent of the physically inhabited environment tends to become more restricted. This represents far more than a developmental regression to the limited realm of space inhabited in childhood. The gestalt of the use and meaning of space may become qualitatively different (Rowles, 1978). As the physical life space becomes smaller and centered around the home, interior spaces and spaces immediately adjacent to the dwelling may once again assume increasing significance (Csikszentmihalyi & Rochberg-Halton, 1981, p. 138; Rowles, 1978, 1981). A sense of emotional attachment to familiar spaces within the home may intensify. Possessions and treasured artifacts, cues to increased vicarious participation in worlds beyond the threshold that are displaced in time and space, may become increasingly central to the preservation of identity (Rowles, 1978).

Divestiture of possessions may be a particularly important aspect of the changing relationship between elders and their interior environments during later life. Characteristically, growing up in a Western society involves the gradual accumulation of possessions (a house, an automobile, furniture, and an array of personal artifacts) that over the years become not only expressions of material culture signifying status but also key symbols of identity (Csikszentmihalyi & Rochberg-Halton, 1981). By late middle age, with the departure of children and entry into the "empty nest" phase of life, many people have accumulated far more possessions than they need to live a comfortable life.

For many elders, the latter stages of life are accompanied by a downsizing of residential space with movement to progressively smaller spaces in parallel with changing needs and capabilities. This generally entails a divestiture of possessions—a process that very often involves not only discarding items but also the socially important and highly selective process of passing them on to heirs. This process is closely related to both maintaining a sense of continuing identity—through the items we choose to retain as transitional objects—and the ordered transference of material elements of this identity to the next generation (Boschetti, 1995; Kalymun, 1985; Morris, 1992; Wapner, Demick, & Redondo, 1990; Whitmore, 2001). But what items do we give up as we move from a family home to a small apartment? What criteria, apart from discarding those items that will not physically fit into the new space, do we use in ceding elements of our persona? For some elders, although by no means all, the process of choosing what to give up and what to retain may be highly stressful (Carp, 1972, pp. 89-90). The need to selectively pass on items that will be retained and appreciated by recipients is manifest in the lengths to which some elders go (for example, marking the names of those who are to receive particular items on the back of the item) to ensure that when they die the artifacts they own are given to heirs who will value them as they do and thus enable them to live on beyond their corporeal existence (Morris, 1992; Rowles & Watkins, 2003).

Placed in broader context, these processes reflect a cultural generativity that surfaces after midlife and that provides for continuity of the family as, with advancing age, a person gradually comes to recognize and assume the role of custodian of family history and ancestral artifacts (Kotre, 1984; Wapner, Demick, & Redondo, 1990).

LOSING CONTROL: DISRUPTION OF RELATIONSHIPS WITH INTERIOR SPACES IN OLD AGE

Elders who are able to exercise choice do not necessarily report negative responses to changes in their home environment or voluntary moves (Oswald, Schilling, Wahl, & Gäng, 2002). Indeed, Rutman and Freedman (1988) reported increases in environmental satisfaction following relocation. Participants in their study reported dealing with stress by exercising personal control over their environment. Nearly all the respondents wanted to see the relocation process as one over which they had choice and control. The interior space of home is a place in which personal control is expected, resulting in a sense of freedom and relaxation in a world where there may be little autonomous power (Csikszentmihalyi & Rochberg-Halton, 1981). An ability to transfer treasured possessions and to recreate interior environments providing a semblance of the abandoned setting through, for example, a similar spatial arrangement of furniture and artifacts, may also significantly reduce the inevitable stress of relocation (Rowles & Ravdal, 2002; Rowles & Watkins, 2003).

Unfortunately, there are many situations in which the ability to control interior environments is diminished during old age. First are the effects of serious illness and disability—a primary reason for abrupt change in and the loss of control over environmental settings. Second, as has been noted, are sudden changes when a spouse retires and existing territorial boundaries within the home are threatened or redefined through redistribution of household activities and reorganization of interior spaces (Szinovacz, 2000). A third common cause of unexpected disruption of relationships with interior environments may be the death of a spouse. Rearranging the interior space of a family home following this event, or, alternatively, leaving the family home and its memories because the widow can no longer afford to maintain it, can be highly stressful (Hartwigsen, 1987). A final example of loss of control and choice in an interior environment is during disaster. Be it through natural or man-made causes, the physical destruction of an elder's residence can be traumatic (Brown & Perkins, 1992; Detzner, Bell, & Stum, 1991; Rutman & Freedman, 1988). Each of these disruptions of relationships with interior spaces threaten deeply embedded personal routines and habits, shatter an established sense of being in place, and can be gravely detrimental to an older person's level of functioning and well-being. They create a sense of being out of control and "out of place."

Involuntary environmental changes (either the need for reconstruction of an existing dwelling or forced relocation to a new residence) can result in increased mortality rates, seriously compromise functional health, reduce life satisfaction, and undermine the psychological well-being of elders. This is especially true if the elders are already vulnerable in terms of declining health or financial problems (Danermark & Ekstrom, 1990; Lawton & Yaffe, 1970; Pruchno & Resch, 1988). Consequently, a need exists for extensive critical review of research on housing-related control beliefs with a view to determining the manner in which an understanding of such beliefs might be utilized in supporting elders who are coping with environmental change (Oswald, Wahl, Martin, & Mollenkopf, 2003).

INTERIOR ENVIRONMENTS AND WELL-BEING

As has been noted throughout this chapter, interior environments are capable of exerting strong influence on the well-being of elders. In this section we briefly summarize this theme in terms of the relationship between interior environments and health, residential satisfaction, and, most important, the maintenance of a nurturing sense of identity and meaning through place.

Interior Environments and Health

Poor quality interior environments have been shown to be a major cause of physical illness and poor health in general (e.g., Lawrence, 2002) as well as in old age (see for an overview Evans, Kantrowitz, & Eshelman, 2002; Gitlin, 1998; Lanspery & Hyde, 1997; Shipp & Branch, 1999; Steinfeld & Danford, 1999; Wahl, 2001). Historically, outbreaks of disease were associated with poor housing conditions of many working-class families and eventually led to the enforcement of systems of health regulation and planning law to improve the quality of housing stock (Jacobs & Stevenson, 1981). There has also been increasing emphasis on design of interior residential environments fostering health and safety, especially to reduce the risk of accidents and falls inside the home (Connell & Wolf, 1997; Sattin, Rodriquez, DeVito, & Wingo, 1998; Tinetti, Doucette, & Claus, 1995).

Concern with the impact of interior environments on physical health has not been paralleled by equivalent consideration of mental health. Yet, work in environmental psychology has shown that the environment can indeed have a direct effect on mental health. Weich, Blanchard, Prince, Burton, and Sproston (2002) found that features of the built environment were associated with poor mental health. Other studies found associations between improvements in the built environment and lower levels of anxiety and depression (Halpern, 1995). Finally, there is evidence that poor mental health, manifest, for example, in environmental stress and depression, can lead to an enhanced susceptibility to disease in general (Freeman, 1986).

The relationship between environment and health in old age is nowhere more apparent than in the plethora of studies on the relationship between relocation and both mortality and morbidity, although it must be acknowledged that this literature is somewhat dated, plagued by methodological pitfalls and somewhat equivocal in its conclusions. Since the seminal research of Aldrich and Mendkoff (1963), studies of this relationship have evolved into a cottage industry. Critical themes in this literature have been a focus on the degree to which moves are voluntary or forced, the degree to which morbidity is a function of age versus other factors, the relationship between the sequence of relocation and the appearance of stress, and interventions to ease the stress of relocation (for reviews of this literature see Danermark & Ekstrom, 1990; Grant, 1997; Pastalan, 1983; Reed, Payton, & Bond, 1998; Reinardy, 1995). We suggest that, consistent with the argument developed throughout this essay, the degree of discordance between interior environmental characteristics of a previous location and a new setting is likely to be a key determinant of outcomes. Research on this topic is surprisingly limited. To what extent might the reconciliation of interior environments between the two settings act as a buffer to stress and serve to reduce both mortality and morbidity?

Interior Environments and Residential Satisfaction

Residential satisfaction is a reflection of perceived environmental quality and subjective well-being. There is neither a precise definition nor a methodological standard to measure residential satisfaction. Indeed:

> Given the complexity of the real world, and the wide range of idiosyncratic factors that might influence the perceptions of individual residents, it probably is unrealistic to expect that any finite set of objective variables can predict even a majority of the variance in the subjective assessments of a community sample. (Christensen, Carp, Cranz, & Wiley, 1992, p. 233)

Nevertheless, research has repeatedly revealed that residential satisfaction is a complex outcome of demographic and health-related circumstances as well as objective and subjective characteristics of the person's environment (Christensen et al., 1987, 1992; Jirovec, Jirovec, & Bosse, 1984; O'Bryant & Wolf, 1983). Residential satisfaction is an important construct in assessing the perceived quality of interior residential environments and their relationship to subjective well-being (see also Pinquart & Burmedi, this volume).

Interpreting residential satisfaction in later life can be particularly problematic because the construct does not embrace experiential and emotional dimensions of place-based well being that may be particularly important to elders. Comparable levels of residential satisfaction have been observed in very different settings, some which are supportive of the needs of elders, and others that are unsupportive and even unsafe. Indeed, high levels of residential satisfaction among elders have frequently been reported in objectively inferior environments (Kivett, 1988; Walden, 1998; Weideman & Anderson, 1985). Older people seem to be particularly adept at adapting to different objective living conditions and sustaining high levels of satisfaction (Diener, Suh, Lucas, & Smith, 1999; Schwarz & Strack, 1991; Staudinger, 2000).

How do we explain this paradox? To answer this question, we suggest that residential satisfaction represents only one facet, one fairly superficial level of interpretation, of elders' environmental experience. Although it provides a useful indicator, it does not adequately capture the richness, subtlety, and complexity of the intensely personal transaction between elders and the interiors of their places of residence that we have attempted to describe in this chapter and that we suggest ultimately contributes to well-being. To capture this richness, subtlety and complexity, well-being within interior environments must be considered using a phenomenological focus on lived experience that seeks to reveal the meaning of being in place.

Interior Environments and Being in Place

As has been noted, a sense of being in place can foster well-being even within what might be considered distinctly suboptimal environments. Dimensions of familiarity and habituation act as a medium of stress reduction and energy conservation. A sense of environmental confidence results from intimate cognitive awareness of the configuration of the interior space of the dwelling. Emotional investment in one's own place may provide a sense of comfort, belonging and control over the space. Personally significant artifacts may act as critical cues to vicarious reimmersion in the places of a person's life. In combination, each of these experiential themes, reinforced by the presence of cherished belongings, rituals of daily life, and the continuing sense of identity imbued by familiar place, may enable the individual to transcend constraints of a contemporary interior physical environment and sustain an ongoing sense of being in the world. As the person ages it is possible that environmental supports, as experienced not only objectively but also, perhaps even more significantly, subjectively, become more and more important for both mental and physical health.

Physical and mental health, residential satisfaction, and being in place are clearly interlinked (Altman & Low, 1992; Sundstrom et al., 1996). However, these constructs have seldom been considered as mutually relevant, nor has their interrelationship been empirically investigated in a systematic way (Bonaiuto, Aiello, Perugini, Bonnes, & Ercolani, 1999). A European multicenter study that is currently in progress may yield important insights in this regard as it integrates these themes in an examination of the role of interior living environments in supporting healthy aging (for details see www.enableage.arb.lu.se).

IMPLICATIONS

In making the argument that interior spaces, especially the spaces of home as experienced, are of great importance to elders, it is important to avoid the dual perils of naive romanticism and dangerously distorting homogenization. It is comforting to think of elders, as they become more physically frail, being able to spend twilight years in the warm comfort of a familiar dwelling surrounded by artifacts that symbolize the richness of their life. However, such a view is a romantic and not entirely positive stereotype for most elders. It is important to counterbalance this view with clear recognition that for many elders their home, particularly if it is not appropriately modified to take into account changing needs, can be a very dangerous place (elders record very high accident rates in their homes; see, for example, Fogel, 1993; Watzke & Kemp, 1992). It is important to acknowledge the loss of control of interior spaces that reduces the quality of life of so many elders. Finally, it is important to acknowledge the insensitivity to need that is a consequence of failure to adequately consider developmental and life course related aspects of elders' experience of interior environments.

There is an increasing propensity for elders to spend time in several different environments as they pass through various phases of late life (Litwak & Longino, 1987). Moreover, many elders remain active and outgoing until very late in life, and the period of their life when they are environmentally vulnerable may be growing progressively shorter. It is also critical to acknowledge the influence of cohort and generational changes that are enabling elders to remain far more mobile than their predecessors. As the baby boom generation moves into its old age, there will be progressively fewer elders who have spent their entire lives residing in the same dwelling or even the same community. Future generations of elders may have very different patterns of both indoor and outdoor activities that in turn may lead to different uses and meanings of interior spaces.

Considering possible interventions and applications, one may argue that understanding of the uses and meanings of interior living environments must be better incorporated into existing programs of environmental adaptation and optimization (e.g., Steinfeld & Danford, 1999). In particular, there is a need to sensitize planners and those responsible for home modifications to the full range of meanings of interior environments and to an appreciation of less obvious aspects of being in place, especially those that become more salient with progressive loss of environmental competence, such as the increasing role of familiarity in sustaining function. In the domain of institutional design it is not enough to put a few wooden chairs and other items of furniture into resident rooms to create an illusion of home. The pretense involved in the creation of such "false homes" must be replaced by genuine concern with making both community and institutional spaces experientially meaningful to their residents. Indeed, it is important to explore the full range of potential environmental interventions that have been proposed in recent literature on "place therapy" (Scheidt & Norris-Baker, 1999).

Finally, it is important to acknowledge that the meaning of an elder's interior environment may be transformed in the coming decades as advances in technology ranging from benign surveillance, through robot maids, smart houses and more sophisticated communications technologies, lead to the transformation of home spaces. The very notion of the residential isolation or withdrawal of elders may become an artifact of the past. Alternatively, it may assume different manifestations as spatial isolation is replaced by even more invidious forms of isolation resulting from inability to use sophisticated highly technical communication systems.

As we embrace new technologies that transform distance and provide rich potential for the support of frail elders in their residences, it is important to be sure that in the process we do not destroy what for many is the essence of being in place at home. We must retain the ability for elders to dwell in places *they create for themselves* (in contrast to places created by others) that will give their life a continued sense of centering and meaning, a sense of oneness with their world.

REFERENCES

Ahrentzen, S. B. (1992). Home as a workplace in the lives of women. In I. Altman & S. M. Low (Eds.), *Place attachment* (pp. 113-138). New York: Plenum Press.

Aldrich, C., & Mendkoff, E. (1963). Relocation of the aged and disabled: A mortality study. *Journal of the American Geriatrics Society, 11*(3), 185-194.

Altman, I. (1970). Territorial behavior in humans: An analysis of the concept. In L. A. Pastalan & D. H. Carson (Eds.), *Spatial behavior of older people* (pp. 1-13). Ann

Arbor: The University of Michigan—Wayne State University Institute of Gerontology.

Altman, I., & Low, S. M. (Eds.). (1992). *Place attachment* (Vol. 12). New York: Plenum Press.

American Association of Retired Persons. (2000). *Fixing to stay. A national survey of housing and home modification issues.* Washington, DC: AARP Independent Living program.

Ardrey, R. (1966). *The territorial imperative.* New York: Atheneum.

Bachelard, G. (1969). *The poetics of space.* Boston: Beacon Press.

Balint, M. (1955). Friendly expanses—horrid empty space. *International Journal of Psychoanalysis, 36*(5), 225-241.

Baltes, M. M., Maas, I., Wilms, H. U., & Borchelt, M. (1999). Everyday competence in old and very old age: Theoretical considerations and empirical findings. In P. B. Baltes & K. U. Mayer (Eds.), *The Berlin aging study* (pp. 384-402). Cambridge, UK: Cambridge University Press.

Baltes, M. M., Wahl, H. W., & Schmid-Furstoss, U. (1990). The daily life of elderly Germans: Activity patterns, personal control, and functional health. *Journal of Gerontology: Psychological Sciences, 45,* 173-179.

Belk, R. W. (1992). Attachment to possessions. In I. Altman & S. M. Low (Eds.), *Place attachment* (pp. 37-62). New York: Plenum Press.

Boesch, E. E. (1991) *Symbolic action theory and cultural psychology.* Berlin, Germany: Springer.

Bonaiuto, M., Aiello, M., Perugini, M., Bonnes, M., & Ercolani, A. P. (1999). Multidimensional perception of residential environment quality and neighbourhood attachment in the urban environment. *Journal of Environmental Psychology, 19,* 331-352.

Boschetti, M. A. (1995). Attachment to personal possessions: An interpretive study of the older person's experience. *Journal of Interior Design, 21*(1), 1-12.

Bronfenbrenner, U. (1979). *The ecology of human development: Experiments by nature and design.* Cambridge, MA: Harvard University Press.

Bronfenbrenner, U. (1999). Environments in developmental perspective: Theoretical and operational models. In S. L. Friedman & T. D. Wachs (Eds.), *Measuring environment across the life span* (pp. 3-28). Washington, DC: American Psychological Association.

Brown, B. B., & Perkins, D. D. (1992). Disruptions in place attachment. In I. Altman & S. M. Low (Eds.), *Place attachment* (pp. 279-304). New York: Plenum Press.

Bundesministerium für Familie Senioren Frauen und Jugend (BMFSFJ) [Federal Ministry for Family Affairs, Senior Citizens, Women and Youth]. (Ed.). (2001). *Dritter Bericht zur Lage der älteren Generation in der Bundesrepublik Deutschland: Alter und Gesellschaft [Third report on the situation of older people. Ageing and society].* Berlin, Germany: BMFSFJ.

Buttimer, A. (1980). Home, reach and the sense of place. In A. Buttimer & D. Seamon (Eds.), *The human experience of space and place* (pp. 166-187). New York: St. Martin's Press.

Callahan, J. J. (1992). Aging in place. *Generations 16*(2), 5-6.

Carp, F. M. (1972). *A future for the aged: Victoria Plaza and its residents.* Austin: University of Texas Press.

Christensen, D. L., & Carp, F. M. (1987). PEQI-based environmental prediction of the residential satisfaction of older women. *Journal of Psychology, 7,* 45-64.

Christensen, D. L., Carp, F. M., Cranz, G. L., & Whiley, J. A. (1992). Objective housing indicators as predictors of the subjective evaluations of elderly residents. *Journal of Environmental Psychology, 12,* 225-236.

Connell, B. R., & Wolf, S. L. (1997). Environmental and behavioural circumstances associated with falls at home among healthy elderly individuals. *Arch Phys Med Rehabilitation, 78,* 179-186.

Csikszentmihalyi, M., & Rochberg-Halton, E. (1981). *The meaning of things: Domestic symbols and the self.* Cambridge, UK: Cambridge University Press.

Danermark, B., & Ekstrom, M. (1990). Relocation and health effects on the elderly: A commented research review. *Journal of Sociology and Social Welfare, 17*(1), 25-49.

Davison, B., Kendig, H., Stephens, F., & Merrill, V. (1993). *"It's my place:" Older people talk about their homes.* Canberra: Australian Government Publishing Service.

Detzner, D. F., Bell, L., & Stum, M. (1991). The meaning of home and possessions to elderly public housing residents displaced by fire. *Housing and Society, 18*(2), 3-12.

Diener, E., Suh, E. M., Lucas, R. E., & Smith, H. L. (1999). Subjective well-being: Three decades of progress. *Psychological Bulletin, 125,* 276-302.

Eliade, M. (1959). *The sacred and the profane.* New York: Harcourt, Brace & World.

Evans, G. E., Kantrowitz, E., & Eshelman, P. (2002). Housing quality and psychological well-being among the elderly population. *Journal of Gerontology: Psychological Sciences, 57B*(4), P381-P384.

Everard, K., Rowles, G. D., & High, D. M. (1994). Nursing home room changes: Toward a decision-making model. *The Gerontologist, 34*(4), 520-527.

Fisk, M. J. (2001). The implications of smart home technologies. In S. M. H. Peace & C. Holland (Eds.), *Inclusive housing in an ageing society* (pp. 101-124). Bristol, UK: The Policy Press.

Fogel, B. S. (1993). Psychological aspects of staying at home. In J. J. Callahan, Jr. (Ed.), *Aging in place* (pp. 19-28). Amityville, NY: Baywood.

Frain, J. P., & Carr, P. H. (1996). Is the typical modern house designed for future adaptation for disabled older people? *Age and Ageing, 25,* 398-401.

Freeman, H. F. (1986). Environmental stress and psychiatric disorder. *Stress Medicine, 2,* 291-299.

Gallimore, R. L., & Lopez, E. M. (2002). Everyday routines, human agency, and eco-cultural context: Construction and maintenance of individual habits. *The Occupational Therapy Journal of Research, 22*(S1), 70S-77S.

Gitlin, L. N. (1998). Testing home modification interventions: Issues of theory, measurement, design and implementation. In R. Schultz, G. Maddox, & M. P. Lawton (Eds.), *Focus on interventions research with older adults. Annual review of gerontology and geriatrics* (Vol. 18, pp. 190-246). New York: Springer.

Gosling, S. D., Ko, S. J., Mannarelli, T., & Morris, M. E. (2002). A room with a cue: Personality judgments based on offices and bedrooms. *Journal of Personality and Social Psychology, 82*(3), 379-398.

Grant, P. R. (1997). The relocation of nursing home residents: An illustration of the advantages gained by planning a new program and designing an implementation evaluation together. *Evaluation and Program Planning, 20*(4), 507-516.

Gurney, C. M. (1997). ". . . Half of me was satisfied": Making sense of home through episodic ethnographies. *Women's Studies International Forum, 20*(3), 373-386.

Halpern, D. (1995). *Mental health and the built environment.* London: Taylor & Francis.

Hartwigsen, G. (1987). Older widows and the transference of home. *International Journal of Aging and Human Development, 25*(3), 195-207.

Hearn, J. (1995). Imaging the aging of men. In M. Featherstone & A. Wernick (Eds.), *Images of aging: Cultural representations of later life* (pp. 97-115). London: Routledge.

Heidegger, M. (1962). *Being and time.* New York: Harper & Row.

Howell, S. (1994). Environment and the aging woman: Domains of choice. In I. Altman & A. Churchman (Eds.), *Women and the environment* (pp. 105-131). New York: Plenum Press.

Jacobs, M., & Stevenson, G. (1981). Health and housing: A historical examination of alternative perspectives. *International Journal of Health Services, 1*(1), 105-122.

Jirovec, R. L., Jirovec, M. M., & Bosse, R. (1984). Environmental determinants of neighborhood satisfaction among urban elderly men. *The Gerontologist, 24*(3), 261-265.

Kalymun, M. (1985). The prevalence of factors influencing decisions among elderly women concerning household possessions during relocation. *Journal of Housing for the Elderly, 3*(3), 81-99.

Kastenbaum, R. J. (1981). Habituation as a model of human aging. *International Journal of Aging and Human Development, 12*(3), 159-169.

Kendig, H., & Pynoos, J. (1996). Housing. In J. E. Birren (Ed.), *Encyclopedia of gerontology. Age, aging, and the aged* (Vol. 1, pp. 703-713). San Diego, CA: Academic Press.

Kivett, V. (1988). Aging in a rural place: The elusive source of well-being. *Journal of Rural Studies, 4,* 125-132.

Kose, S. (1998). From barrier free to universal design: An international perspective. *Assistive Technology, 10*(1), 44-50.

Kotre, J. (1984). *Outliving the Self: Generativity and the interpretation of lives.* Baltimore: Johns Hopkins University Press.

Küster, C. (1998). Zeitverwendung und Wohnen im Alter. [Use of time and housing in old age.] In Deutsches Zentrum für Altersfragen (Ed.), *Wohnbedürfnisse, Zeitverwendung und soziale Netzwerke älterer Menschen. Expertisenband 1 zum Zweiten Altenbericht der Bundesregierung [Housing needs, use of time, and social networks of older adults]* (pp. 51-175). Frankfurt/Main, Germany: Campus.

Lanspery, S., & Hyde, J. (Eds.). (1997). *Staying put: Adapting the places instead of the people.* Amityville, NY: Baywood.

Lawrence, R. (1982). Domestic space and society: A cross-cultural study. *Comparative Studies in Society and History, 24,* 104-130.

Lawrence, R. J. (1987). What makes a house a home? *Environment and Behavior, 19*(2), 154-168.

Lawton, M. P. (1985). Housing and living environments of older people. In R. H. Binstock & E. Shanas (Eds.), *Handbook of aging and the social sciences* (pp. 450-478). New York: Van Nostrand Reinhold.

Lawton, M. P. (1987). Environment and the need satisfaction of the aging. In L. L. Carstensen & B. A. Edelstein (Eds.), *Handbook of clinical gerontology* (pp. 33-40). New York: Pergamon Press.

Lawton, M. P. (1989). Environmental proactivity in older people. In V. L. Bengtson & K. W. Schaie (Eds.), *The course of later life* (pp. 15-23). New York: Springer.

Lawton, M. P. (1998). Environment and aging: Theory revisited. In R. J. Scheidt & P. G. Windley (Eds.), *Environment and aging theory. A focus on housing* (pp. 1-31). Westport, CT: Greenwood Press.

Lawton, M. P., & Nahemow, L. (1973). Ecology and the aging process. In C. Eisdorfer & M. P. Lawton (Eds.), *The psychology of adult development and aging* (pp. 619-674). Washington, DC: American Psychological Association.

Lawton, M. P., & Simon, B. B. (1968). The ecology of social relationships in housing for the elderly. *The Gerontologist, 8*, 108-115.

Lawton, M. P., & Yaffe, S. (1970). Mortality, morbidity and voluntary change of residence by older people. *Journal of the American Geriatrics Society, 18*(10), 823-831.

Lawrence, R. J. (2002). Healthy residential environments. In R. B. Bechtel & A. Churchman (Eds.), *Handbook of environmental psychology* (pp. 394-412). New York: John Wiley & Sons.

Litwak, E., & Longino, C. F., Jr. (1987). Migration patterns among the elderly: A developmental perspective. *The Gerontologist, 27*(3), 266-272.

Mace, R. L. (1998). Universal design in housing. *Assistive Technology, 10*(1), 21-28.

Mann, W. C. (2001). Potential of technology to ease the care provider's burden. *Generations, 25*(1), 44-48.

Marcus, C. C. (1995). *House as a mirror of self.* Berkeley, CA: Conari Press.

McHugh, K. E., & Mings, R. C. (1996). The circle of migration: Attachment to place in aging. *Annals of the Association of American Geographers, 86*(3), 530-550.

Miller, D. (Ed.).(2001). *Home possessions: Material culture behind closed doors.* Oxford, UK: Berg.

Morris, B. R. (1992). Reducing inventory: Divestiture of personal possessions. *Journal of Women & Aging, 4*(2), 79-92.

Moss, M. S., & Lawton, M. P. (1982). Time budgets of older people: A window of four lifestyles. *Journal of Gerontology, 37*, 115-123.

Motel, A., Künemund, H., & Bode, C. (2000). Wohnen und Wohnumfeld älterer Menschen [Housing and living arrangements of older adults]. In M. Kohli & H. Künemund (Eds.), *Die zweite Lebenshälfte—Gesellschaftliche Lage und Partizipation im Spiegel des Alters-Survey [The second half of life—Societal stage and participation in the light of the Alters-Survey]* (pp. 124-175). Opladen, Germany: Leske & Budrich.

Niepel, T. (1999). *Wohnberatung: Erfolge, Wirkungsmechanismen und Qualitätssicherung. [Housing counselling: Success, mechanisms and quality assurance.]* (Vol. Berichte im Projekt "Wohnberatung für Bürgerinnen und Bürger in NRW" im Auftrag des Ministeriums für Arbeit, Soziales und Stadtentwicklung, Kultur und Sport des Landes Nordrhein-Westfalen und der Landesverbände der Pflegekassen NRW.) Bielefeld, Germany: Universität.

Norris-Baker, C., & Scheidt, R. J. (1989). Habituation theory and environment-aging research: Ennui to joie de vivre. *International Journal of Aging and Human Development 29*(4), 241-257.

O'Bryant, S. L. (1982). The value of home to older persons. *Research on Aging, 4*, 349-363.

O'Bryant, S. L., & Wolf, S. M. (1983). Explanation of housing satisfaction of older homeowners and renters. *Research on Aging, 5*(2), 217-233.

Oswald, F. (2003). Linking subjective housing needs to objective living conditions among older adults in Germany. In K. W. Schaie, H. W. Wahl, H. Mollenkopf, & F. Oswald (Eds.), *Aging independently: Living arrangements and mobility* (pp. 130-147). New York: Springer.

Oswald, F., Schilling, O., Wahl, H. W., & Gäng, K. (2002). Trouble in paradise? Reasons to relocate and objective environmental changes among well-off older adults. *Journal of Environmental Psychology, 22* (3), 273–288.

Oswald, F., & Wahl, H. W. (2001). Housing in old age: Conceptual remarks and empirical data on place attachment. *Bulletin on People-Environment Studies, 19,* 8-12.

Oswald, F., & Wahl, H. W. (in press a). Dimensions of the meaning of home. In G. D. Rowles & H. Chaudhury (Eds.), *Coming home: International perspectives on place, time and identity in old age.* New York: Springer.

Oswald, F., & Wahl, H. W. (in press b). Place attachment across the life span. In J. R. Miller, R. M. Lerner, L. B. Schiamberg, & P. M. Anderson (Eds.), *Human ecology: An encyclopedia of children, families, communities, and environments.* Santa Barbara, CA: ABC-Clio.

Oswald, F., Wahl, H. W., Martin, M., & Mollenkopf, H. (2003). Toward measuring proactivity in person-environment transactions in late adulthood: The housing-related Control Beliefs Questionnaire. *Journal of Housing for the Elderly, 17*(1/2), 135-152.

Pastalan, L. A. (1983). Environmental displacement: A literature reflecting old-person-environment transactions. In G. D. Rowles & R. J. Ohta (Eds.), *Aging and milieu: Environmental perspectives on growing old* (pp. 189-203). New York: Academic Press.

Paton, H. C., & Cram, F. (1992). Personal possessions and environmental control: The experiences of elderly women in three residential settings. *Journal of Women & Aging, 4*(2), 61-78.

Peterson, W. (1998). Public policy affecting universal design. *Assistive Technology, 10*(1).

Porteous, J. D. (1970). Home: The territorial core. *The Geographical Review, 66,* 383-390.

Pruchno, R. A., Dempsey, N. P., Carder, P., & Koropeckyj-Cox, T. (1993). Multigenerational households of caregiving families: Negotiating shared space. *Environment and Behavior, 25*(3), 349-366.

Pruchno, R. A., & Resch, M. L. (1988). Intrainstitutional relocation: Mortality effects. *The Gerontologist, 28*(3), 311-317.

Pynoos, J. (1995). Home modifications. In G. L. Maddox (Ed.), *The encyclopedia of aging. A comprehensive resource in gerontology and geriatrics* (2nd ed., pp. 466-469). New York: Springer.

Redfoot, D. L., & Back, K. W. (1988). The perceptual presence of the life course. *International Journal of Aging and Human Development 27*(3), 155–170.

Reed, J., Payton, V. R., & Bond, S. (1998). The importance of place for older people moving into care homes. *Social Science and Medicine, 46*(7), 859-867.

Reinardy, J. (1995). Relocation to a new environment: Decisional control and the move to a nursing home. *Health and Social Work, 20*(1), 31-37.

Regnier, V. (1994). *Assisted living housing for the elderly: Design innovations from the United States and Europe.* New York: John Wiley & Sons.

Regnier, V. (2003). Purpose-built housing and home adaptations for older adults: The American perspective. In K. W. Schaie, H. W. Wahl, H. Mollenkopf, and F. Oswald (Eds.), *Aging independently: living arrangements and mobility* (pp. 99-117). New York: Springer.

Relph, E. (1976). *Place and Placelessness.* London: Pion Limited.

Reschovsky, J. D., & Newman, S. J. (1990). Adaptations for independent living by older frail households. *The Gerontologist. 30,* 543-552.

Rowles, G. D. (1978). *Prisoners of space? Exploring the geographical experience of older people.* Boulder, CO: Westview Press.

Rowles, G. D. (1981). The surveillance zone as meaningful space for the aged. *The Gerontologist, 21*(3), 304-311.

Rowles, G. D. (1983). Between worlds: A relocation dilemma for the Appalachian elderly. *International Journal of Aging and Human Development, 17*(4), 301-314.

Rowles, G. D. (1993). Evolving images of place in aging and "aging in place." *Generations, 17*(2), 65-70.

Rowles, G. D. (2000). Habituation and being in place. *The Occupational Therapy Journal of Research, 20* (Suppl. 1), 52S-67S.

Rowles, G. D. (2003). The meaning of place as a component of self. In E. B. Crepeau, E. S. Cohn, & B. A. Schell, (Eds.), *Willard & Spackman's Occupational Therapy* (pp. 111-119). Philadelphia: Lippincott, Williams & Wilkins.

Rowles, G. D., & Ravdal, H. (2002). Age, place and meaning in the face of changing circumstances. In R. S. Weiss & S. A. Bass (Eds.), *Challenges of the third age: Meaning and purpose in later life* (pp. 81-114). New York: Oxford University Press.

Rowles, G. D., & Watkins, J. F. (2003). History, habit, heart and hearth: On making spaces into places. In K. W. Schaie, H. W. Wahl, H. Mollenkopf, & F. Oswald (Eds.), *Aging independently: Living arrangements and mobility* (pp. 77-96). New York: Springer.

Rubinstein, R. L. (1986). The construction of a day by elderly widowers. *International Journal of Aging and Human Development, 23,* 161-193.

Rubinstein, R. L. (1987). Significance of personal objects to older people. *Journal of Aging Studies, 1*(3), 225-238.

Rubinstein, R. L. (1989). The home environments of older people: A description of the psychosocial processes linking person to place. *Journals of Gerontology: Social Sciences, 44*(2), S45-S53.

Rubinstein, R. L., & Parmelee, P. A. (1992). Attachment to place and representation of life course by the elderly. In I. Altman & S. M. Low (Eds.), *Human behavior and environment: Vol. 12, Place attachment* (pp. 139-163). New York: Plenum Press.

Russell, C. (1999). Meanings of home in the lives of older women (and men). In M. Poole & S. Feldman (Eds.), *A certain age* (pp. 36-55). St. Leonards NSW, Australia: Allen and Unwin.

Rutman, D. L., & Freedman, J. L. (1988). Anticipating relocation: Coping strategies and the meaning of home for older people. *Canadian Journal on Aging, 7*(1), 17-31.

Saegert, S., & McCarthy, D. E. (1998). Gender and housing for the elderly: Sorting through the accumulations of a lifetime. In R. J. Scheidt & P. G. Windley (Eds.), *Environment and aging theory. A focus on housing* (pp. 61-87). Westport, CT: Greenwood Press.

Sattin, R. W., Rodriquez, J. G., DeVito, C. A., & Wingo, P. A. (1998). Home environmental hazards and the risk of fall injury events among community-dwelling older persons. *Journal of the American Geriatric Society, 46,* 669-676.

Scheidt, R. J., & Norris-Baker, C. (1999). Place therapies for older adults: Conceptual and interventive approaches. *International Journal of Aging and Human Development, 48*(1), 1-15.

Schwarz, N., & Strack, F. (1991). Evaluating one's life: A judgement model of subjective well-being. In F. Strack, M. Argyle, & N. Schwarz (Eds.), *Subjective well-being. An interdisciplinary perspective* (pp. 27-47). Oxford, UK: Pergamon Press.

Seamon, D. (2002). Physical comminglings: Body, habit, and space transformed into place. *The Occupational Therapy Journal of Research, 22*(S1), 42S-51S.

Sherman, E. N., & Newman, E. S. (1977). The meaning of cherished personal possessions for the elderly. *International Journal of Aging and Human Development, 8*(2), 181-192.

Shipp, K. M., & Branch, L. G. (1999). The physical environment as a determinant of the health status of older populations. *Canadian Journal on Aging, 18*(3), 313-327.

Sit, M. (1992). With elders in mind: A home can be made more suitable. *Generations, 16*(2), 73.

Statistisches Bundesamt (StBA). (2000). *Datenreport 1999. Ergebnisse des Wohlfahrtssurvey [Data report 1999. Findings from the "Wohlfahrtssurvey"].* Stuttgart, Germany: Metzler-Poeschel.

Staudinger, U. M. (2000). Viele Gründe sprechen dagegen, und trotzdem geht es vielen Menschen gut: Das Paradox des subjektiven Wohlbefindens [Many reasons speak against it, yet many people feel good: The paradox of subjective well-being]. *Psychologische Rundschau, 51*(4), 185-197.

Steinfeld, E., & Danford, G. S. (Eds.). (1999). Enabling environments. *Measuring the impact of environment on disability and rehabilitation.* New York: Plenum.

Story, M. F. (1998). Maximizing usability: The principles of universal design. *Assistive Technology, 10*(1), 4-12.

Sundstrom, E., Bell, P. A., Busby, P. L., & Asmus, C. (1996). Environmental psychology 1989-1994. *Annual Review of Psychology, 47,* 485-512.

Swenson, M. M. (1998). The meaning of home to five elderly women. *Health Care for Women International, 19*(5), 381-394.

Szinovacz, M. E. (2000). Changes in housework after retirement: A panel analysis. *Journal of Marriage and the Family, 62*(1), 78-92.

Thomas, D. W. (1996). Case study on the effects of a retrofitted dementia special care unit on resident behaviors. *American Journal of Alzheimer's Disease, 11*(3), 8-10.

Tilson, D. (Ed.). 1990. *Aging in place: Supporting the frail elderly in residential environments.* Glenview, IL: Scott Foresman.

Tinetti, M. E., Doucette, J. T., & Claus, E. B. (1995). The contribution of predisposing and situational risk factors to serious fall injuries. *Journal of the American Geriatric Society, 43,* 1207-1213.

Toyama, T. (1988). *Identity and milieu: A study of relocation focusing on reciprocal changes in elderly people and their environment.* Stockholm, Sweden: Department for Building Function Analysis, the Royal Institute of Technology.

Treas, J. (1995). Older Americans in the 1990s and beyond. *Population Bulletin,* Vol. 50, No. 2. Washington, DC: Population Reference Bureau.

U.S. Bureau of the Census (1996). Current Population Reports, Special studies, P23-10, *65+* in the United States. Washington, DC: U.S. Government Printing Office.

Wahl, H. W. (2001). Environmental influences on aging and behavior. In J. E. Birren & K. W. Schaie (Eds.), *Handbook of the psychology of aging* (5th ed., pp. 215-237). San Diego, CA: Academic Press.

Wahl, H. W., Oswald, F., & Zimprich, D. (1999). Everyday competence in visually impaired older adults: A case for person-environment perspectives. *The Gerontologist, 39,* 140-149.

Wahl, H. W., Schilling, O., Oswald, F., & Heyl, V. (1999). Psychosocial consequences of age-related visual impairment: Comparison with mobility-impaired older adults and long-term outcome. *Journal of Gerontology: Psychological Sciences, 54B,* P304-P316.

Walden, R. (1998). Wohnzufriedenheit, Wohlbefinden und Wohnqualität [Residential satisfaction, well-being, and housing quality]. In F. Dieckmann, A. Flade, R. Schuemer, G. Ströhlein, & R. Walden (Eds.), *Psychologie und gebaute Umwelt. Konzepte, Methoden, Anwendungsbeispiele. [Psychology and the built environment: Concepts, methods, application examples.]* Darmstadt, Germany: Institut Wohnen und Umwelt.

Wapner, S., Demick, J., & Redondo, J. P. (1990). Cherished possessions and adaptation of older people to nursing homes. *International Journal of Aging and Human Development, 31*(3), 219-235.

Watzke, J. R., & Kemp, B. (1992). Safety for older adults: The role of technology and the home environment. *Topics in Geriatric Rehabilitation, 7*(4), 9-21.

Weich, S., Blanchard, M., Prince, M., Burton, E., & Sproston, K. (2002). Mental health and the built environment: Cross-sectional survey of individual and contextual risk factors for depression. *The British Journal of Psychiatry, 180,* 428-433.

Weideman, S., & Anderson, J. R. (1985). A conceptual framework for residential satisfaction. In I. Altman & C. M. Werner (Eds.), *Human behavior and environment: Vol. 8. Home environments* (pp. 153-182). New York: Plenum Press.

Wheeler, W. M. (1995). *Elderly residential experience: The evolution of places as residence.* New York: Garland.

Whitmore, H. (2001). Value that marketing cannot manufacture: Cherished possessions as links to identity and wisdom. *Generations, 25*(3), 57-63.

CHAPTER 8

Correlates of Residential Satisfaction in Adulthood and Old Age: A Meta-Analysis

MARTIN PINQUART
UNIVERSITY OF JENA

DAVID BURMEDI
GERMAN CENTER FOR RESEARCH ON AGING AT THE UNIVERSITY OF HEIDELBERG

The present meta-analysis integrates results from 121 studies on housing satisfaction and neighborhood satisfaction in adulthood and old age. An age-associated increase in housing satisfaction was found in cross-sectional and longitudinal studies. This effect was stronger in younger age groups, probably reflecting proactive improvements of housing conditions. However, whereas older respondents reported higher levels of neighborhood satisfaction in cross-sectional studies, no change in this variable appeared in longitudinal studies. Aesthetic qualities of the home showed the strongest associations with housing satisfaction, whereas the level of maintenance, safety, good relationships with neighbors, and aesthetic characteristics of the neighborhood were most strongly related to neighborhood satisfaction. Associations between environmental characteristics and residential satisfaction were stronger in younger adults, which may indicate that older adults have adapted their evaluation standards to their present living conditions.

Residential satisfaction has become a critical subject matter for human ecology (e.g., LaGory, Ward, & Sherman, 1985). It can be defined as an emotional response to the dwelling, the positive or negative feeling the respondents have for the place where they live (Weideman & Anderson, 1985). Residential satisfaction can be further divided into satisfaction with one's house or apartment (housing satisfaction), satisfaction with the immediate neighborhood (neighborhood satisfaction), and general satisfaction with the town or village one lives in (community satisfaction). In the present chapter, we focus on housing satisfaction and neighborhood satisfaction because these represent the most personal and immediate home environments. In addition, individuals, and older adults in particular, spend a great deal of time in their apartment and their immediate neighborhood rather than in the wider community (e.g., Moss & Lawton, 1982; Lawton, Moss, & Fulcomer, 1986).

We used meta-analysis to integrate the results of studies on residential satisfaction by focusing on three research questions. First, because environmental needs and environmental conditions may change across adulthood, we examine whether residential satisfaction changes with age. Second, we examine which factors contribute to environmental satisfaction, such as other sociodemographic variables and aspects of the environment. Third, we analyze whether the size of these correlations varies with the age of the respondent.

AGE DIFFERENCES IN HOUSING SATISFACTION AND NEIGHBORHOOD SATISFACTION

In old age, the life space of the individual tends to contract with more activities focused in and around the home (Pynoos, 1995, Moss & Lawton, 1982). Thus, the immediate environment becomes more important to satisfying one's needs. In addition, age-associated losses in competence make the older adults more vulnerable to environmental press (Wahl, Oswald, & Zimprich, 1999). There are theoretical reasons to suggest that residential satisfaction might vary with age. At least six arguments support the assumption of an age-associated increase in housing satisfaction and neighborhood satisfaction.

Age Differences in Objective Housing Quality

Older adults may have had more time to select a favorable environment and to build better living conditions for themselves (e.g., Campbell, Converse, & Rodgers, 1976). In the American Housing Survey (U.S. Census Bureau, 2001), older adults had fewer physical problems with their housing than younger adults (e.g., problems with plumbing, heating, or upkeep; $r = -.07$), and crime in their neighborhood ($r = -.07$). Similarly, they had more available living space ($r = .08$) and more basic and nice household amenities ($r = .07$ and $r = .06$, respectively). In addition, they were more likely to be homeowners (82 percent versus 64 percent), which may be a source of housing satisfaction. However, correlations of age with objective housing quality are usually small, and many older adults show high levels of residential satisfaction even when their housing appears to be quite deficient to outside observers (Campbell et al., 1976). Moreover, housing that has been carefully selected and improved by young or middle-aged adults may become less optimal as the resident ages and experiences decline in day-to-day functioning.

Lower Aspirations

Older adults may be more satisfied with their environment than younger adults as a result of cohort-specific lower aspiration levels (Golant, 1984) or age-associated changes. First, older adults have lived a greater share of their lives before the arrival of modern amenities, and thus may have grown accustomed to certain forms of hardship and adversity. Traditional religious and ideological beliefs may also lead the older adult to stoically endure a lack of material wants (Johnson, 1995). Second, because, on average, older adults have been living in their home for a longer period than younger adults, they may have had more time to adapt their needs to their existing environment (Golant, 1984). In fact, older adults have lower standards with regard to their housing than younger adults, which results in lower discrepancies between their perceived present housing conditions and their housing aspirations (e.g., Glatzer & Volkert, 1980; Siara, 1980).

Lack of Alternatives

Satisfaction with housing in later life may be interpreted as a reduction of cognitive dissonance: due to the lack of housing alternatives and age-associated limitations in physical and/or financial resources, moving to a better apartment or remodeling one's home may become difficult (e.g., LaGory et al., 1985; Golant, 1984). In one study (Carp, 1975b), applicants for public housing tended to rate their present home as satisfactory, even though most of them were actually living in crowded or substandard housing. However, after being accepted for the housing project and realizing that they had a better alternative, the subjects rated their present housing conditions less favorably.

Relative Weight of Residential Problems

Older adults may interpret environmental stress as minor, relative to life's other difficulties, such as widowhood, chronic illness, and disability, which may result in relatively high levels of residential satisfaction (Golant, 1984).

Environment as a Trigger of Memories

Older adults have lived for a longer period of time in their homes (e.g., $r = .60$, U.S. Census Bureau, 2001). Over the years, the home becomes a reservoir of memories, and arguably even a part of the self (Neisser, 1988). Fond memories of one's home may reinforce positive feelings regarding the present environment. In fact, Golant (1984) showed that fond memories of one's home are positively correlated with housing satisfaction ($r = .23$). Furthermore, a home that remains the same from year to year may contribute to a sense of continuity despite age-associated losses (Gonyea, Hudson, & Seltzer, 1990). However, the higher residential satisfaction among older adults cannot be explained by longer duration of residence per se, because age differences in housing satisfaction remain significant after statistically controlling for length of residence (Herzog & Rodgers, 1986).

Age Differences in Social Desirability

Older adults may be more likely to give socially desirable answers and less likely to report negative feelings. In fact, Wood and Johnson (1979) reported that interviewers judge the housing satisfaction of older adults more negatively compared to older adults' self-ratings. However, in a large study by Herzog and Rodgers (1986), the association of age and housing satisfaction did not change after statistically controlling for social desirability.

Despite the arguments for higher levels of residential satisfaction in older adults, some factors may contribute to lower levels of residential satisfaction in older adults or may at least attenuate the age-associated increase in residential satisfaction suggested above.

HIGHER RISK OF UNFULFILLED NEEDS

With declining health, older adults become increasingly dependent on their environment (environmental docility hypothesis; Lawton & Simon, 1968). It may become increasingly difficult to climb stairs or maintain a yard, and the growing misfit between environmental conditions and individual needs might cause an age-associated decrease in residential satisfaction. Nonetheless, impaired elders employ a wide variety of compensation strategies to reduce the gaps between environmental demands and individual competence (e.g., Wahl et al., 1999); thus, this argument may only hold true for the severely impaired older adult who is no longer able to compensate for environmental deficits.

MOVE TO LONG-TERM CARE FACILITIES

Due to declining health, a minority of older adults is more or less forced to move to nursing homes, which permit less space and privacy. One might thus expect a concomitant decline in residential satisfaction. However, most older adults live in the community, and most studies on residential satisfaction focused exclusively on community-dwelling adults; thus, it is doubtful that such concerns will alter the association between age and residential satisfaction in the present analysis.

Many studies reported that older adults are more satisfied with their housing and neighborhood than younger adults (e.g., Campbell et al., 1976), but some other studies could not replicate these findings (e.g., Biewas-Diener & Diener, 2001). Therefore, the first goal of the present meta-analysis was to integrate these heterogeneous findings.

The association of age with residential satisfaction has mainly been investigated in cross-sectional research. However, cross-sectional studies cannot reveal whether the observed age differences reflect an aging process (age-associated change) or differences between cohorts. Thus, we analyzed whether similar age-differences in residential satisfaction are found in both cross-sectional and longitudinal studies.

ASSOCIATIONS OF RESIDENTIAL SATISFACTION WITH ENVIRONMENTAL CHARACTERISTICS

Age is only one variable of interest in the present study, however. There are many other variables that might plausibly be related to housing satisfaction, such as specific amenities (the presence of a garden or balcony) or maintenance concerns (adequate plumbing and heating). Neighborhood satisfaction can be expected to correlate with access to shops and services, the presence of friends in the immediate area, or perceptions of safety.

HOUSING CONDITIONS

- **Tenure status:**   Home ownership implies security and stability, provides a visual symbol of social status, signalizes considerable personal investment, and may, therefore, contribute to residential satisfaction (e.g., O'Bryant, 1982). In addition, owners are less likely to report housing problems such as physical inadequacy, overcrowding, and excessive expenditures (e.g., Newman & Struyck, 1984).
- **Size of the home (number of rooms per resident):**   Having enough space for activities and possessions may be a source of housing satisfaction. However, the relationship with housing satisfaction may not be linear because very large homes are difficult to maintain (Baillie & Peart, 1992).
- **Basic household amenities:**   These amenities, such as the availability of cold and hot running water, a modern heating system, a working stove or oven, refrigerator, and tub, may be necessary preconditions of housing satisfaction.

- **Maintenance:** The upkeep of a dwelling, that is the lack of serious, permanent defects (e.g., specific electrical problems or inadequately vented heating facilities), indicates a lack of housing-related stress and may, therefore, be a precondition of housing satisfaction.
- **Aesthetics:** Having a charming and attractive home and nice amenities in the home (such as a useable fireplace, a balcony or patio, or attractive furniture) may be a source of comfort and pride and contribute, therefore, to residential satisfaction (e.g., Butterfield & Weideman, 1987).
- **Year of construction:** Residents of older homes may show lower levels of residential satisfaction than residents of newly built homes because the former are more likely to be faced with housing deficits, such as defective electricity or heating. In addition, because housing standards and construction guidelines have improved over time, newly built homes are more likely to be better designed and better built.
- **Living in a nursing home:** Nursing home residents may report lower levels of residential satisfaction than community dwelling older adults because of restricted space, reduced control, and privacy (e.g., Saup, 1993).

NEIGHBORHOOD CHARACTERISTICS

Other variables focus on aspects of the neighborhood and may subsequently show stronger associations with neighborhood satisfaction than with housing satisfaction. Some examples are

- **Availability of services:** The availability of services (e.g., good schools, shops, senior centers, etc.) may be a source of residential satisfaction and neighborhood satisfaction in particular, because essential needs are met by the environment.
- **Safety:** Every home should provide its occupants with safety from crime, fire, accident, and health hazards. These are among the most essential characteristics of any form of shelter, and thus are arguably important sources of residential satisfaction (e.g., Carp & Christensen, 1986).
- **Maintenance (e.g., no signs of vandalism or litter):** A well-maintained neighborhood may contribute to residential satisfaction because it gives the impression that the residents care about their homes and may motivate the residents to contribute toward keeping the environment attractive and functional (e.g., Butterfield & Weideman, 1987).
- **Aesthetics:** The beauty of one's neighborhood (e.g., architectural quality, presence of greenery) is expected to contribute to residential satisfaction (Carp & Christensen, 1986) because it promotes identification with one's neighborhood.
- **Urbanization:** On the one hand, services such as shopping facilities, health care, and public transport are more easily available in urban than in

rural areas, which may contribute to environmental satisfaction. On the other hand, environmental satisfaction may be impaired in urban areas due to higher levels of environmental stress (e.g., higher crime, more noise and air pollution; e.g., Davis & Fine-Davis, 1981). Both of these trends counteract each other, so that differences in residential satisfaction between rural and urban areas may be small.

• **Neighbor characteristics:**   A supportive neighborhood may well contribute to residential satisfaction (Weideman & Anderson, 1985). In line with this, Rosow (1967) has shown that the ease of making friends in a neighborhood and community is related to housing satisfaction. In addition, it has been suggested that the age-homogeneity of the community may contribute to residential satisfaction, since older peers share much in common. Older adults may also profit from age-homogeneity of the neighborhood because of a lower risk of unpredictable and disruptive teenager behavior (Normoyle, 1987).

INDIVIDUAL CHARACTERISTICS

• **Length of residence:**   Longer residence may lead to better integration into the local milieu, and, therefore, higher residential satisfaction (e.g., Speare, 1974). Conversely, high levels of residential satisfaction produce longer duration of residence.

• **Socioeconomic status:**   Residential satisfaction may be positively related to socioeconomic status because richer individuals are able to select better neighborhoods and have the financial means to improve both the comfort and appearance of their home, which, again, contributes to residential satisfaction (Gonyea et al., 1990).

• **Physical health/competence:**   Individuals in poor health will have a more difficult time managing their household and taking advantage of all their neighborhood has to offer. Thus, one would expect them to experience the inadequacies of substandard housing and neighborhood deficits more keenly and report lower levels of residential satisfaction.

• **General subjective well-being:**   According to the top-down view of subjective well-being and life satisfaction, subdomains of life satisfaction (e.g., residential satisfaction) are determined largely by one's general life satisfaction. Conversely, the bottom-up view suggests that subdomains of life satisfaction are determined by objective living conditions, which in turn influence general life satisfaction (e.g., Veenhoven, 1996). Top-down processes may be an important reason for discrepancies between residential satisfaction and the objective quality of residential conditions.

• **Other variables:**   It is less clear whether other demographic variables, such as sex and marital status, are related to residential satisfaction. Because some of the studies reported relevant information on these variables, they were included in the present meta-analysis. Although individual aspiration levels (e.g., Campbell et al., 1976) and social comparisons (Carp, Carp, & Millsap, 1982) have been included in models of predictors of residential satisfaction, there were almost no studies on these variables to include them in the analysis.

AGE DIFFERENCES IN THE ASSOCIATIONS OF ENVIRONMENTAL VARIABLES WITH RESIDENTIAL SATISFACTION

The predictors of residential satisfaction might vary with age. For instance, it is easy to imagine that elderly persons are more concerned with crime in the neighborhood because they might become victimized, than in the quality of kindergartens and schools that they do not need to use any more. It is less clear whether other aspects of environmental quality would show stronger or weaker associations with residential satisfaction in old age. On the one hand, older adults are more dependent on their environment than younger adults. Their residential satisfaction may, therefore, show stronger associations with environmental quality. On the other hand, older people have had more time to adjust their needs to their existing environment and may have learned to be satisfied with their environment irrespective of its present quality. There is empirical evidence that older adults are more likely than younger adults to adapt their general evaluation standards when confronted with unfulfilled needs (e.g., Brandtstädter, Wentura, & Greve, 1993). This may cause an age-associated decline in the relationship between environmental quality and residential satisfaction. There is—with one exception—almost no research on age differences in predictors of residential satisfaction. Bohland and Davis (1979) found that the effect of physical conditions on neighborhood satisfaction declined between the ages of 18 and 64 and increased thereafter. The importance of safety for neighborhood satisfaction increased with age until 64 years and declined thereafter. Having good neighbors had highest importance for neighborhood satisfaction for those aged 25–44 and 65+ years. In order to solve these contradictions, the third goal of the present meta-analysis was to analyze whether the size of the relationship between environmental quality and residential satisfaction varies with the age of the respondents.

METHODS

We used meta-analysis to analyze the associations between environmental and individual variables and residential satisfaction. Meta-analysis is a statistical analysis of results from existing studies in order to achieve a systematic integration of the results.

SAMPLE

We identified studies investigating the relation of housing satisfaction and neighborhood satisfaction with age, other demographic variables, characteristics of the home and the neighborhood, and general psychological well-being. Our survey was based upon a review of the gerontological and psychological literature available in electronic databases (Psycinfo, Psyndex) and a nonsystematic search of the literature. Criteria for inclusion of studies in the meta-analysis were as follows:

a. the respondents were adults (> 18 years)
b. bivariate associations with residential satisfaction could be computed.

Furthermore, in order to obtain a sufficient data base, variables were only included in the analysis if four or more studies were available on associations with at least one indicator of residential satisfaction. About 15 percent of the total number of studies had to be eliminated, for the most part due to insufficient information about the magnitude of the relationships (zero-order effect sizes) of interest.

We were able to include 121 empirical papers in the meta-analysis. The majority was published in English-language journals; an additional seven German papers were also used. The majority of studies were drawn from books (20), *Social Indicators Research* (14), the *International Journal of Aging and Human Development* (8), *Housing and Society* (6), the *Journal of Gerontology* (5), the *Gerontologist* (5), and other journals (49). In addition, we included 13 unpublished studies in the meta-analysis. With regard to eight of them, we were able to use the original electronic raw data file. The studies are listed in the References.

Fifty-nine percent of the studies used probability samples and 41 percent convenience samples. About 37 percent of the studies exclusively focused on older adults (lowest age: 60 or 65 years, respectively), 10 percent on adults younger than 60 or 65 years, and 53 percent included both younger and older adults in their samples. Fifty-one percent of the studies included respondents from urban and rural areas; another 37 percent were exclusively focused on urban respondents and 12 percent on respondents from rural areas.

MEASURES

• **Residential satisfaction:** Housing satisfaction was most often assessed with single-item indicators (67 studies). Twenty-eight papers used sum-scales, and two others qualitative interviews. Similarly, 48 studies measured neighborhood satisfaction with single-item indicators, and 19 with sum-scales.

- **Age differences:** Thirty-six studies analyzed age differences in housing satisfaction, and 26 in neighborhood satisfaction. In addition, 12 longitudinal studies were used.
- **Environmental characteristics:** Most studies used respondents' self-reports of environmental quality (35 studies). Other studies used interviewer ratings (nine studies).
- **Health/competence:** This was assessed with scales of *activities of daily living* (ADLs) and *instrumental activities of daily living* (IADLs; eight studies), symptom checklists (three studies), and single-item indicators of perceived health (eight studies).
- **General subjective well-being:** This was measured with life-satisfaction scales (15 studies), single-item indicators on happiness (six studies), and other well-being scales (14 studies).
- **Sex** (woman = 1, men = 0), **marital status** (married = 1, others = 0), **and ethnicity** (1 = Caucasian, 0 = others): These factors were measured with single-item indicators.

Additional information on the assessment of the variables is available from the first author.

STATISTICAL INTEGRATION OF THE FINDINGS

Two common groups of statistical procedures are used in meta-analysis: fixed- and random-effects models (e.g., Hedges & Vevea, 1998). If a common effect size is hypothesized for all studies, fixed-effects models are appropriate. If effect sizes vary systematically between studies according to moderator variables (e.g., between older and younger respondents), random-effects models are more appropriate because fixed-effects models can lead to inflated Type I errors. Thus, the random-effect model was used, primarily based on procedures outlined by Hedges and Vevea (1998) and Raudenbush (1994).

1. We computed effect sizes d for each study, for example, by transforming correlational coefficients, t values, and F values. In four cases where the direction of the statistical effect but no effect size was reported, we used vote counts to estimate the effect size (Bushman & Wang, 1996). If in one study effect sizes were reported for more than one subsample (e.g., younger versus older adults), separate effect sizes were computed for these subsamples rather than computing an average effect size for the whole sample.

2. The homogeneity of effect sizes was tested by using the homogeneity statistics Q, which is distributed approximately as X^2. In the case of heterogeneous effect sizes, we estimated the between-study variance of the effects, based on Hedges and Vevea (1998).

3. Studies were weighted by the reciprocal of the sum of the between-study variance component and the random sampling error of the study.

4. The significance of the mean effect size was tested by dividing the weighted mean effect size by the estimation of the standard deviation. Then, confidence intervals that include 95 percent of the effects were computed for each effect size. Differences between two conditions were interpreted as significant when the 95 percent intervals did not overlap.

RESULTS

Our first research question addressed age differences in residential satisfaction. As shown in Table 8.1, older adults reported higher levels of housing satisfaction and neighborhood satisfaction. Age explained 0.7 percent of the variance of housing satisfaction and 1.9 percent of the variance of neighborhood satisfaction. According to Cohen's (1992) criteria, observed age differences have to be interpreted as small. The positive association of age and housing satisfaction was found for both cross-sectional and longitudinal data. As shown by the overlap of the confidence intervals, longitudinal and cross-sectional studies on housing satisfaction did not vary significantly in their effect sizes. With regard to neighborhood satisfaction, significant effects appeared in cross-sectional studies, but not in longitudinal studies. In addition, age differences in neighborhood satisfaction were significantly stronger in cross-sectional studies than in longitudinal studies.

It has been suggested that reasons specific to old age may cause the age-associated increase in residential satisfaction (e.g., the relative lack of housing alternatives in advanced age, LaGory et al., 1985). If this holds true, there should be a stronger association of age with residential satisfaction in older than in younger samples. In order to test this, we computed a weighted ordinary least squares regression analysis with the mean age of the sample as the independent variable and the association of age and residential satisfaction as the dependent variable (Raudenbush, 1994). Contrary to the previous suggestion, we found a stronger age-associated increase of housing satisfaction ($\beta = -.08$, $t = -3.06$, $p < .01$) and neighborhood satisfaction ($\beta = -.30$, $t = -6.24$, $p < .001$) in younger samples. For example, in samples that exclusively focused on younger adults (18 to 59 years), the size of the association of age with housing satisfaction and neighborhood satisfaction was $d = .20$ and $d = .18$, respectively, compared to $d = .10$ and $d = .09$ in older samples (60+ years).

The associations between residential satisfaction and objective aspects of the environment, as well as with individual variables, were the topic of our second research question. As shown in Table 8.1, homeowners were more satisfied with their homes and their neighborhoods than renters.

TABLE 8.1. Correlates of Housing Satisfaction and Neighborhood Satisfaction

	Housing Satisfaction						Neighborhood Satisfaction						Sign. diff. between groups
	k	N	d	C.I.		Z	Hetero-geneity	k	N	d	C.I.		Z	Hetero-geneity	
Associations with age															
All studies	158	773,299	.17	.14	.19	13.63***	3,108.76***	54	676,160	.28	.23	.32	11.82***	3,719.19***	H>N
Cross-sectional studies	139	755,741	.16	.14	.18	13.65***	2,764.29***	49	664,427	.29	.25	.34	12.29	3,488.67***	H>N
Longitudinal studies	19	17,558	.23	.10	.35	3.70***	175.18***	5	11,733	-.01	-.26	.24	-.09	7.71	
Associations with housing characteristics															
Tenure status (1=owner, 0=renter)	37	790,302	.35	.28	.42	10.02***	7,083.28***	31	799,167	.33	.27	.39	10.00***	5,149.54***	
Size of the home	30	108,497	.42	.34	.50	10.68***	799.89***	14	48,080	.16	.15	.17	3.01**	449.53***	H > N
# Basic household amenities	16	68,805	.48	.40	.56	11.12***	245.39***	8	51,013	.26	.17	.38	5.50***	87.85***	H > N
Maintenance of home	14	604,986	.35	.30	.40	14.51***	1,105.04***	15	605,542	.19	.16	.21	11.78***	492.97***	H > N
Year of construction	19	580,051	.13	.07	.20	4.01***	2,400.09***	15	573,772	.07	.03	.11	3.02*	855.96***	
Aesthetics (convenience/ pleasantness/nice household amenities)	13	96,849	.64	.55	.73	14.35***	345.43***	8	51,013	.40	.28	.52	6.27***	167.05***	H > N
Nursing home (1=yes, 0=no)	4	4,229	-.32	-.66	.02	-1.86	91.12***	—	—	—	—	—	—	—	
Associations with neighborhood characteristics															
Availability of services	15	55,076	.14	.06	.22	3.43***	123.58***	25	78,415	.31	.23	.39	7.49***	440.94***	H < N
Maintenance of neighborhood	12	50,779	.53	.43	.63	10.63***	106.46***	12	60,377	1.00	.78	1.21	9.11***	1,271.48***	H < N
Safety	16	57,040	.31	.23	.39	7.92***	138.38***	34	147,651	.81	.72	.89	19.10***	1,488.54***	H < N
Aesthetics of neighborhood	8	2,560	1.02	.57	1.47	4.46***	176.97***	7	4,844	.75	.50	1.00	5.82***	112.02***	

	k	N	d			Z	Heterog.		k	N	d			Z	Heterog.	
Greenery (e.g., parks nearby)	8	50,519	.51	.32	.70	5.21***	309.37***		12	69,666	.52	.36	.68	6.17***	812.90***	
Urbanization	106	1,204,385	-.06	-.08	-.04	-5.59***	2,874.10***		49	1,168,910	-.22	-.27	-.18	-10.33***	5,098.70***	H > N
Age homogeneity of neighborhood	1	945	.18	.05	.31	2.76**	0.00		5	7,955	.10	-.19	.39	0.68	123.63***	
Perceived quality of relations with neighbors	8	6,025	.18	.12	.24	5.18***	9.57		13	11,415	.81	.53	1.08	5.77***	491.06***	H < N
Association with individual variables																
Length of residence	21	149,960	.06	.01	.11	2.27*	278.63***		19	169,730	.32	.19	.45	3.07**	2,576.75***	H < N
Income	137	647,529	.19	.17	.21	16.22***	2,266.93***		56	566,059	.14	.11	.17	8.59***	1,231.71***	
Physical health	16	10,196	.22	.14	.30	5.15***	60.55***		5	4,824	.16	.07	.26	3.38***	8.42	
Physical competence	10	8,598	.16	.07	.25	3.48***	32.11***		6	4,228	.13	.04	.22	2.84**	7.00	
Being female	116	178,388	-.02	-.04	.005	-1.54	474.52***		37	99,802	-.00	-.03	.03	-0.21	128.61***	
Being married	117	195,526	.28	.24	.32	14.44***	1,929.65***		31	75,630	.13	.08	.18	5.18***	261.87***	H > N
Ethnic minority	12	28,493	-.40	-.51	-.29	-7.18***	177.52***		9	43,316	-.24	-.33	-.15	-5.08***	138.45***	
Associations between aspects of satisfaction/subjective well-being																
Subj. well-being	106	112,430	.68	.62	.74	23.05***	2,439.29***		39	31,652	.55	.42	.68	8.80***	1,001.67***	
Neighborhood satisfaction	45	78,677	1.48	1.35	1.61	22.02***	2,247.55***									

Note. k = number of studies, N= pooled sample size, d = effect size, C.I. 95% confidence interval, Z = Test of the significance of the mean, Heterog. = Heterogeneity of effects, H > N stronger positive association with housing satisfaction than with neighborhood satisfaction. *** p<.001, ** p<.01, * p<.05.

Similarly, residential satisfaction was positively associated with the size of the home, the number of basic household amenities, the maintenance of the home, living in a newer home, and the perceived aesthetics of the home. Housing satisfaction was not significantly lower among nursing home residents, probably due to the small number of studies available. Housing satisfaction was more strongly related with the perceived aesthetics of the home than with the number of basic household amenities, tenure status, the maintenance of the home, and the year of construction of the building. In addition, the number of basic household amenities and the size of the home showed stronger associations with housing satisfaction than the maintenance of the home and the year of construction. Furthermore, housing satisfaction was more positively correlated with tenure status than with the year of construction of the building. The perceived aesthetics of the home shared 7.4 percent of variance with housing satisfaction, and the number of basic household amenities and the size of the home shared about 4.5 percent of their variance with housing satisfaction.

Housing satisfaction should be tied closely to housing characteristics and neighborhood satisfaction less so. As shown by the non-overlap of the confidence intervals, this was the case for home size, the number of basic household amenities, maintenance of the home, and aesthetic qualities of the home.

In the next step, we analyzed associations between residential satisfaction and neighborhood characteristics. As shown in Table 8.1, residential satisfaction was related to the presence of services, a well-maintained neighborhood, greenery, higher perceived safety, rural areas (as opposed to urban areas), and having good neighborhood relationships. In addition, an age-homogeneous neighborhood was associated with a higher level of housing satisfaction, but not neighborhood satisfaction. With regard to neighborhood satisfaction, the strongest associations were found with the maintenance of neighborhood, safety, good relations with neighbors, and the perceived aesthetic quality of the neighborhood. These variables shared between 9.4 and 12.5 percent of their variance with neighborhood satisfaction. In addition, these associations were significantly stronger than the associations with the availability of services, age homogeneity of the neighborhood, and the level of urbanization. With regard to housing satisfaction, the strongest association was found with the perceived aesthetics of the neighborhood, and the weakest with the availability of services and the level of urbanization. As shown by the non-overlap of the confidence intervals, five out of eight neighborhood characteristics showed significantly stronger associations with neighborhood satisfaction than with housing satisfaction.

With regard to individual variables, we found that the length of residence, the level of income, being married, Caucasian origin, and having good health and high levels of competence were positively related to both indicators of residential satisfaction (Table 8.1). However, no gender differences in residential satisfaction were observed. The associations with individual variables were generally small, explaining four percent (ethnic minority status—housing satisfaction) to 0.4 percent (length of residence—housing satisfaction) of the variance of residential satisfaction.

As shown in the lower part of Table 8.1, housing satisfaction and neighborhood satisfaction showed a strong positive association with indicators of general subjective well-being (e.g., global life satisfaction, happiness). The indicators of residential satisfaction shared 8.8 percent and 5.6 percent of variance, respectively, with general subjective well-being. In addition, housing satisfaction and neighborhood satisfaction were positively correlated and shared 28.3 percent of their variance.

Some of the studies employed in the present analysis reported results from multivariate analyses. They usually included individual variables in the first step of a regression analysis, and environmental characteristics in the second step. However, most studies included only a very small number of environmental variables. With regard to housing satisfaction, individual variables explained on average 3.6 percent of the variance of the dependent variable, and housing characteristics an additional 12.3 percent ($N = 36,453$). With regard to neighborhood satisfaction, individual variables explained 2.9 percent of the variance and characteristics of the neighborhood 10.9 percent ($N = 23,938$).

Our third research question addressed whether the association between environmental characteristics and residential satisfaction varies with the age of the respondents. We compared studies in which the age of the participants was less than 60 or 65 years with studies that included only older participants. Comparisons were only computed if at least two independent studies were available for each age group. With regard to housing satisfaction we found that home ownership, the maintenance of the home, the year of construction, and the length of residence showed stronger associations with the dependent variable in younger than in older groups (Table 8.2). Similarly, the maintenance of neighborhood, the level of safety, and the length of residence showed stronger associations with neighborhood satisfaction in younger than in older samples. Between-group differences with regard to urbanization were in the same direction, but not statistically significant.

DISCUSSION

In the present study, we analyzed how age, other sociodemographic variables, and characteristics of housing and the neighborhood are related to residential satisfaction. We found that cross-sectional studies showed a positive association of age with housing satisfaction and neighborhood

TABLE 8.2. Age Differences in the Association Between Home and Neighborhood Characteristics and Residential Satisfaction

	Younger Participants (< 60/65 years)						Older Participants (≥ 60/65 years)						Sign. diff. between groups
	k	N	d	C.I.		Z	Hetero-geneity	k	N	d	C.I.		Z	Hetero-geneity	

	k	N	d	C.I.	Z	Hetero-geneity	k	N	d	C.I.	Z	Hetero-geneity	Sign. diff. between groups
Associations with housing characteristics with housing satisfaction													
Tenure status													
(1=owner, 0=renter)	9	440,454	.60	.58 .62	69.19***	42.30**	19	145,284	.24	.19 .31	10.19***	261.82***	Y > O
Size of the home	5	68,322	.43	.30 .55	6.77***	146.65***	11	29,679	.28	.21 .35	7.94***	44.98***	
# of basic household													
amenities	4	34,687	.55	.29 .81	4.09***	26.04***	9	29,387	.47	.34 .60	7.13***	103.47***	
Maintenance of home	7	473,481	.42	.37 .47	16.63***	445.21***	7	131,505	.29	.23 .34	9.55***	176.20***	Y > O
Year of construction	6	442,715	.25	.22 .28	15.05***	148.55***	9	133,619	-.01	-.14 .12	-0.20	1,111.25***	Y > O
Aesthetics													
(nice household													
amenities)	4	68,249	.67	.59 .75	16.69***	48.06**	8	26,581	.58	.48 .68	11.24***	51.68***	
Length of residence	5	105,404	.18	.16 .20	18.78***	5.47	12	40,454	.01	-.03 .05	0.67	21.69*	Y > O
Associations with neighborhood characteristics with neighborhood satisfaction													
Availability of services	4	37,438	.12	-.25 .49	0.63	203.70***	8	32,537	.11	-.03 .25	1.49	37.32***	
Safety	3	67,348	.93	.81 1.04	15.64***	86.26***	12	46,011	.58	.53 .64	20.97***	46.85***	Y > O
Maintenance of													
neighborhood	2	33,771	.95	.93 .97	82.73***	4.00	2	27,338	.60	.38 .82	5.33***	83.69***	Y > O
Urbanization	10	441,855	-.27	-.30 -.24	-16.75***	165.77***	10	146,840	-.20	-.27 -.13	-5.46***	450.00***	Y > O
Length of residence	4	105,926	.11	.07 .14	6.21**	9.70*	7	37,509	-.05	-.09 -.02	-2.83**	11.40	Y > O

Note.:k = number of studies, N= pooled sample size, d = effect size, C.I. 95% confidence interval, Z = Test of the significance of the mean, Y > O stronger association in younger than in older samples. *** p<.001, ** p<.01, * p<.05.

210

satisfaction, as did longitudinal studies with regard to housing satisfaction. When focusing on environmental characteristics, the perceived aesthetic quality of the home showed the strongest association with housing satisfaction, whereas the level of maintenance of the neighborhood, safety, the quality of relationships with neighbors, and the aesthetics of the neighborhood showed the strongest relationship with neighborhood satisfaction. In addition, we found that environmental characteristics were more closely related to residential satisfaction in younger than in older respondents.

Given the theoretical considerations discussed at the beginning of our paper, it may not be surprising to find a positive association of age with residential satisfaction. However, the present meta-analysis revealed that similar age-associated increases in housing satisfaction were found in cross-sectional and longitudinal studies, whereas age differences in neighborhood satisfaction were only found in cross-sectional studies. If there were only cohort differences but no age-associated change, effects of age would only be observed in cross-sectional studies but not in longitudinal studies. Because longitudinal studies found age-associated change in housing satisfaction, we have to conclude that housing satisfaction changes with increasing age, although we were not able to test whether the size of longitudinal changes would also vary between cohorts.

In addition, our meta-analysis does not support the suggestion that the higher residential satisfaction of older adults can be traced back to the lack of housing alternatives of the oldest age groups due to limited resources (e.g., LaGory et al., 1985) or the relative low weight of residential problems in old age, given other, more severe problems (such as bad health; Golant, 1984). To the contrary, stronger age-associated improvements in residential satisfaction were observed in younger adults, for whom the search for a better home or the remodeling of one's home is not yet restricted by limited health or financial concerns. This effect was probably not based on a restriction of variance in older samples because younger and older samples showed similar levels of inter-individual variability. A stringent test would be to statistically control for the variance of age and residential satisfaction. Unfortunately, this was not possible because many studies did not provide this information.

Nonetheless, the current findings are very plausible: middle-aged adults have the financial and physical resources to create or select residential conditions that fit their needs. Their resources are considerably greater compared to young adults and, through home improvement, they become more satisfied with their current housing conditions. Although one can improve one's place of residence by remodeling, improving one's neighborhood often presupposes a move to a new location. Thus, environmental proactivity plays a greater role with regard to housing conditions and housing satisfaction than with regard to neighborhood conditions and neighborhood satisfaction. Indeed, the stability of neighborhood satisfaction over longitudinal intervals may reflect natural limitations to improving one's neighborhood. Note that the largest available longitudinal study on neighborhood satisfaction was based on a sample that did not relocate between the two points of measurement, so improvements in neighborhood conditions and their effect on neighborhood satisfaction were quite unlikely. Thus, improvements in neighborhood satisfaction are more likely to be found in samples that include a share of residents who moved to a better neighborhood between points of measurement. However, based on the present data, we can not rule out completely that age differences in neighborhood satisfaction simply reflect cohort differences.

Associations between residential satisfaction and characteristics of housing and neighborhood were the focus of our second research question. The perceived aesthetics and pleasantness of the home showed the strongest relationship with housing satisfaction. This may indicate that nice household amenities provide pleasure and enjoyment (e.g., Butterfield & Weideman, 1987) and are more important for residential satisfaction than basic housing characteristics. In fact, due to an improvement of general housing conditions in the last decades, severe deficits in the maintenance of the home became less common, so that the restricted variance of this variable may have attenuated the observed relationship with housing satisfaction. For example, in the American Housing Survey, only about seven percent of the respondents reported moderate or severe physical housing problems (U.S. Census Bureau, 2001). A second interpretation would be that the association between the perceived aesthetics of the home and housing satisfaction may have been enlarged by a response bias because some studies on the aesthetic quality of the home used highly subjective measures, such as the residents' perception of pleasantness of their home, which may have been influenced by their mood states and social desirability. Basic household amenities and housing deficits rely upon more objective information and are less prone to such bias.

The level of maintenance of the neighborhood (e.g., no vandalism), perceived safety, good social relations with neighbors, and the perceived aesthetic quality of the neighborhood (e.g., enough public space) showed the strongest associations with neighborhood satisfaction, thus indicating that the absence of environmental stress was as important as aesthetic characteristics of the neighborhood. With regard to the controversy whether rural or urban residents report higher levels of residential satisfaction, we found rural residents to be more satisfied, especially with their neighborhood. This probably reflects the fact that environmental stressors—such as crime, litter, and noise—that are related to low residential satisfaction are much more prevalent in urban areas (e.g., Davis & Fine-Davis, 1981).

We did not find empirical support for the suggestion that a higher age-homogeneity of the neighborhood is associated with higher levels of neighborhood satisfaction, although the results have to be interpreted with caution due to the fact that only five studies were available on that question. However, there is other empirical evidence that people may derive satisfaction from age-homogeneous as well as age-heterogeneous neighborhoods, for example, depending on individual residential preferences (e.g., LaGory et al., 1985).

Associations between residential satisfaction and sociodemographic variables were small. The higher satisfaction of Caucasians and individuals with higher income probably reflect their better objective residential conditions (U.S. Census Bureau, 2001). However, the association between income and residential satisfaction was weaker than might be expected, perhaps due to the fact that housing aspirations vary by income, and prices for buying or renting a home of similar quality can vary considerably between different areas.

The strong positive association between housing satisfaction and neighborhood satisfaction may indicate that high quality homes are often located in better neighborhoods. Moreover, ratings of different aspects of residential satisfaction may be influenced by general subjective well-being and individual coping styles, such as the tendency to downgrade problems and to adapt to one's living conditions. However, because we found meaningful correlates between residential satisfaction and objective housing and neighborhood conditions, associations between housing satisfaction and neighborhood satisfaction cannot exclusively be interpreted as effects of a general coping style. The strong positive association between housing satisfaction and neighborhood satisfaction may indicate that a sum-measure of residential satisfaction may be preferable. However, because housing satisfaction shows stronger associations with the quality of the home and neighborhood satisfaction with neighborhood quality, it is useful to separate both concepts.

When interpreting the observed bivariate associations, one has to be aware that housing characteristics and neighborhood characteristics are correlated. For example, homeowners may have higher income, more available living space, and may be more likely to have built or remodeled their homes to suit their aesthetic preferences. Unfortunately, studies seldom include a full matrix of these variables and we were thus unable to compute multivariate analyses.

With regard to our third research question, we found that the association between objective residential conditions and residential satisfaction is stronger in younger than in older samples. Although older adults may become more dependent on their environment due to age-associated losses of competence, they base their environmental satisfaction less strongly on objective characteristics of their environment. We conclude that older adults had more time to adapt their criteria for evaluating their environment so that environmental deficits lose part of their significance for residential satisfaction. However, despite decreasing associations with residential satisfaction, it is still true that good housing and neighborhood conditions are associated with higher residential satisfaction in old age.

LIMITATIONS AND CONCLUSIONS

The present study has some limitations. First, for some research questions we found only a very limited number of studies. For example, some housing and neighborhood characteristics could not be included in our meta-analysis due to the lack of sufficient data (e.g., room configuration, lighting levels etc.). Second, different aspects of housing quality and neighborhood quality may be interrelated. Because the studies usually did not provide a fully correlational matrix of the variables, we had to focus on bivariate associations with residential satisfaction. Third, we tested for linear associations between environmental characteristics and satisfaction. There may also be curvilinear relationships (e.g., Bohland & Davis, 1979; Lawton, 1980a). Fourth, meta-analytic random-effects models may slightly overestimate the actual between-study variability of effect sizes and make the identification of moderators more difficult (e.g., Hedges & Vevea, 1998). Nevertheless, this more conservative approach is appropriate for low information situations (Overton, 1998). Such is the case in our study because other potential moderators can not be controlled for, and because only very few studies were available for some research questions. Fifth, analyses on how sample characteristics other than age (e.g., the representativeness of the sample) and aspects of measurement (e.g., residents' self-ratings versus observer ratings) influence the size of the associations with residential satisfaction still have to be done.

Despite these limitations, several conclusions can be drawn from the present study. First, we conclude that higher levels of housing satisfaction in older adults reflect age-associated changes rather than cohort differences. Second, increases in residential satisfaction are more likely to be found in middle-age than in older adults, probably because the former group is more likely to improve their housing conditions, and the latter group has often already found or created their preferred residential conditions. Third, we conclude that aesthetic qualities of the home are more important for housing satisfaction than basic housing conditions, at least as long as most basic housing needs are met. Fourth, we conclude that with increasing age objective housing conditions become less important for residential satisfaction, thus indicating that older adults have adapted their evaluation standards to their present living conditions. Thus, high levels of residential satisfaction become a less valid indicator of objective deficits, and older adults' subjective assessments of residential satisfaction should be accompanied by objective evaluations of their housing conditions. Fifth, further research is needed on whether this adaptation of standards is mainly found with regard to mild environmental deficits or whether some older adults may even be satisfied with their home and neighborhood despite severe objective deficits. Sixth, because environmental variables explained less variance of residential satisfaction in older samples, we would encourage researchers to examine variables that might account for the "missing share" of residential satisfaction in the elderly. For example, place attachment, such as the autobiographical significance of the environment and the familiarity with the place, may be one such variable. Seventh, Weideman and Anderson's (1985) critique that only a small number of environmental variables has been related to residential satisfaction still holds true. Thus, we recommend the incorporation of a greater number of variables in research on residential satisfaction, such as layout, the uniqueness of the home, the view afforded from the windows, the amount of sunshine the house gets, and so on. This is especially true given the fact that we have shown *aesthetics* to be critical to satisfaction. Finally, given the fact that most studies on residential satisfaction are cross-sectional, we recommend more longitudinal research. For example, these studies could investigate how changes in environmental conditions (e.g., remodeling one's home, moves) and changes in individual resources (e.g., declines in physical competence) are related to changes in residential satisfaction.

ACKNOWLEDGMENTS

Special thanks to Pasqualina Perrig-Chiello and Karin Poppelaars for giving access to their unpublished data.

REFERENCES

References marked with an asterisk indicate studies included in the meta-analysis.

*Adams, R. E. (1992). Is happiness a home in the suburbs? The influence of urban versus suburban neighborhoods on psychological health. *Journal of Community Psychology, 20,* 353-371.

*Altus, D. E., & Mathews, R. M. (2000). Examining satisfaction of older home owners with intergenerational homesharing. *Journal of Clinical Geropsychology, 6,* 139-147.

*Altus, D. E., Xaverius, P. K., & Kosloski, K. D. (2002). Evaluating the impact of elder cottage housing on residents and their hosts. *Journal of Clinical Geropsychology, 8,* 117-137.

*Alvi, S., Schwartz, M. D., DeKeseredy, W. S., & Maue, M. O. (2001). Women's fear of crime in Canadian public housing. *Violence Against Women, 7*, 638-661.

*Andrews, F. M., & Whitey, S. B. (1976). *Social indicators of well-being: Americans' perception of life quality.* New York: Plenum Press.

*Baillie, S. (1990). Dwelling features as intervening variables in housing satisfaction and propensity to move. *Housing and Society, 17*, 1-15.

*Baillie, S. T., & Peart, V. (1992). Determinants of housing satisfaction for older married and unmarried women in Florida. *Housing and Society, 19*, 101-116.

*Baldassare, M. (1979). *Residential crowding in urban America.* Berkeley: University of California Press.

*Barresi, C. M., Ferraro, K. F., & Hobey, L. L. (1983-84). Environmental satisfaction, sociability, and well-being among urban elderly. *International Journal of Aging and Human Development, 18*, 277-293.

*Berghorn, F. J., Schafer, D. E., Steere. G. H., & Wiseman, R. F. (1978). *The urban elderly: A study of life satisfaction.* New York: Universe Books.

*Biwas-Diener, R., & Diener, E. (2001). Making the best of a bad situation: Satisfaction in the slums of Calcutta. *Social Indicators Research, 55*, 329-352.

*Bohland, J. R., & Davis, L. (1979). Sources of residential satisfaction amongst the elderly: An age comparative analysis. In S. M. Golant (Ed.), *Location and environment of elderly population* (pp. 95-109). New York: Wiley.

Brandtstädter, J., Wentura, D., & Greve, W. (1993). Adaptive resources of the aging self. *International Journal of Behavioral Development, 16*, 323-349.

Bushman, B. J., & Wang, M. C. (1996). A procedure for combining sample standardized mean differences and vote counts to estimate the population standardized mean difference in fixed effects models. *Psychological Methods, 1*, 66-80.

*Butterfield, D., & Weideman, S. (1987). Housing satisfaction of the elderly. In V. Regnier & J. Pynoos (Eds.), *Housing the aged: Design directives and policy considerations* (pp. 133-150). New York: Elsevier.

*Campbell, A. P., Converse, P. E., & Rodgers, W. L. (1976). *The quality of American life: Perceptions, evaluations and satisfactions.* New York: Sage.

*Carp, F. M. (1975a). Long-range satisfaction with housing. *Gerontologist, 15*, 68-72.

Carp, F. M. (1975b). Ego defense and cognitive consistency in evaluations of living environments. *Journal of Gerontology, 30*, 707-711.

*Carp, F. M., & Carp, A. (1982). A role for technical environmental assessment in perceptions of environmental quality and well-being. *Journal of Environmental Psychology, 2*, 171-191.

Carp, F. M., Carp, A., & Millsap, R. (1982). Equity and satisfaction among the elderly. *International Journal of Aging and Human Development, 15*, 151-166.

*Carp, F. M., & Christensen, D. L. (1986). Older women living alone: Technical environmental assessment of psychological well-being. *Research on Aging, 8*, 407-425.

*Chou, S. C., Boldy, D. P., & Lee, A. H. (2002). Resident satisfaction and its components in residential aged care. *The Gerontologist, 42*, 188-198.

*Christakopolou, S., Dawson, J., & Gari, A. (2001). The community well-being questionnaire: Theoretical context and initial assessment of its reliability and validity. *Social Indicators Research, 56*, 321-351.

*Christensen, D. L., & Carp, F. M. (1987). PEQI-based environmental predictors of the residential satisfaction of older women. *Journal of Environmental Psychology*, 7, 45-64.
*Churchman, A., & Ginsberg, Y. (1984). The image and experience of high rise housing in Israel. *Journal of Environmental Psychology*, 4, 27-41.
Cohen, J. (1992). A power primer. *Psychological Bulletin*, 112, 155-159.
*Cook, C. C. (1988). Components of neighborhood satisfaction: Responses from urban and suburban single-parent women. *Environment and Behavior*, 20, 115-149.
*Currie, R. D., & Thacker, C. (1986). Quality of the urban environment as perceived by residents of slow and fast growth cities. *Social Indicators Research*, 18, 95-118.
*Cutter, S. (1982). Residential satisfaction and the suburban homeowner. *Urban Geography*, 3, 315-327.
*Davis, E. E., & Fine-Davis, M. (1981). Predictors of satisfaction with housing and neighborhood. *Social Indicators Research*, 9, 477-494.
*Devlin, A. S. (1980). Housing for the elderly: Cognitive considerations. *Environment and Behavior*, 12, 451-466.
*Droettboom, T., McAllister, R. J., Kaiser, E. J., & Butler, E. W. (1971). Urban violence and residential mobility. *Journal of the American Institute of Planners*, 37, 319-325.
*Eurobarometer cumulaltive data files (1973-6). Köln: GESIS.
*Foote, N. N., & Abu-Loghod, Foley, M. M., & Winnick, L. (1969). *Housing choices and housing constraints*. New York: McGraw-Hill.
*Fried, M. (1973). *The world of the urban working class*. Cambridge, MA: Harvard University Press.
*Fried, M. (1984). The structure and significance of community satisfaction. *Population and Environment*, 7, 61-86.
*Fuhrer, U., & Kaiser, F. (1991). Ortsbindung und Verkehrsdichte [Place attachment and traffic intensity]. *Zeitschrift für experimentelle und angewandte Psychologie*, 38, 365-378.
*Gilderbloom, J., & Mullins, R. (1995). Elderly housing needs: An examination of the American Housing Survey. *International Journal of Aging and Human Development*, 40, 57-72.
Glatzer, W., & Volkert, M. (1980). Lebensbedingungen und Lebensqualität alter Menschen [Living conditions and quality of life in old age]. *Zeitschrift für Gerontologie*, 13, 247-260.
*Glatzer, W., & Zapf, W. (1984). *Lebensqualität in der Bundesrepublik Deutschland* [Quality of life in the Federal Republic of Germany]. Frankfurt/Main, Germany: Campus.
*Godman, A. C., & Hankin, J. R. (1984). Elderly Jews and happiness with locale. *Population and Environment*, 7, 87-102.
*Golant, S. (1984). *A place to grow old: The meaning of environment in old age*. New York: Columbia University Press.
*Gonyea, J. G., Hudson, R. B., & Seltzer, G. B. (1990). Housing preferences of vulnerable elders in suburbia. *Journal of Housing for the Elderly*, 7, 79-95.
*Gruber, K. J., & Shelton, G. G. (1987). Assessment of neighborhood satisfaction by residents of three housing types. *Social Indicators Research*, 19, 303-315.

218   PINQUART & BURMEDI

*Ha, M., & Weber, M. J. (1994). Residential quality and satisfaction: Toward developing residential quality indexes. *Home Economics Research Journal, 22,* 296-308.

*Hampe, G. D., & Blevins, A. L. (1976). Primary group interaction of residents in a retirement hotel. *International Journal of Aging and Human Development, 6,* 309-319.

*Handal, P. J., Barling, P. W., & Morrissy, E. (1981). Development of perceived and preferred measures of physical and social characteristics of the residential environment and their relationship to satisfaction. *Journal of Community Psychology, 9,* 118-124.

Hedges, L. V., & Vevea, J. L. (1998). Fixed- and random-effects models in meta-analysis. *Psychological Methods, 3,* 486-504.

Herzog, A., & Rodgers, W. (1986). Satisfaction among older adults. In F. Andrews (Ed.), *Research on the quality of life* (pp. 235-251). Ann Arbor, MI: Institute of Social Research.

*Inglehart, R. (2000). *World values surveys and European values surveys 1981-1984, and 1990-1993* [Computer file]. Ann Arbor, MI: Institute for Social Research.

*Jelinkova, Z., & Picek, M. (1984). Physical and psychological factors determining population responses to environment. *Activitas Nervosa Superior, 26,* 144-146.

*Jirovec, R. L., Jirovec, M. M., & Bosse, R. (1985). Residential satisfaction as a function of micro and macro environmental conditions. *Research on Aging, 7,* 601-616.

Johnson, C. L. (1996). Determinants of adaptation of oldest old Black Americans, *Journal of Aging Studies, 9,* 23-244.

*Johnson, M. K., Lovingood, R. P., & Goss, R. C. (1993). Satisfaction of elderly residents in subsidized housing: The effect of the manager's leadership style. *Housing and Society, 20(2),* 51-60.

*Johnson, P. J., & Abernathy, T. J. (1983). Sources of urban multifamily housing satisfaction. *Housing and Society, 10(1),* 36-42.

*Kasl, S. V., & Harburg, E. (1972). Perceptions of the neighborhood and the desire to move out. *Journal of the American Institute of Planners, (38),* 318-324.

*Kearns, R. A., Smith, C. J., & Abbott, M. W. (1991). Another day in paradise? Life on the margins in urban New Zealand. *Social Science and Medicine, 33,* 369-379.

*LaGory, M., Ward, R., & Sherman, S. (1985). The ecology of aging: Neighborhood satisfaction in an older population. *Sociological Quarterly, 26,* 405-418.

*Lansing, J. B., & Merans, R. W. (1969). Evaluation of neighborhood quality. *Journal of the American Institute of Planners, 35,* 195-199.

*Lawton, M. P. (1980a). Housing the elderly: Residential quality and residential satisfaction. *Research on Aging, 2,* 309-328.

*Lawton, M. P. (1980b). Neighborhood environment and the wellbeing of older tenants in planned housing. *International Journal of Aging and Human Development, 11,* 211-227.

*Lawton, M. P., Brody, E. M., & Turner-Massey, P. (1978). The relationship of environmental factors to changes in well-being. *The Gerontologist, 18,* 133-137.

*Lawton, M. P., & Cohen, J. (1974). The generality of housing impact on the well-being of older people. *Journal of Gerontology, 29,* 194-204.

Lawton, M. P., Moss, M., & Fulcomer, M. (1986). Objective and subjective uses of time by older people. *International Journal of Aging and Human Development, 24,* 171-188.

*Lawton, M. P., & Nahemow, L. (1979). Social areas and the well-being of tenants in housing for the elderly. *Multivariate Behavioral Research, 14*, 463-484.

*Lawton, M. P., Nahemow, L., & Teaff, J. (1975). Housing characteristics and the well-being of elderly tenants in federally assisted housing. *Journal of Gerontology, 30*, 601-607.

*Lawton, M. P., Nahemow, L., & Yeh, T. M. (1980). Neighborhood environment and the well-being of older tenants in planned housing. *International Journal of Aging and Human Development, 11*, 211-227.

Lawton, M. P., & Simon, B. B. (1968). The ecology of social relationships in housing for the elderly. *The Gerontologist, 8*, 108-115.

*Leonardi, F., Spazzafumo, L., Marcellini, F., & Gagliardi, C. (1999). The top-down/bottom-up controversy from a constructivist approach. *Social Indicator Research, 48*, 187-216.

*Levy-Leboyer, C. (1983). The need for space and residential satisfaction. *Architecture & Behavior, 9*, 475-490.

*Lija, M., & Borell, L. (1997). Elderly people's daily activities and need for mobility support. *Scandinavian Journal of Caring Sciences, 11*, 73-80.

*McAuley, W. J., & Offerle, J. M. (1983). Perceived suitability of residence and life satisfaction among the elderly and handicapped. *Journal of Housing for the Elderly, 1*, 63-75.

*McNeil, J. K., Stones, M. J., & Kozma, A. (1986). Longitudinal variation in domain indicators of happiness. *Social Indicators Research, 18*, 119-124.

*Merans, R., & Rodgers, W. (1975). Toward an understanding of community satisfaction. In A. H. Hawley & V. P. Rock (Eds.), *Metropolitan America in contemporary perspective* (pp. 299-352). New York: Wiley.

*Michalos, A. C. (1980). Satisfaction and happiness. *Social Indicators Research, 8*, 385-422.

*Michalos, A. C., Hubley, A. M., Zumbo, B. D., & Hemingway, D. (2001). Health and other aspects of quality of life of older people. *Social Indicators Research, 54*, 239-274.

*Michalos, A. C., & Zumbo, B. D. (2000). Criminal victimization and the quality of life. *Social Indicators Research, 50*, 245-295.

*Miller, F. D., Tsemberis, S., Malia, G. P., & Grega, D. (1980). Neighborhood satisfaction among urban dwellers. *Journal of Social Issues, 3*, 101-117.

*Mollenkopf, H., Oswald, F., Schilling, O., & Wahl, H. W. (2001). Aspekte der außerhäuslichen Mobilität älterer Menschen in der Stadt und auf dem Land [Aspects of mobility of older urban and rural residents]. *Sozialer Fortschritt, 50*, 214-220.

*Moller, V., & Saris, W. (2001). The relationship between subjective well-being and domain satisfaction in South Africa. *Social Indicators Research, 55*, 97-114.

*Montgomery, J. E., Stubbs, A. C., & Day, S. S. (1980). The housing environment of the rural elderly. *The Gerontologist, 20*, 444-451.

*Morris, E. W., Crull, S. R., & Winter, M. (1976). Housing norms, housing satisfaction and the propensity to move. *Journal of Marriage and the Family, 39*, 309-320.

Moss, M. S., & Lawton, M. P. (1982). Time budgets of older people: A window of four lifestyles. *Journal of Gerontology, 37*, 115-123.

*Nathanson, C. A., Newman, J. S., Moen, E., & Hiltabiddle, H. (1976). Moving plans among residents of a new town. *Journal of the American Institute of Planners, 42*, 295-302.

*Nelson, F. L. (1979). Residential dissatisfaction in the crowded urban neighborhood. *International Review of Modern Sociology, 8,* 227-238.

Neisser, U. (1988). Five kinds of self-knowledge. *Philosophical Psychology, 1,* 35-59.

Newman, S. J., & Struyck, R. J. (1984). An alternative targeting strategy for housing assistance. *The Gerontologist, 24,* 584-592.

*Normoyle, J. B. (1987). Fear of crime and satisfaction among elderly public housing residents: The impact of residential segregation. *Basic and Applied Social Psychology, 8,* 193-207.

O'Bryant, S. L. (1982). The value of home to older persons. *Research on Aging, 4,* 349-363.

*O'Bryant, S. L., & Wolf, S. M. (1983). Explanations of housing satisfaction of older homeowners and renters. *Research on Aging, 5,* 217-233.

*Okun, M. A. (1993). Predictors of volunteer status in a retirement community. *International Journal of Aging and Human Development, 36,* 57-74.

*Onibokun, A. G. (1976). Social system correlates of residential satisfaction. *Environment and Behavior, 8,* 323-344.

*Oswald, F., Schmitt, M., Sperling, U., & Wahl, H. W. (2000). Wohnen als Entwicklungskontext: Objektive Wohnbedingungen, Wohnzufriedenheit und Formen der Auseinandersetzung mit dem Wohnen in Ost- und Westdeutschland [Housing as developmental context: Objective housing conditions, housing satisfaction, and ways of coping with housing conditions in East and West Germany]. In P. Martin, U. Lehr, D. Roether, M. Martin, & A. Fischer-Cyrulis (Eds.), *Aspekte der Entwicklung im mittleren und höheren Lebensalter* (pp. 201-219). Darmstadt, Germany: Steinkopff.

Overton, R. C. (1998). A comparison of fixed-effects and mixed (random-effects) models for meta-analysis. *Psychological Methods, 3,* 354-379.

*Paulus, P. B., Nagar, D., Larey, T. S., & Camacho, L. M. (1996). Environmental, lifestyle, and psychological factors in the health and well-being of military families. *Journal of Applied Social Psychology, 26,* 2053-2075.

*Perrig-Chiello, P. (1997). *Wohlbefinden im Alter* [Well-being in old age]. Weinheim, Germany: Juventa.

*Potter, R. B. (1984). Perceived life domain satisfaction and social status. *Journal of Social Psychology, 124,* 259-260.

*Potter, R. B., & Coshall, J. T. (1987). Socio-economic variations in perceived life domain satisfaction: A southwest Wales case study. *Journal of Psychology, 127,* 77-82.

Pynoos, J. (1995). Home modifications. In G. L. Maddox (Ed.), *The encyclopedia of aging* (2nd ed., pp. 466-469). New York: Springer.

Raudenbush, S. W. (1994). Random effect models. In H. Cooper & L. V. Hedges (Eds.), *Handbook of research synthesis* (pp. 301-321). New York: Sage.

*Riemer, S. (1945). Maladjustment to family home. *American Sociological Review, 10,* 642-648.

*Ringel, N. B., & Finkelstein, J. C. (1991). Differentiating neighborhood satisfaction and neighborhood attachment among urban residents. *Basic and Applied Social Psychology, 12,* 177-193.

*Rogers, E. C., & Nikkel, S. R. (1979). The housing satisfaction of large urban families. *Housing and Society, 6,* 83-87.

*Rosow, I. (1967). *Social integration of the aged*. New York: Free Press.
*Rossi, P. H. (1955). *Why families move*. Glencoe, IL: Free Press.
*Rutman, D. L., & Freedman, J. L. (1988). Anticipating relocation: Coping strategies and the meaning for older people. *Canadian Journal on Aging, 7*, 17-31.
Saup, W. (1993). *Alter und Umwelt: Eine Einführung in die ökologische Gerontologie* [Aging and environment: An introduction into ecological gerontology]. Stuttgart, Germany: Kohlhammer.
*Scheidt, R. J., & Windley, P. G. (1983). The mental health of small-town rural elderly residents: An expanded ecological model. *Journal of Gerontology, 38*, 472-479.
*Schumacher, J., Gunzelmann, T., & Brähler, E. (1996). Lebenszufriedenheit im Alter [Life satisfaction in old age]. *Zeitschrift für Gerontopsychologie und -psychiatrie, 1*, 1-17.
*Sherman, S. R. (1972). Satisfaction with retirement housing: Attitudes, recommendations and moves. *Aging and Human Development, 3*, 339-366.
*Siara, C. S. (1980). *Komponenten der Wohlfahrt* [Components of welfare]. Frankfurt/Main, Germany: Campus.
*Sikorska, E. (1999). Organizational determinants of resident satisfaction with assisted living. *The Gerontologist, 39*, 450-456.
*Sirgy, M. J., & Cornwell, T. (2002). How neighborhood features affect quality of life. *Social Indicators Research, 59*, 79-114.
*Snider, E. L. (1980). Some social indicators for multiple family housing. *Social Indicators Research, 8*, 157-173.
*Speare, A. (1974). Residential satisfaction as an intervening variable in residential mobility. *Demography, 11*, 173-188.
*Stationery Office, The (2001). *Housing in England 1999/00*. London. Available online at www.housing.dtlr.gov.uk.
*Sweaney, A. L., Pittman, J. F., & Montgomery, J. E. (1984). The influence of marital status and age on the housing behavior of older southern women. *Journal of Housing for the Elderly, 2(3)*, 25-36.
*Talbott, J. F., & Kaplan, R. (1991). The benefits of nearby nature for elderly apartment residents. *International Journal of Aging and Human Development, 33*, 119-130.
*Teaff, J., Lawton, M. P., Nahemow, L., & Carlson, D. (1978). Impact of age integration on the well-being of elderly tenants in public homes. *Journal of Gerontology, 33*, 126-133.
*Thomae, H. (1983). *Alternsstile und Altersschicksale* [Patterns and fates of aging]. Bern, Germany: Huber.
*U.S. Census Bureau (1985-2001). *American housing survey for the United States: 1983-1999*. Washington, DC: U.S. Government Printing Office.
*U.S. Department of Agriculture Section 502 single family household survey (1998). Available online: www.ers.usda.gov/data/ruralhousing.
Veenhoven, R. (1996). Developments in satisfaction research. *Social Indicator Research, 37*, 1-46.
Wahl, H. W., Oswald, F., & Zimprich, D. (1999). Everyday competence in visually impaired older adults: A case for person-environment perspectives. *Gerontologist, 39*, 140-149.

*Weideman, S., & Anderson, J. R. (1982). Residents' perceptions of satisfaction and safety: A basis for change in multifamily housing. *Environment and Behavior, 14*, 695-724.

Weideman, S., & Anderson, J. R. (1985). A conceptual framework for residential satisfaction. In I. Altman (Ed.), *Home environments* (pp. 153-182). New York: Plenum.

*Wilner, D., Walkey, R., Pinkerton, T., & Tayback, M. (1962). *Housing environment and family life*. Baltimore: John Hopkins Press.

*Windley, P. G., & Scheidt, R. J. (1982). An ecological model of mental health among small-town rural elderly. *Journal of Gerontology, 37*, 235-242.

*Wood, L. A., & Johnson, J. (1979). Life satisfaction among the rural elderly: What do the numbers mean? *Social Indicators Research, 21*, 379-408.

*Zehner, R. B. (1976). Neighborhood and community satisfaction: A report on new towns and less planned suburbs. In J. F. Wohlwill, & D. Carlson (Eds.), *Environment and the social science: Perspectives and applications* (pp. 169-183). Washington, DC: APA.

CHAPTER 9

Neighborhoods, Health, and Well-Being in Late Life

NEAL KRAUSE
SCHOOL OF PUBLIC HEALTH AND THE INSTITUTE OF GERONTOLOGY
THE UNIVERSITY OF MICHIGAN

Sociologists have been studying neighborhoods for at least eight decades (Burgess, 1929). A good deal of this early research focused on how various aspects of the neighborhood environment affect physical and (especially) mental health (Faris & Dunham, 1939). Recently, there has been renewed interest in the health-related effects of neighborhoods. This research has been driven, in part, by the desire to learn more about how social inequalities influence health (Robert, 1999). Toward this end, a rapidly growing number of studies indicate that run-down and economically challenged neighborhoods exert an adverse effect on a wide array of health-related outcomes, including acute and chronic health conditions (Ross & Mirowsky, 2001), all-cause mortality (Kaplan, 1996), cognitive functioning (Espino, Lichtenstein, Palmer, & Hazuda, 2001), mental health (Ross, 2000), and a range of health behaviors, such as smoking, alcohol use, and dietary intake (see Pickett & Pearl, 2001, for a review of this research). However, with some notable exceptions (Krause, 1996; Lawton, 1989), a good deal of the research on neighborhoods and health has taken place outside social and behavioral gerontology. This has prompted some investigators to examine why gerontological research on the physical environment is in such a " . . . languishing state" (Parmelee & Lawton, 1990).

The purpose of this chapter is to rekindle interest in neighborhood conditions and health in late life. The discussion that follows is divided into six main sections. Issues in defining neighborhoods are examined first. Following this, various approaches to measuring neighborhood characteristics are evaluated in section two. Section three contains a discussion of age variations in the relationship between neighborhood characteristics and health. The fourth section provides an overview of theoretical perspectives that attempt to explain why neighborhoods may influence health

223

and well-being. Fifth, methodological and statistical issues in the assessment of neighborhood conditions are identified. Finally, suggestions for further research and additional issues for consideration are provided in the Discussion section.

DEFINING NEIGHBORHOODS

As Gutman and Popenoe observed some time ago, "The term 'neighborhood' . . . has become one of the most used, and also abused, terms in the lexicon of urban sociological analysis" (1970, p. 568). Two factors have contributed to this problem. The first involves the widespread practice of using a number of terms interchangeably with the neighborhood. For example, some researchers refer to local communities, others claim to be investigating physical, residential, or built environments, while yet others say they are studying the effects of residential locations (see Diez-Roux, 2001, for a detailed discussion of this problem). Second, some researchers plunge directly into the study of neighborhoods and health without carefully defining neighborhoods in the first place (Krause, 1993). This is unfortunate, because the lack of clear definitions makes it more difficult to develop good measures of neighborhoods, and it impedes the development of sound theories to explain how neighborhoods may influence health in late life.

Many years ago, Burgess (1929) spoke of neighborhoods as "natural areas" in the city that have well-recognized historical names, dividing lines (e.g., streets) that are jointly acknowledged by local residents, and boundaries that are claimed by local organizations, such as improvement associations, local newspapers, or political entities. There are, however, a number of problems with this definition. First, local residents may not recognize or use the same boundaries to define the same neighborhood. Second, some neighborhoods may not have well-recognized historical names. Third, it is difficult to see why the neighborhood characteristics identified by Burgess might be related to health. However, in fairness to Burgess, he was not primarily interested in studying the health-related effects of neighborhoods.

The last criticism of Burgess's (1929) research gets right to the heart of the matter. Maybe there is no one best way to define the neighborhood. Instead, as Diez-Roux (2001) argues, different definitions may be needed to study different research questions. So, for example, it makes sense to focus on geographically defined boundaries when assessing exposure to environmental toxins. But it might make more sense to focus on residents' subjective definitions of the neighborhood when evaluating factors that influence mental health.

This later strategy is captured in the work of Ross and Mirowsky, who set out to study the relationships between the neighborhood, physical health, and mental health by focusing on subjective perceptions of neighborhood disorder (Ross, 2000; Ross & Mirowsky, 2001). They define perceived neighborhood disorder as, " . . . visible cues indicating a lack of order and social control in a community" (Ross & Mirowsky, 1999). Visible signs of social disorder include the presence of people hanging out in the streets, panhandling, and public consumption of alcohol and drugs. In contrast, signs of physical disorder include the presence of rundown and abandoned buildings, vandalism, graffiti, and a high level of street noise. This approach to defining the neighborhood is useful because it begins to more clearly pinpoint factors that might be related to physical and mental health. However, it sidesteps the important issue of boundaries. Neighborhoods have either physical or psychological boundaries (Pickett & Pearl, 2001). If these boundaries are not specified clearly, then study participants may not be using the same referent when they answer questions about the neighborhood. This makes it more difficult for researchers to identify and explain the underlying causal factors that may be at work.

MEASURING NEIGHBORHOODS

Focusing on different ways of measuring or assessing neighborhoods provides another way of getting a handle on this elusive construct. More specifically, the process of devising sound operational definitions of the neighborhood forces researchers to think more deeply about the essential characteristics of neighborhood environments. Blalock's (1982) seminal work on auxiliary measurement theories highlights the importance of this process. He argues that theoretical statements and assumptions about the essential nature of the phenomena under study are embedded in measures of a construct. In addition, because measures are inherently selective, and emphasize some dimensions of a phenomenon over others, these auxiliary measurement theories set the stage for shaping the way that key constructs (e.g., the neighborhood) are related to other variables of interest (e.g., health). This means that if a researcher measures neighborhoods solely in terms of traffic noise levels (Ouis, 2001), he or she is likely to see very different results than if measures of psychological sense of community were used instead (Obst, Smith, & Zinkiewicz, 2002).

The literature contains a bewildering range of ways to measure neighborhoods. A simple way to organize this research is to think in terms of objective and subjective neighborhood measures.

OBJECTIVE NEIGHBORHOOD MEASURES

The most straightforward objective neighborhood measures consist of laboratory assessments of exposure to physical aspects of the neighborhood, such as environmental toxins or traffic noise. In the process of conducting this type of research, investigators may, for example, go to different geographical locations and measure traffic noise levels (Ouis, 2001). Then, once measurements are taken at a number of locations, geographical areas are clustered together based on their relative levels of traffic noise. After this has been accomplished, areas with different noise levels are compared to see if they exert a differential effect on health and well-being. These bench science measures of the neighborhood are quite valuable because they are highly standardized and can be replicated easily. Moreover, direct physiological connections can be made between things like exposure to environmental toxins and biochemical changes in the body. However, there are also some limitations associated with the use of this measurement strategy. More specifically, these bench science measures provide very narrow operational definitions of the neighborhood and overlook wider psychosocial factors that may be at work. For example, laboratory measures of the physical environment are not capable of capturing wider social structural influences (e.g., *socioeconomic status* [SES]) that shape exposure to environmental toxins and traffic noise in the first place.

Official public records constitute what is perhaps the most widely used approach to measuring neighborhoods. As Pickett and Pearl (2001) point out, researchers use these public records in a number of different ways. Some investigators operationally define neighborhoods in terms of census tracts or adjacent census blocks. Others focus instead on using census data to create areas that are homogeneous with respect to income, home ownership, housing values, the proportion of mother-only households, or the proportion of people who own a car. Yet, other investigators use federal poverty areas to define neighborhoods. In contrast to using census data, some researchers simply rely on existing political boundaries to delimit different neighborhoods. Finally, taking a somewhat different approach, Lawton, Nahemow, and Yeh (1980) focused on the availability of resources in the community, such as access to public transportation and health care.

There are several advantages associated with using official public records to devise neighborhood measures. First, they are relatively easy to obtain or create. Second, by using official data, there are some assurances that the measures are standardized across different neighborhoods, thereby facilitating the process of comparison. However, there are also some limitations involved in using these objective indicators. First, it is not clear whether local residents define neighborhoods in terms of things like census tracts. Second, many of the measures identified above are primarily economic in nature. This may create selection problems. More specifically, some investigators argue that people are sorted into neighborhoods based on their individual economic characteristics, and it is these individual economic characteristics that drive the observed relationship between aggregate measures of neighborhood income and health (Diez-Roux, 2001). Finally, administrative records do not capture certain neighborhood characteristics, such as unreported crime, that may affect the health and well-being of local residents.

SUBJECTIVE NEIGHBORHOOD MEASURES

A number of different strategies have been devised to assess residents' perceptions of the neighborhoods in which they live. Two are discussed below. The first deals with subjective ratings of a psychological sense of community, whereas the second involves subjective ratings of specific neighborhood characteristics.

There is a fairly substantial amount of research on the psychological sense of community. This construct is typically assessed with a fairly wide range of measures. For example, some studies use items that are designed to gauge the quality and character of interpersonal relationships that arise within specific communities. Other scales contain indicators that assess whether people feel they belong in their community and whether they are able to identify with the other people who live there (Obst et al., 2002). Evaluating the psychological sense of community is important because social identity theory suggests that psychological well-being is enhanced when individuals are committed to social groups, value them highly, and find emotional significance in being associated with them (Hogg & Abrams, 1988).

However, researchers must reflect carefully on the potential limitations associated with measures of the psychological sense of community. Obst and her associates use the following indicator to assess one aspect of the psychological sense of community: "I find it difficult to form a bond with other people who live in my local neighborhood" (Obst et al., 2002, p. 129). Several issues arise with the use of this item. First, because the local neighborhood is never defined, the respondent must determine what it means for himself or herself. As a result, it is likely that people residing in the same neighborhood will have different geographical locations in mind when they respond to this item. Second, this indicator may be confounded with psychological distress. More specifically, some people have difficulty forming close bonds with their neighbors because they have mental health problems (Joiner & Coyne, 1999). This could lead to obvious limitations in studies that attempt to assess the relationship between a psychological sense of community and measures of psychological distress, such as depressive symptoms.

Ross and Mirowsky (2001) take a different approach to measuring subjective neighborhood characteristics. More specifically, these investigators asked respondents to rate a number of different neighborhood conditions including the amount of graffiti that was present, whether the neighborhood was safe and clean, and whether there was too much alcohol use in the neighborhood. This measurement strategy is based on longstanding social psychological principles, which stipulate that we cannot study phenomena, such as neighborhoods, without first understanding how they are perceived by the people who live in them. As W. I. Thomas (1951) argued some time ago, adjustment is not a simply mechanical process in which cause and effect can be assessed by identifying objective conditions and studying objective responses to them. Instead, intervening between the two are subjective definitions of the situation.

Although many subjective aspects of neighborhood life have not been examined extensively in studies of older adults, one facet has been the object of considerable attention—the fear of crime (Krause, 1993; Lawton & Yafee, 1980). In fact, the study of the fear of neighborhood crime in late life has become a separate area of interest in its own right (Ferraro & LaGrange, 1992). The fear of crime has been shown to affect the lives of older adults in a number of ways. For example, some gerontologists maintain that the fear of crime among older people is so great that many live in a state of virtual self-imposed house arrest (Dowd, Sisson, & Kern, 1981). There is some evidence to support this concern. More specifically, research by Thompson and Krause (1998) suggests that the fear of crime is related to diminished social support in late life, especially among older people who live alone. This is important, because an extensive literature indicates that social support exerts a significant influence on the health of older people (Krause, 2001).

The study by Thompson and Krause (1998) makes a second useful contribution to the literature on subjective neighborhood measures by assessing something that is known as the incivility hypothesis (Burby & Rohe, 1989). This perspective states that physical disorder (i.e., incivility) in the neighborhood, such as abandoned buildings, graffiti, and broken or barricaded windows provide nonverbal cues to people, suggesting an area is dangerous. Subsequent empirical analysis by Thompson and Krause (1998) highlights the social implications of these unfavorable evaluations. More specifically, findings from this study indicate that subjective assessments of the quality of the neighborhood (e.g., subjective ratings of noise and air pollution, as well as the general conditions of buildings in the neighborhood) are strongly related to the fear of crime. These results are significant because they point to an essential issue that researchers should keep in mind when working with subjective neighborhood measures: In addition to assessing whether these indicators are related to health, it is important to look for potentially meaningful causal relationships among the various measures of subjective neighborhood characteristics.

Regardless of the specific subjective neighborhood measures that are used, it is also important for researchers to keep the potential limitations of these indicators in mind. Two especially important problems arise from having respondents rate the characteristics of their own neighborhoods. First, some subjective dimensions of the neighborhood might be confounded with psychological distress. For example, respondents who are suffering from a psychological disorder may be more fearful of neighborhood crime than study participants who are not struggling with mental health problems. Second, and in contrast, there is some evidence that respondents rate other aspects of the neighborhood, such as the condition of buildings, sidewalks, and other homes in an overly positive manner (Carp, 1994).

In an effort to deal with these problems, Krause (1998) tried a different approach to assessing neighborhood characteristics. Instead of relying on respondent reports, he had interviewers rate various aspects of the neighborhood, including the condition of other building and houses, as well as the condition of roads and sidewalks. Although this strategy may help eliminate the problems discussed, it presents a different set of challenges. In particular, Krause did not assess the inter-rater reliability of neighborhood assessments that were made by the interviewers. As a result, it cannot be determined if different interviewers would rate the same neighborhood in the same way. Fortunately, this problem has been addressed in recent research by Raudenbush and Sampson (1999). Using systematic social observation techniques, these investigators had trained personnel view videotapes of neighborhoods and rate them according to a set of prespecified criteria. The criteria rated in this study were similar to those used by Krause (1993) and Ross and Mirowsky (1999) (e.g., the amount of graffiti, litter on sidewalks, public use of alcohol).

Although the systematic social observation approach devised by Raudenbush and Sampson (1999) addresses concerns about obtaining acceptable levels of inter-rater reliability, it is not without its own limitations. First, this approach appears to be fairly time consuming and expensive. Moreover, it would be difficult to implement when studying the relationship between neighborhoods and health on a nationwide level. Finally, and perhaps most important, it makes subtle theoretical assumptions about how neighborhoods affect health. More specifically, this measurement strategy assumes that it is possible to obtain assessments of neighborhood conditions independently of the people who live there. However, other researchers maintain that in order to describe a neighborhood, and fully grasp its effects on health and well-being, we must see the neighborhood through the eyes of the local residents (Taylor, 2001). Simply put, in order to understand how neighborhoods influence physical and mental health, the people who live there must be aware of local conditions, perceive them, and evaluate them as problematic in some way (Ross & Mirowsky, 1999). The difference between these two points of view cuts right to the heart of Blalock's (1982) discussion of auxiliary measurement theory: All measures have embedded in them subtle theoretical assumptions about the fundamental nature of the phenomenon under study and the way in which it may influence outcomes, such as health.

But arguing that subjective self-rated aspects of the neighborhood are crucial does not mean that objective assessments are irrelevant, nor does it mean the two broad measurement strategies are inherently at odds with each other. Instead of pitting these different measurement strategies against each other in an effort to see which exerts the greatest direct effect on health, a more productive strategy might be to see how the two work together. Taking a causal modeling approach, it would be helpful to see how objective neighborhood characteristics influence subjective neighborhood ratings, and how both factors are, in turn, related to health. Ross and Mirowsky (1999) briefly review research on the relationship between self-rated neighborhood assessments and independent assessments made by research personnel. They report that the correlations across different studies and different measures range from .20 to .76. This suggests that while objective and subjective assessments of neighborhood characteristics are clearly related, objective ratings do not fully explain the variance in subjective evaluations. We need to know more about why this is so. More specifically, we need to know why some residents rate a given neighborhood characteristic as problematic whereas others fail to rate the same factor in the same way. Doing so may provide valuable clues and insight into how neighborhoods may influence the physical and mental health of the people who reside in them.

NEIGHBORHOODS, HEALTH, AND WELL-BEING IN LATE LIFE

There are two reasons why neighborhoods are more likely to play a larger role in shaping the health and well-being of older than younger people. The first is relatively straightforward and has to do with the length of time that older people spend in their neighborhoods. Data gathered in 1999 indicate that only 28.5 percent of men and 18.4 percent of women between the ages of 65 and 69 were employed outside the home (Federal Interagency Forum on Aging Related Statistics, 2000). By age 70, these labor force participation rates drop to 11.7 percent and 5.5 percent, respectively. Since many older people are no longer employed outside the home, they are likely to spend more time each day in their neighborhoods than individuals who are still in the labor force. In fact, one study of people aged 70 and over revealed that approximately 80 percent of the time in a typical day was spent in the home (Horgas, Wilms, & Baltes, 1998). This research is important because if neighborhoods affect physical and mental health, then these effects should be especially evident among the people who spend the most time in them.

Research on attachment to place represents a second way of showing why neighborhood effects may be more pronounced in late life. This concept is closely akin to the psychological sense of community. Attachment to place is not well defined, but it generally refers to affective bonds or linkages between people and specific geographical locations (Hidalgo & Hernandez, 2001). These geographical locations could refer either to specific residential locations (i.e., one's own home) or to the wider neighborhood environment. It is important to reflect on why attachment to place may become especially important as people grow older. Erikson's (1959) well-known theory of lifespan development provides a useful point of departure for showing why this may be so. In his view, the final stage of development deals with resolving the crisis of integrity versus despair. This is a time of deep introspection, when a person looks back over the life he or she has lived and attempts to accept the way things have turned out. Similar views may be found in Butler's research on the life review process (Butler & Lewis, 1982). He argues that as people enter late life, they invest a significant amount of time reviewing experiences they have had with an eye toward weaving their life stories into a more coherent whole.

There is some evidence that attachment to place may play a significant role in the important developmental process described by Erikson (1959). More specifically, the cumulative memories associated with specific places such as the neighborhood may play an important role in the life review process, thereby providing one way for resolving the crisis of integrity versus despair. In addition, neighborhoods represent the place where major roles in life, such as child rearing, are enacted. Finally, living in a neighborhood for an extended period of time may provide a sense of continuity that cannot be gleaned from other life domains, such as employment. Taken together, these factors may help explain why research shows that attachment to place becomes stronger as people grow older (Hidalgo & Hernandez, 2001) and why it appears to exert an important influence on their sense of well-being (Taylor, 2001).

Although research on attachment to place is helpful, most of the work that has been done focuses on how "good" neighborhood characteristics promote positive feelings of attachment. We need to know whether neighborhoods that are dilapidated and run-down have the opposite effect. More specifically, research is needed to see whether older people who reside in neighborhoods with a large number of abandoned or run-down buildings and high levels of crime fail to develop a strong sense of attachment to place, and if a weak sense of attachment to place is, in turn, associated with poor health and well-being.

Taken together, the theory and research reviewed in this section would appear to suggest that the relationship between neighborhoods and health should be more evident among older than younger people. Even so, recent reviews of the literature suggest that the potentially deleterious effects of run-down and economically depressed neighborhoods on health may actually become less evident with advancing age (Pickett & Pearl, 2001). Pickett and Pearl attribute these findings to survivor effects. In their view, years of living in disadvantaged neighborhoods have weeded out those who are less fit, leaving a core of relatively hardy survivors. However, most of the studies in their review define neighborhoods solely in terms of census tract data, and most do not consider subjective assessments of neighborhood conditions, like the ones devised by Ross and Mirowsky (1999). Clearly, more research is needed to explore age differences in the relationship between a full complement of objective and subjective neighborhood indicators and health.

THEORETICAL PERSPECTIVES ON NEIGHBORHOODS AND HEALTH

In his insightful discussion of causality, Suppes (1970) argues that, "The analysis of causes and their identification must always be relative to a conceptual framework" (p. 90). This means that empirically demonstrating that run-down neighborhoods are associated with physical health problems is not enough. Instead, researchers hoping to uncover a causal relationship must also devise well-articulated theories that identify the intervening mechanisms that link neighborhoods with health, and provide convincing explanations of how they operate. Unfortunately, theoretical explanations and conceptual frameworks in the study of neighborhoods and health are underdeveloped. In fact, a good deal of the work in this field provides little or no theory at all. In order to move the literature forward, more fully developed theoretical models are needed.

Four broad approaches to explaining the health-related effects of the neighborhood are reviewed below. The first involves specifying direct linkages between objective characteristics of the neighborhood and health; the second is concerned with explaining the effects of neighborhoods on health behavior; the third has to do with showing how subjective perceptions of neighborhoods may influence physical health status; and the fourth involves casting the study of neighborhood and health within a stress framework.

OBJECTIVE NEIGHBORHOOD CHARACTERISTICS AND HEALTH

As noted earlier, a good deal of research focuses on how exposure to environmental toxins influences the health of neighborhood residents (for reviews of this research, see Diez-Roux, 2001; Pickett & Pearl, 2001).

Relatively little theory is used in this work because most investigators merely correlate exposure to things like air pollution and respiratory disease. However, as noted earlier, this research typically overlooks the fact that wider social forces may exert an important influence on this relationship. More specifically, levels of exposure to environmental toxins are influenced by socioeconomic status (SES) because people with few economic resources are more likely to live in neighborhoods with high levels of air pollution (Lynch & Kaplan, 2000). In addition, there is a vast literature relating SES and health. Consequently, those who focus solely on exposure to environmental toxins and health are often unaware they are providing evidence of one way in which the social structure influences health.

When measures of objective neighborhood conditions were discussed above, it was noted that the majority of investigators in the field focus primarily on the effects of neighborhood economic conditions on health. Census data are typically used by these investigators to derive aggregate estimates of neighborhood economic well-being. However, these researchers often fail to provide an adequate explanation for why the neighborhood, instead of individual income, is an important factor. A large number of studies have been conducted that explain why a person's own income may influence his or her health (Marmot & Wilkinson, 1999), but it is harder to find clearly articulated models that explain why the aggregate income level of a person's neighborhood should have a similar, or even more important, effect.

NEIGHBORHOODS AND HEALTH BEHAVIORS

Other researchers turn to the assessment of health behaviors in an effort to explain how neighborhood conditions may affect health. For example, Reijneveld (1998) assessed the relationship between living in economically deprived neighborhoods, cigarette smoking, and health. The findings indicate that people who live in economically disadvantaged neighborhoods are more likely to smoke, and have more health problems than individuals who reside in more well-to-do neighborhoods. Unfortunately, these investigators do not fully explain why living in low-income neighborhoods might influence the use of tobacco. Some insight is provided by Jarvis and Wardle (1999). These investigators point out that the pattern of increased tobacco use among lower SES people may be explained by social modeling effects. In particular, they argue that because smoking rates are higher in lower SES areas, an individual is more likely to have significant others who smoke, and who serve as role models reinforcing the use of tobacco. However, this role-modeling mechanism has not been measured or evaluated directly in studies of neighborhood effects on cigarette smoking. Moreover, the utility of the social modeling perspective for studying tobacco use in late life has yet to be determined. Few people smoke for the first time when they reach late life. As a result, it seems unlikely that social modeling is a major factor for older people because this explanation appears to be more useful for explaining why people first decide to take up cigarette smoking.

Fortunately, Jarvis and Wardle (1999) provide additional evidence that may be more directly relevant to the older smoker. They provide data showing that although lower SES people are more likely to become smokers, they are substantially more likely to continue smoking than upper SES individuals. Moreover, they provide compelling data that show that levels of plasma continine (a measure of total nicotine intake) are dramatically higher in lower SES people, suggesting that they not only smoke more, but that they smoke each cigarette more intensively than upper SES persons. A key question is why this may be so. Jarvis and Wardle (1999) provide several potential explanations, but one appears to be especially relevant for the study of neighborhood effects. In particular, they suggest that lower SES people may smoke more for the euphoriant effects. According to this perspective, cigarette use becomes a form of self-medication that is pursued in an effort to regulate mood and cope with the hassles and strains arising from material deprivation. Because older people are less likely than younger people to move out of poverty areas (South & Crowder, 1997), they may be more likely to continue the use of tobacco for this reason. Unfortunately, no one has empirically evaluated this potentially important explanation in studies of older adults.

SUBJECTIVE NEIGHBORHOOD CHARACTERISTICS AND HEALTH

There are a number of ways in which subjective assessments of neighborhood characteristics may influence health and well-being in late life. For example, some investigators ask local residents to rate the conditions of sidewalks and roads in their neighborhoods (Krause, 1998). There may be relatively straightforward reasons why these fundamental aspects of the neighborhood infrastructure are related to health. More specifically, sidewalks that are in poor condition or stairways in apartments that are poorly maintained may increase the odds of falls or accidents, which is a major concern in late life. However, researchers who use these subjective ratings of the physical environment have yet to empirically evaluate the relationship between things like poorly maintained sidewalks and falls, per se. But, more important, empirically relating poorly maintained sidewalks to accidents and health status hardly constitutes a theory. Instead, like research with other more objective neighborhood characteristics, it merely represents the test of specific hypothesis.

Ross and Mirowsky (1999, 2001) provide what is probably the most well-developed theoretical rationale for why subjectively rated neighborhood characteristics may be related to physical and mental health. As discussed earlier, they focus on the notion of neighborhood disorder. They maintain that economically disadvantaged individuals are clustered in geographically defined areas or neighborhoods that have clear characteristics, including widespread poverty and a high proportion of mother-only households. These visible cues are perceived and evaluated by local residents as threatening and undesirable. As a result, alienation is widespread, informal social control weakens, and crime as well as other forms of social disorder (e.g., public consumption of alcohol) increase. This perspective makes a good deal of sense theoretically. Moreover, it relates neighborhood characteristics with a range of factors that are related to physical and mental health in late life (e.g., social isolation; see Berkman & Glass, 2000). Although their research shows that various characteristics of neighborhood disorder are related to physical (Ross & Mirowsky, 2001) and mental disorder (Ross, 2000), a number of the intervening linkages specified in their theory have not been empirically evaluated.

Fortunately, other investigators have assessed some of the intervening linkages identified by Ross and Mirowsky (1999). For example, research by Krause (1993) assessed the relationship between ratings of neighborhood characteristics by interviewers and study participants, distrust, and social isolation. His research reveals that older people who reside in run-down and dilapidated neighborhoods are more likely to be distrustful of others, and are more likely to be socially isolated than older people who live in more well-to-do neighborhoods.

A second problem with the perspective devised by Ross and Mirowsky (1999) arises from the fact that it doesn't explain why some, but not all, people who reside in disordered neighborhood environments subsequently experience physical or mental health problems. As their empirical research shows, there is no one-to-one correspondence between living in run-down neighborhoods and health. Researchers need to devise a theoretical scheme that can help explain why some older adults are vulnerable to undesirable neighborhood conditions whereas others do not appear to suffer any adverse effects even though they live in the same area. Some preliminary thoughts on how to approach this issue are provided in the next section.

NEIGHBORHOOD CHARACTERISTICS AS SOCIAL STRESSORS

The theoretical perspectives that have been examined so far point to a range of factors that may help explain how neighborhoods influence both physical and mental health. However, the number of mechanisms that have been identified is bewildering, and there appears to be no common thread that serves to bind them together in a more coherent whole. For example, some investigators attribute the health-related effects of neighborhoods to aggregate income levels, others suggest that self-medication with harmful substances such as tobacco or alcohol might be involved, yet other researchers argue that a wide range of subjective factors, like the fear of crime, may be important. A major goal of this chapter is to argue that researchers will be able to devise a more coherent and tightly integrated theory of neighborhood conditions and health if they take advantage of insights provided by research on stress.

Many of the subjective, and even a good number of the objective, neighborhood characteristics that have been identified in the literature may be construed as forms of stress. In some cases, the link is fairly obvious. For example, having an inadequate income or the fear of crime is certainly a stressful experience that impacts the lives of many older people. However, it may be less evident why other key neighborhood characteristics can be viewed within the context of stress. More specifically, it is important to specify why things like run-down and abandoned buildings or roads and sidewalks in a state of disrepair would be stressful. A number of researchers argue that local residents read the different physical characteristics of the neighborhood like a lexicon. When buildings are dilapidated and covered with graffiti, and when people hang out on street corners and openly consume alcohol, local residents may feel overwhelmed by the neighborhood environment and find it difficult to live comfortably within it (Krause, 1993).

But merely identifying neighborhood characteristics as potential sources of stress does not go far enough. For some time, researchers have argued that there are qualitatively different kinds of stressors (Pearlin, Menaghan, Lieberman, & Mullan, 1981). The distinction between acute stressors and chronic strains is especially useful when thinking about neighborhood stress. Acute stressors are events that are fairly short lived —they typically have a clear beginning and end, and they tend to peak and dissipate relatively quickly. In contrast, chronic strains are continuous and ongoing. As Lepore (1997) and others argue, deteriorated living environments constitute a significant source of ongoing chronic strain. This makes sense because neighborhood conditions typically do not change rapidly over time.

Viewing neighborhood characteristics as specific types of chronic strain is important because an extensive amount of research indicates that chronic strains tend to have a more deleterious effect on health than acute stressors. More specifically, research by McEwen (1998) and his colleagues indicates that repeated or persistent exposure to stress slowly exerts wear and tear on body organs that eventually leads to dysfunction and disease.

There is also some evidence that exposure to chronic strains compromises immune functioning, as well (Kiecolt-Glaser & Glaser, 1995).

In addition to creating physical health problems, chronic strains have important psychological consequences. For example, as Krause (1998) points out, people frequently lose hope when chronic strains are encountered because it seems as if there is no end in sight to their problems. This is especially true for people who live in deteriorated living conditions. More specifically, the lack of hope and optimism that arises from living in dilapidated neighborhoods has been documented in quantitative (Greenberg & Schneider, 1997) as well as qualitative studies, alike (Hughes, Tremblay, Rapoport, & Leighton, 1960; Stephens, 1976). The loss of hope and optimism is noteworthy because a number of researchers suspect they contribute to mental health problems (Nunn, 1996).

Although viewing neighborhood characteristics as specific types of chronic strain is useful, the stress perspective provides additional ways to help researchers better understand the effects of the neighborhood environment on health. Soon after researchers began working in the stress field, it became evident that people who were exposed to stress do not all subsequently become ill. This led investigators to hypothesize that some individuals are able to avoid the deleterious effects of stress because they rely on certain social and psychological resources to help them cope effectively with the events that arise in their lives (see Snyder, 2001, for a recent review of research on coping with stress). The same appears to be true with respect to neighborhood stressors as well (Krause, 1998). Not everyone who lives in deteriorated neighborhood conditions subsequently suffers from a physical or mental health problem. As a result, it is important for researchers to identify those who are at risk. Assessing the effects of coping resources represents an important point of departure. Yet, it is surprising to find very few studies in social and behavioral gerontology that explicitly evaluate the relationships among neighborhood conditions, coping resources, and health. This issue is explored in some detail below, by assessing the potentially important relationships among chronic neighborhood strain, social support, and health.

An extensive literature indicates that older people who have strong social support systems tend to cope more effectively with stress, and tend to enjoy better physical and mental health, than older adults who do not maintain close ties with others (Krause, 2001). Although a number of studies have evaluated social support in specific neighborhood settings, this literature suffers from at least four problems. First, most of this research has been done with adults of all ages, whereas very few studies focus specifically on older people. Second, most of the studies in this field don't explicitly correlate measures of neighborhood characteristics with neighborhood social support systems. As a result, it is more difficult to see how neighborhood conditions actually influence the social relationships of local residents. Third, many researchers do not attempt to evaluate the relationships among neighborhood social support systems, physical, and mental health. Finally, even when support is assessed in the study of neighborhood environments, most researchers rely on global measures that are designed to capture support provided by all social network members taken together, including those who do and do not reside in the same neighborhood as the study participant. But it may be important to take the source of support into consideration. More specifically, researchers need to know whether support provided specifically by one's neighbors is more efficacious than assistance that is obtained from other social network members who do not reside in the same neighborhood. Although no one has examined this issue in samples composed of older people, the discussion that follows shows why this may be an important issue to consider.

It is difficult to determine whether support provided specifically by one's neighbors would be more beneficial than assistance obtained from those outside the neighborhood. On the one hand, research indicates there are costs associated with seeking assistance from significant others. More specifically, some people are concerned that seeking and accepting help makes them appear weak or vulnerable, and unable to handle problems on their own (Eckenrode & Wethington, 1990). Moreover, in order for support to be effective, support providers must fully understand the situation of the support recipient, know what kind of assistance would work best, and determine the best way to provide it. Unfortunately, this does not always happen and as a result, sincere efforts to help may be miscarried (Coyne, Wortman, & Lehman, 1988). Based on this literature, it appears that assistance provided by neighbors is better for dealing with neighborhood problems because those who live close by are better able to understand the nature of the problem, and have a better insight into the specific types of assistance most helpful in dealing with it. Moreover, because neighbors are likely to be grappling with the same neighborhood stressors, it is unlikely they will blame the help recipient for not being able to deal with the problem in an effective manner.

But it is also possible to take the opposite position, and argue that people who reside in the same neighborhood as an older focal person may not be the best support providers. Hobfoll's (1998) social support deterioration model helps show why this may be so. This perspective is best understood within the context of economic problems, although it can be generalized to other stressful situations as well. Hobfoll argues that social networks are relatively homogeneous and comprise individuals who have access to similar resources. When people are economically challenged, they may turn to significant others for assistance. However, because potential help providers are likely to be faced with economic problems of their own, they are placed in the difficult situation of having to choose between keeping scarce resources for their own needs, or giving them to a needy other.

Hobfoll (1998) argues that when demands for assistance become too great, and resources are stretched too thin, support in these fragile networks may ultimately be withdrawn. It is important to point out that this problem is especially likely to arise when stressors are persistent and ongoing. As the work of Coyne et al. (1988) suggests, stressors that are intractable gradually wear down or burn out support providers, resulting in assistance that is ineffective at best, and openly hostile at its worst.

Given the current state of the literature, it is not possible to determine which of the two perspectives on the efficacy of neighborhood social support is more accurate. However, some insight into this issue is provided by two sources. First, Lepore, Evans, and Schneider (1991) conducted one of the few studies that assess the relationships among neighborhood strain, support from local residents, and psychological distress. These investigators focused on the effect of a neighborhood stressor that has not been discussed to this point—residential overcrowding. Their findings reveal that, initially, support from coresidents tended to offset the noxious effects of residential overcrowding on psychological distress. However, over time, the stress-buffering function of social support disappeared. This finding points to a critical feature of chronic neighborhood stressors. More specifically, it suggests that run-down and economically challenged neighborhoods may have a pernicious effect on health because they erode the very resources that are needed to cope effectively with them.

A small cluster of studies on social support in poverty areas provides further evidence that neighborhood support systems may not always be the most efficacious source of coping assistance. Belle (1982) conducted an empirical study of social support in a Boston poverty area. Consistent with the perspective devised by Hobfoll (1998), she found that local residents were reluctant to accept assistance from others because they were concerned they would not be able to reciprocate if current support providers needed help in the future. Some of the more dramatic evidence of the problems with social support systems in lower SES areas is provided by a qualitative study by Hughes et al. (1960). Referring to the residents of the lower SES area they studied, these investigators note that, "They find difficulties in family and community social relationships and expect inconsistency of affection and support from their fellows. Meeting hostility from their nearest human contacts, they react in many situations with avoidance and antipathy" (Hughes et al., 1960, p. 250; see also Stephens, 1976).

Even though the evidence appears to suggest that social support systems in run-down and economically challenged neighborhoods may not be functioning at an optimal level, it is important to keep two points in mind. First, this research suffers from a number of the problems that were identified earlier. More specifically, a good deal of this literature does not focus explicitly on older people. In addition, a careful examination of this work reveals that it was done in the most impoverished neighborhoods.

This raises an important but largely unexamined research question. Perhaps the problems identified by Hughes et al. (1960) and others apply only to the worst poverty areas, and that the same findings would not emerge if neighborhoods at the next SES level (i.e., working-class neighborhoods) were evaluated instead. Stated in more technical terms, perhaps there is a nonlinear relationship between neighborhood conditions and neighborhood support systems such that social network problems arise only in the most impoverished settings, but improve rapidly beyond that point.

Viewed more broadly, the research reviewed in this section indicates that casting the study of neighborhood conditions and health in a stress perspective provides several advantages. First, a diverse array of neighborhood characteristics can be pulled together into a single conceptual rubric (i.e., chronic strains) that helps more clearly identify why they might be associated with physical and mental health in late life. Second, assuming a stress perspective makes it possible to directly confront a longstanding problem in the literature. Rather than reacting passively to the neighborhood stressors that confront them, older people may take active steps to improve their situation. This is done, in part, by turning to coping resources that are at their disposal. This is especially important because virtually all the studies on neighborhood conditions and health have not made an effort to identify the steps local residents take in an effort to eradicate the neighborhood problems that confront them.

METHODOLOGICAL AND STATISTICAL ISSUES

In order to improve further the quality of research on neighborhood conditions and health in late life, it would be useful if researchers paid attention to three methodological and statistical issues that are often overlooked in gerontological research on the neighborhood. The first deals with the need to consider the influence of key confounding variables, the second is concerned with incorporating potentially valuable insights from the life course perspective, and the third has to do with the advantages afforded by multilevel modeling techniques.

It seems reasonable to argue that most of the problems faced by older people in their neighborhoods are economically driven. More specifically, SES appears to be the root cause of run-down and dilapidated buildings, poorly maintained streets and sidewalks, graffiti, public consumption of alcohol, and the fear of crime. But SES influences spread far beyond the neighborhood and touch the lives of older people in many other ways. For example, SES is clearly related to the occupations that people enter. This is important because people with low levels of educational attainment (one marker of SES) are more likely to take jobs that expose them to unsafe levels of toxic materials and solvents. Prolonged exposure to these environmental toxins has been shown to have a deleterious effect on health. Evidence of this may be found in a compelling study of nearly 4,000 older people in France. Dartigues and his colleagues found that lower SES elders were more likely than their upper SES counterparts to have worked in occupations that exposed them to unsafe levels of toxins (Dartigues et al., 1992). Moreover, these researchers report that people who worked in unsafe jobs when they were younger had a much higher risk of becoming cognitively impaired when they reached late life. These findings are important for the following reason. Earlier, research was reviewed which showed that older people who live in disadvantaged neighborhoods have higher levels of cognitive impairment than older adults who live in more well-to-do neighborhoods (Espino et al., 2001). But if the findings by Dartigues et al. (1992) are valid, then it becomes difficult to tell whether high levels of cognitive impairment are due to neighborhood effects, per se, or whether they reflect the influence of lifelong exposure to environmental toxins at work.

This dilemma presents two ways of thinking about occupations, neighborhoods, and health in late life. First, one might argue that because occupations typically determine where people live, findings that link neighborhood conditions with health-related outcomes (e.g., cognitive impairment) might be spurious. But there is a second, more profitable, way to approach this issue. More specifically, it is possible that occupations work synergistically with neighborhood characteristics to influence health. According to this view, there may be a statistical interaction effect between lifetime occupations and neighborhood characteristics on health, and the joint effects of these factors may be greater than their individual impact on health. Regardless of which perspective one assumes, the discussion of occupations, neighborhoods, and health reveals that neighborhoods do not exist in isolation from wider social structural influences, and as a result, it is important to consider the potentially important influence of the wider social context.

The need to consider lifelong occupations points to a second issue that has been overlooked in the study of neighborhoods and health in late life. Most researchers merely assess the relationship between neighborhood characteristics and health without attempting to determine how long study participants have resided in their current neighborhood. Unfortunately, this overlooks the fact that there may be significant variations in a person's residential history: Some older people may be lifelong residents whereas others may have moved into the neighborhood only recently. As a result, pooling subjects who have lived in a neighborhood for different lengths of time must be handled with care. If people have lived in a neighborhood for a relatively short period of time, then their current health status may reflect the influence of where they lived in the past.

Although people who are born into poor neighborhoods generally remain in poor neighborhoods for most of their lives, there are substantial variations in this process by age and race (South & Crowder, 1997). To the extent that this is true, the impact of current neighborhood characteristics on health may be contingent upon the characteristics of previous residential locations. This suggests that it may be useful to see if the current neighborhood environment interacts with the characteristics of previous residential locations to influence health. In order to perform this type of analysis, researchers must obviously obtain residential history data. This compounds the problems of doing research in this field, but it holds out the promise of more accurately specifying the relationship between current neighborhood conditions and health. Viewed in a more general way, this issue provides yet another reason why a life course perspective is essential in research with older adults (George, 1996).

Finally, the study of neighborhood effects is challenging because researchers are attempting to show that a larger social entity called the "neighborhood" has effects on health above and beyond the influence of individual respondent characteristics. In essence, the intent is to show that the whole (i.e., the neighborhood) is larger than the sum of the parts (i.e., the individuals who reside in them). This research is exciting because it represents an important step toward conducting research that is truly sociological in nature. But it is difficult to tease apart aggregate and individual-level influences. The problem arises because, as Ross and Mirowsky point out, "Disadvantaged neighborhoods contain persons who, on average, are disadvantaged themselves; thus it is possible that the geographically-defined places have no effect independent of the demographic characteristics of their residents" (Ross & Mirowsky, 2001, p. 262). One way to approach this problem is to develop multilevel data sets in which data on individual cases (e.g., individual income) are nested with aggregate-level data on the neighborhood (e.g., census block-level income). Then, by including both aggregate and individual-level variables in the same regression equation, net neighborhood effects of the individual-level influences on health can be estimated. These sophisticated multilevel modeling techniques have been used fairly widely in research with younger people (see Pickett & Pearl, 2001, for a review of 25 studies), but few researchers in social and behavioral gerontology appear to have taken advantage of them. Doing so should be a high priority for the future.

DISCUSSION

Many older people spend a good deal of time at home, in their neighborhoods (Horgas et al., 1998). In addition, many have lived in the same neighborhood for decades: They have raised their children there and they have grown old there. Consequently, as some investigators have pointed out, attachment to these places runs deep in late life (Taylor, 2001). Yet, we know so little about neighborhood effects in late life. In particular, social and behavioral gerontologists do not know enough about how important neighborhood characteristics may affect physical and mental health, even though research with younger adults suggests this may be an important area of inquiry (Pickett & Pearl, 2001). Outside of the pioneering work of Lawton and a few others (Lawton et al., 1980), papers that assess the effects of the neighborhood in late life are hard to find in the gerontological literature. So it was out of necessity that a good deal of the empirical research that was reviewed in this chapter was conducted with adults of all ages. This situation is compounded by problems in the measurement of neighborhoods, as well as the lack of adequate theoretical frameworks for explaining neighborhood effects.

With respect to measurement, researchers have yet to successfully grapple with the distinction between objective and subjective neighborhood indices. A central premise in this chapter is that the two are not inherently at odds, and that a greater understanding of neighborhood characteristics may be obtained by studying how objective conditions influence subjective assessments of the neighborhood environment. But, when taken down to the most fundamental level, it was assumed that it is subjective assessments of the neighborhood that are likely to exert the most significant direct effects on health and well-being. This notion is hardly new in the literature. In his classic work on the city, Park (1923) argued that the city, " . . . is something more than a congeries of individual men and social conveniences—streets, buildings, electric lights, tramways, and telephones, etc.; something more than a mere constellation of institutions and administrative devices. . . . The city is, rather, a state of mind" (p. 577). Just like cities, neighborhoods are, in the final analysis, a state of mind. They are a set of subjective perceptions, beliefs, and reactions that older people construct in order to negotiate their immediate physical and social environment. But they are more than just individual perceptions. As Burgess (1929) pointed out in his definition of natural areas, neighborhoods are determined in part by agreed upon natural boundaries (e.g., roads). This suggests that instead of being an entirely individual matter, a subjective sense of the neighborhood is socially constructed, both by the people who live there, and by those who reside in other places. This means that merely assessing the interface between objective and individual subject assessments of the neighborhood doesn't go far enough. Instead, we must learn more about how subjective perceptions of the neighborhood are socially constructed.

Earlier, research was reviewed which suggests that the social support systems in run-down and dilapidated neighborhoods are underdeveloped. Yet, Argyle's (1994) review of research conducted primarily in the United Kingdom indicates that, " . . . the effects of neighbors and neighborhood groups on happiness and mental health are actually greater for those who are lower-class, old, and living alone" (p. 73). This suggests there may be significant variation in the efficacy of lower SES neighborhood networks. We need to learn more about why this may be so. Why is it that residents in some local areas develop strong social networks that foster a sense of collective self-efficacy (i.e., empowerment—see Zimmerman, 2000) whereas others do not? Earlier, research using multilevel analyses was hailed as a significant advance in the literature on neighborhood effects. Yet, researchers who use this technique typically focus on objective aggregate data, such as average neighborhood income. Aggregate measures of subjective neighborhood perceptions should be evaluated in the same way as well. For example, does an aggregate or collective sense of empowerment help explain variance in health outcomes above and beyond the influence of individual feelings of self-efficacy?

With respect to theory, a major goal of this study was to emphasize the relative contributions of the life stress perspective. Here, the intent was to show that many objective and subjective characteristics can be profitably viewed as chronic strains, thereby providing one way of pulling a wide array of seemingly disparate indicators into a more coherent whole. Moreover, it was argued that the stress perspective holds out the promise of being able to explain individual variations in response to neighborhood conditions through the study of coping resources. Social support figured prominently in this respect, but it is only one of a range of potentially important resources that are worthy of further consideration. For example, a growing number of studies suggest that religion helps some people deal more effectively with stress (Pargament, 1997), that people may become more religious as they grow older (Wink & Dillon, 2001), and that lower SES people tend to be more religious than their upper SES counterparts (Koenig, McCullough, & Larson, 2001). If all this is true, then perhaps involvement in religion also helps older people cope more effectively with neighborhoods that are dilapidated and run down. In fact, a recent study by Krause (1998) suggests this may be the case. Clearly, the study of this, as well as other potentially important coping resources may help to move the literature on undesirable neighborhood conditions and health further along.

In addition to these issues, a host of other factors should be examined. For example, we need to know more about racial, ethnic, and cultural variations in response to neighborhood conditions. So far, most of the work that has been done on this issue focuses on how neighborhood racial and socioeconomic conditions influence things like adolescent premarital childbearing (South & Baumer, 2000) or the fear of crime (Chiricos, McEntire, & Gertz, 2001), but very little empirical work has focused specifically on older groups of racial minorities. We need to know whether centuries of racial prejudice and discrimination have fostered a deeper sense of community and social solidarity than is typically found in Caucasian majority neighborhoods. For example, does the realization that social structural constraints have created and maintained disordered neighborhood conditions change the way older African Americans evaluate the places in which they live, and do these external causal attributions serve to blunt the potentially deleterious effects of run-down neighborhoods on physical and mental health? Or, alternatively, do social structural barriers supported by prejudice and discrimination exacerbate the effects of deteriorated neighborhood conditions and lead, instead, to the loss of hope and the collapse of ethnic support systems? In the process, more research is needed on how historical and economic factors may shape the way members of different ethnic groups react to their local neighborhood environments. For example, Cuban Americans came to the United States under very different historical and economic circumstances than Mexican Americans (Boswell & Curtis, 1984). We need to know more about how these wider social forces shape the way neighborhoods are perceived and utilized by members of different ethnic and minority group members.

So far, the wide majority of studies on neighborhood conditions and health have focused on the potential influence of urban neighborhoods. This probably reflects the early and pervasive influence of Burgess (1929) and others. Although the study of urban neighborhoods has provided many valuable insights, we need to know more about the ways in which rural neighborhoods may influence the health and well-being of older residents. More specifically, we need to know if the problems faced by rural neighborhood residents differ from those that confront older people living in urban neighborhoods, and we need to know if these relatively unique rural circumstances also influence health and well-being. For example, more research is needed to compare and contrast the effects of economically driven population loss in urban and rural neighborhoods (Norris-Baker & Scheidt, 1994).

Clearly, research on the neighborhood in late life remains in its infancy. Yet, as this chapter has revealed, perhaps no area of social gerontology holds greater promise for showing how macrolevel social forces can shape individual perceptions, behaviors, and health. Research on neighborhoods and health is progressing rapidly in the wider literature on younger adults (Diez-Roux, 2001). It is time for social and behavioral gerontologists to pick up the pace.

ACKNOWLEDGEMENTS

This research was supported by the following grant from the National Institute on Aging: RO1 AG09221 (Neal Krause, Principal Investigator). Address all communications to Neal Krause, Department of Health Behavior and Health Education, School of Public Health, the University of Michigan, 1420 Washington Heights, Ann Arbor, MI 48109-2029; e-mail: nkrause@umich.edu.

246   KRAUSE

REFERENCES

Argyle, M. (1994). *The psychology of social class.* London: Routledge.
Belle, D. (1982). *Lives in stress: Women and depression.* Beverly Hills, CA: Sage.
Berkman, L. F., & Glass, T. (2000). Social integration, social networks, social support, and health. In L. F. Berkman & I. Kawachi, I. (Eds.), *Social epidemiology* (pp. 137-173). New York: Oxford University Press.
Blalock, H. M. (1982). *Conceptualization and measurement in the social sciences.* Beverly Hills, CA: Sage.
Boswell, T. D., & Curtis, J. R. (1984). *The Cuban-American experience: Culture, images, and perspectives.* Totawa, NJ: Rowman and Allanheld.
Burby, R. J., & Rohe, W. M. (1989). Deconcentration of public housing: Effects on residents' satisfaction and their living environments, and their fear of crime. *Urban Affairs Quarterly, 25,* 117-141.
Burgess, E. W. (1929). Basic social data. In T. V. Smith & L. D. White (Eds.), *Chicago: An experiment in social science research* (pp. 47-66). Chicago: University of Chicago Press.
Butler, R. N., & Lewis, M. I. (1982). *Aging and mental health.* St. Louis, MO: Mosby.
Carp, F. M. (1994). Assessing the environment. *Annual Review of Gerontology and Geriatrics, 14,* 302-323.
Chiricos, T., McEntire, Ranee, & Gertz, M. (2001). Perceived racial and ethnic composition of neighborhood and perceived risk of crime. *Social Problems, 48,* 322-340.
Coyne, J. C., Wortman, C. B., & Lehman, D. R. (1988). The other side of support: Emotional overinvolvement and miscarried helping. In B. H. Gottlieb (Ed.), *Marshaling social support: Formats, processes, and effects* (pp. 305-330). Newbury Park, CA: Sage.
Dartigues, J. F., Gagnon, M., Letenneur, L., Barberger-Gateau, P., Commenges, D., Evaldre, M., & Salamon, R. (1992). Principal lifetime occupation and cognitive impairment in a French elderly cohort (Paquid). *American Journal of Epidemiology, 135,* 981-988.
Diez-Roux, A. V. (2001). Investigating neighborhood and area effects on health. *American Journal of Public Health, 91,* 1783-1789.
Dowd, J., Sisson, R., & Kern, D. (1981). Socialization to violence among the aged. *Journal of Gerontology, 36,* 350-361.
Eckenrode, J., & Wethington, E. (1990). The process and outcome of mobilizing social support. In S. Duck & R. C. Silver (Eds.), *Personal relationships and social support* (pp. 83-103). London: Sage.
Erikson, E. (1959). *Identity and the life cycle.* New York: International University Press.
Espino, D. V., Lichtenstein, M. J., Palmer, R. F., & Hazuda, H. P. (2001). Ethnic differences in Mini-Mental State Examination (MMSE) scores: Where you live makes a difference. *Journal of the American Geriatrics Society, 49,* 538-548.
Faris, R. E., & Dunham, H. W. (1939). *Mental disorders in urban areas: An ecological study of schizophrenia and other psychoses.* Chicago: University of Chicago Press.
Federal Interagency Forum on Aging Related Statistics. (2000). Older Americans 2000: Key indicators of well-being. Hyattsville, MD: Federal Interagency Forum on Aging Related Statistics.

Ferraro, K. F., & LaGrange, R. L. (1992). Are older people most afraid of crime? Reconsidering age differences in the fear of victimization. *Journal of Gerontology: Social Sciences, 47,* S233-S244.

George, L. K. (1996). Missing links: The case for a social psychology of the life course. *The Gerontologist, 36,* 248-255.

Greenberg, M., & Schneider, D. (1997). Neighborhood quality, environmental hazards, personality traits, and residential actions. *Risk Analysis, 17,* 169-175.

Gutman, R., & Popenoe, D. (1970). *Neighborhood, city, and metropolis: An integrated reader in urban sociology.* New York: Random House.

Hidalgo, M. C., & Hernandez, B. (2001). Place attachment: Conceptual and empirical questions. *Journal of Environmental Psychology, 21,* 273-281.

Hobfoll, S. E. (1998). *Stress, culture, and community: The psychology and philosophy of stress.* New York: Plenum.

Hogg, M. A., & Abrams, D. (1988). *Social identifications: A social psychology of intergroup relations and group processes.* London: Routledge.

Horgas, A. L., Wilms, H. U., & Baltes, M. M. (1998). Daily life in very old age: Everyday activities as expression of successful living. *The Gerontologist, 38,* 556-568.

Hughes, C. C., Tremblay, M. A., Rapoport, R. N., & Leighton, A. (1960). *People of Cove and Woodlot.* New York: Basic Books.

Jarvis, M. J., & Wardle, J. (1999). Social patterning of individual health behaviors: The case of cigarette smoking. In M. Marmot & R. G. Wilkinson (Eds.), *Social determinants of health* (pp. 240-255). New York: Oxford University Press.

Joiner, T., & Coyne, J. C. (1999). *The interactional nature of depression.* Washington, DC: American Psychological Association.

Kaplan, G. (1996). People and places: Contrasting perspectives on the association between social class and health. *International Journal of Health Services, 26,* 989-998.

Kiecolt-Glaser, J. K., & Glaser, R. (1995). Psychoneuroimmunology and health consequences: Data and shared mechanisms. *Psychosomatic Medicine, 57,* 269-274.

Koenig, H. G., McCullough, M. E., & Larson, D. B. (2001). *Handbook of religion and health.* New York: Oxford University Press.

Krause, N. (1993). Neighborhood deterioration and social isolation in later life. *International Journal of Aging and Human Development, 36,* 9-38.

Krause, N. (1996). Neighborhood deterioration and self-rated health in late life. *Psychology and Aging, 11,* 342-352.

Krause, N. (1998). Neighborhood deterioration, religious coping, and changes in health during late life. *The Gerontologist, 38,* 653-664.

Krause, N. (2001). Social support. In R. H. Binstock & L. K. George (Eds.), *Handbook of aging and the social sciences,* (5th ed., pp. 272-294). San Diego, CA: Academic Press.

Lawton, M. P. (1989). Three functions of the residential environment. *Journal of Housing for the Elderly, 5,* 35-50.

Lawton, M. P., Nahemow, L., & Yeh, T. M. (1980). Neighborhood environments and the well-being of older tenants in planned housing. *International Journal of Aging and Human Development, 11,* 211-227.

Lawton, M. P., & Yaffe, S. (1980). Victimization and fear of crime in elderly public housing tenants. *Journal of Gerontology, 35,* 768-779.

Lepore, S. J. (1997). Social-environmental influences on the chronic stress process. In B. H. Gottlieb (Ed.), *Coping with chronic stress* (pp. 133-160). New York: Plenum.

Lepore, S. J., Evans, G. W., & Schneider, M. L. (1991). Dynamic role of social support in the link between chronic stress and psychological distress. *Journal of Personality and Social Psychology, 61*, 899-909.

Lynch, J., & Kaplan, G. (2000). Socioeconomic position. In L. F. Berkman & I. Kawachi (Eds.), *Social epidemiology* (pp. 13-35). New York: Oxford University Press.

Marmot, M., & Wilkinson, R. G. (Eds.). (1999). *Social determinants of health.* New York: Oxford University Press.

McEwen, B. S. (1998). Protective and damaging effects of stress mediators. *New England Journal of Medicine, 338*, 171-179.

Norris-Baker, C., & Scheidt, R. J. (1994). From "Our Town" to "Ghost Town"? The changing context of home for rural elders. *International Journal of Aging and Human Development, 38*, 181-202.

Nunn, K. P. (1996). Personal hopefulness: A conceptual overview of the relevance of the perceived future to psychiatry. *British Journal of Medical Psychology, 69*, 227-245.

Obst, P., Smith, S. G., & Zinkiewicz, L. (2002). An exploration of sense of community, part 3: Dimensions and predictors of psychological sense of community in geographical communities. *Journal of Community Psychology, 30*, 119-133.

Ouis, D. (2001). Annoyance from road traffic noise: A review. *Journal of Environmental Psychology, 21*, 101-120.

Pargament, K. I. (1997). *Psychology of religious coping: Theory, research, and practice.* New York: Guilford.

Park, R. E. (1923). The city: Suggestions for the investigation of human behavior in the urban environment. *American Journal of Sociology, 20*, 577-612.

Parmelee, P. A., & Lawton, M. P. (1990). The design of special environments for the aged. In J. E. Birren & K. W. Schaie (Eds.), *Handbook of the psychology of aging* (pp. 464-488). New York: Academic Press.

Pearlin, L. I., Menaghan, E., Lieberman, M., & Mullan, J. (1981). The stress process. *Journal of Health and Social Behavior, 19*, 2-21.

Pickett, K. E., & Pearl, M. (2001). Multilevel analysis of neighborhood socioeconomic context and health outcomes: A critical review. *Journal of Epidemiology and Community Health, 55*, 111-122.

Raudenbush, S. W., & Sampson, R. J. (1999). Econometrics: Toward a science of assessing ecological settings with application to the systematic observation of neighborhoods. *Sociological Methodology, 29*, 1-41.

Reijneveld, S. A. (1998). The impact of individual and area characteristics on urban socioeconomic differences in smoking and health. *International Journal of Epidemiology, 27*, 33-40.

Robert, S. A. (1999). Socioeconomic position and health: The independent contribution of community economic context. *Annual Review of Sociology, 25*, 489-516.

Ross, C. E. (2000). Neighborhood disadvantage and adult depression. *Journal of Health and Social Behavior, 41*, 177-187.

Ross, C. E., & Mirowsky, J. (1999). Disorder and decay: The concept and measurement of perceived neighborhood disorder. *Urban Affairs Review, 34*, 412-432.

Ross, C. E., & Mirowsky, J. (2001). Neighborhood disadvantage, disorder, and health. *Journal of Health and Social Behavior, 42,* 258-276.

Snyder, C. R. (2001). *Coping with stress: Effective people and processes.* New York: Oxford University Press.

South, S. J., & Baumer, E. P. (2000). Deciphering community and race effects on adolescent premarital childbearing. *Social Forces, 78,* 1379-1408.

South, S. J., & Crowder, K. D. (1997). Escaping distressed neighborhoods: Individual, community, and metropolitan influences. *American Journal of Sociology, 102,* 1040-1084.

Stephens, J. (1976). *Loners, losers, and lovers: Elderly tenants in a slum hotel.* Seattle: University of Washington Press.

Suppes, P. (1970). *A probabilistic theory of causality.* Amsterdam: North-Holland Publishing.

Taylor, S. A. (2001). Place identification and positive realities of aging. *Journal of Cross-Cultural Gerontology, 16,* 5-20.

Thomas, W. I. (1951). *Social behavior and personality: Contributions of W. I. Thomas to theory and research* (edited by E. H. Volkart). New York: Social Science Research Council.

Thompson, E. E., & Krause, N. (1998). Living alone and neighborhood characteristics as predictors of social support in late life. *Journal of Gerontology: Social Sciences, 53B,* S354-S364.

Wink, P., & Dillon, M. (2001). Religious involvement and health outcomes in late adulthood: Findings from a longitudinal study of women and men. In T. G. Plante & A. C. Sherman (Eds.), *Faith and health: Psychological perspectives* (pp. 75-106). New York: Guilford.

Zimmerman, M. A. (2000). Empowerment theory: Psychological, organizational, and community level analysis. In J. Rappaport & E. Seidman (Eds.), *Handbook of community psychology* (pp. 43-63). New York: Plenum.

CHAPTER 10

Technology and the Good Life: Challenges for Current and Future Generations of Aging People

HEIDRUN MOLLENKOPF
GERMAN CENTER FOR RESEARCH ON AGING AT THE UNIVERSITY OF HEIDELBERG

JAMES L. FOZARD
FLORIDA GERONTOLOGICAL RESEARCH AND
TRAINING SERVICES, PALM HARBOR

At a rapidly increasing rate, technology has proliferated into all domains of private and public life, both in the form of new products and in the electronic user interfaces of contemporary versions of familiar products. Technologies have become an essential part of the environment in the domain of industrial manufacturing and the organization of work, the creation and communication of information, and the rationalization of services and interactions between producers and consumers. The impact of technology on the private everyday world in which aging individuals live is also growing constantly. As pointed out by Lawton (1998), the changing interactions between persons and their (mechanized) environments can either support or deter persons in their activities. The way older people lead their daily lives and take part in society can be facilitated or complicated by continuing developments in household technology, residential infrastructure, public and private means of transportation, communications technologies, rehabilitation aids, and the increasing automation of services, depending on the design, ease of handling, proliferation, and accessibility of all these things. Ongoing advances in technology have enormous potential for improving how people age at any point in their lives. However, adaptations to the technologically based environment may create frustrating restrictions and dependencies in behavior that result in inequalities of access and use by subgroups of the population—including various cohorts of aging persons.

The remainder of this chapter has four parts. The first is a condensed overview of the emerging literature on technology and aging. The second part discusses the various functions technology can fulfill for older people's everyday life: prevention of or compensation for age-related losses in function; enhancement of new social, educational and artistic activities; and technical support to caregivers of persons needing care. It will focus on the options of technologies in the domains of housekeeping (domestic appliances), communication, information, and entertainment, collectively, *information and communication technology* (ICT), mobility, assistive and medical technologies, and integrated "intelligent" systems. Collectively, these are the opportunities afforded by advances in technology. But the increasing pace of technology developments inside and outside the home provides challenges to its users, challenges that are often greater for older than for younger persons. Therefore, the third part concerns the dynamics of accessibility and the affordability of technologies and its acceptability by older persons. The analysis will indicate that innovative applied *person-environment* (P-E) research and consistent efforts to use consumer input into product design and distribution will be needed to assess the significance of the product environment for the autonomy and self-awareness of aging men and women. The fourth part of the chapter examines how recent technological developments will continue to change the traditional categorization of functions and lead to new definitions of what is near or far, healthy or impaired, autonomous or dependent. Changes in technology will continue to create both positive options as well as social risks for the coming generations of older adults. It will be argued that prevailing tendencies of focusing on the microperspective of person-technology interactions must be complemented by macrosociological and social policy viewpoints.

THE EMERGING TOPIC OF TECHNOLOGY AND AGING

The meaning that technology's progressive infiltration of the environment has for people in old age has been addressed for about three decades. The options that "low" technologies and "high" technologies offer for the autonomous living of aging men and women was probably first stressed in the *Office of Technology Assessment's* (OTA) 1984 report, *Technology and Aging in America* (OTA, 1984; see also Festervand & Wylde, 1988; Haber, 1986). Lesnoff-Caravaglia (1988) pointed to the simultaneous progression of population aging and technological advancements. Technical aids have always been utilized where the anthropological prerequisites of human beings, their strength and their skill, did not suffice to deal with the demands of specific environments or in historical or life history situations.

However, the particular weakness of the *conditio humana* in old and very old age defines a new potential for technology.

The life history aspect of aging-technology interaction has been accorded little attention in theoretical discussion thus far, and the nature of its treatment in empirical studies has been more practical than theoretical. Research interest in the topic tends to be problem centered, usually relating to specific areas of technology (Kruse, 1992). For example, researchers are looking for ways in which technology can help people overcome socio-structural difficulties stemming from the population's growing share of elderly people, particularly the very old. The development and use of technical aids, for instance, is being studied primarily with an eye to reducing costs by giving outpatient care rather than hospitalizing the individual. Other major subjects of inquiry are home furnishings, home adaptation, and the use of technical aids to help elderly people run their homes independently if they come to require help or care; the general accessibility of the dwelling's immediate vicinity; means of transportation, and the infrastructure as a whole; and the use of computers and "new media" (Czaja, 1996; Czaja & Sharit, 1998; Fisk & Rogers, 2002). The spotlight in recent years has been on user-friendly technological design, especially the competencies, ergonomic context, and needs of old people (Coleman, 1998; Freudenthal, 1998), and on the acceptance and use of modern technologies and integrated systems (Fozard, Rietsema, Bouma, & Graafmans, 2000; Rogers, Meyer, Walker, & Fisk, 1998; Rudinger, 1996).

Since the beginning of the 1990s, a new scientific discipline called *gerontechnology* has been established to address the broad scope of issues related to technology and aging (Charness, Czaja, Fisk, & Rogers, 2001; Fabris, Marcellini, & Brizioli, 1996; Fozard, Graafmans, Rietsema, et al., 1997; Harrington & Harrington, 2000; Reents, 1996; van Berlo, Bouma, Ekberg, et al., 1997).[1] Among the major features of this scientific approach is its focus on all day-to-day life domains of older people, not exclusively on illness and chronic conditions, as was the case with more traditional rehabilitation and assistive technology approaches.

A specific direction in research looks at the growing information networks in society and the possibility of establishing new forms of relationships, information, and counseling based on ICT. This includes both a technology implementation to meet individual needs for safety, information, and contact, as well as possible ways to provide emergency and long-term care (Charness, Park, & Sabel, 2001; Campbell, Dries, & Gilligan, 1999;

---

[1] The basic ideas and contributions of this interdisciplinary discipline are described in the proceedings of its four international meetings of the International Society of Gerontechnology, a textbook, and a peer-reviewed journal, *Gerontechnology* (Bouma & Graafmans, 1992; Graafmans, Taipale, & Charness, 1998; Pieper, Vaarama, & Fozard, 2002; Gerontechnology vol. 2, 1). The journal may be viewed online at gerontechjournal.net.

PROMISE, 1998). The European TIDE (*Telematics for the Integration of Disabled & Older People in Europe*) and IST (*Information Society Technologies*) programs, in particular, placed, and still place, great emphasis on how to use ICT to provide assistance and services to the elderly and disabled to help them maintain an autonomous lifestyle (Bühler & Knops, 1999; Placencia Porrero & Ballabio, 1998).

A final area of growing research is the networking of previously isolated devices and systems into an "intelligent house" or "Smart Home." What is of particular interest here is the extent to which networking, both in and outside the home, can open up new, independent areas of action to old people in the future, and/or place new restrictions or dependencies on them. Advantages of networked systems are seen in terms of ecology and economy, comfort, and safety (Bonner, 1998; Glatzer, Fleischmann, Heimer, et al., 1998; Meyer, Schulze, Helten, & Fischer, 2001; van Berlo, 2002).

OPPORTUNITIES OF TECHNOLOGY FOR EVERYDAY LIFE IN OLD AGE

Technical products offer a multitude of positive opportunities for the preservation of independence, mobility, and social participation, as well as for supporting people in need of care.

HOUSEHOLD TECHNOLOGY

In the domestic environment, appropriate household technology can reduce physical hardship and thus make dealing with tiresome tasks easier, particularly for persons with failing strength who face a steady increase in problems with everyday demands. An increasing number of products are being developed favored by concepts of optimal user-friendliness and barrier-free design (Coleman, 1998; TNO, 1998). Although these products are interesting to users from all age groups, they are particularly significant to older people with sensory or motor limitations due to the high degree of operational comfort and safety they offer (Czaja, 1997).

COMMUNICATIONS AND INFORMATION TECHNOLOGY

With the help of technical communications equipment, such as the traditional telephone or cell phones, it is possible to ensure that a connection to the important people in one's life can be established at all times, over long distances and despite limited physical mobility. New ICT devices and systems, such as interactive modes of video communication and email, Internet access, multimedia, and information services, can open up a number of communication possibilities to older people as well. They enable interactive and horizontal communication without having to overcome spatial barriers, thereby strengthening the social contacts one already has, creating new ones, and providing opportunities to learn about issues of interest for older persons who are home bound. Technology can protect single living or sensory- and mobility-impaired elders from severe isolation. Safety-alarm systems provide the assurance that help can be obtained quickly in an emergency, and in case of special impairments, speech computers and electronic reading aids serve to compensate for seeing and hearing handicaps (Charness, Park, & Sabel, 2001; PROMISE, 1998; Smith, Czaja, & Sharit; 1999; Mynatt & Rogers, in press).

TRANSPORT TECHNOLOGIES AND MOBILITY AIDS

The mobility of elderly people is supported by various technical means of transportation, such as private cars, busses, and trains from the regional mass transport authorities, as well as by mobility aids that were developed for special function losses. The private automobile plays an ever-greater role in this because the proportion of older drivers will clearly rise in the future. The statistics are increasing particularly rapidly among women, slowly diminishing the current gender gap (Hjorthol & Sagberg, 2000; Oxley, 2000). For the coming generations of elderly men and women, driving a car will be a natural part of their everyday life experience. Older adults with an impaired ability to walk, especially those living in rural areas and suburbs with reduced local public transport services, are frequently in need of a private car to deal with daily demands. Thus, travel trends in Europe are moving in the same direction as in the U.S., albeit with a certain time lag (Mollenkopf, Marcellini, Ruoppila, et al., 2002; Rosenbloom, 2000). At least as long as mass transit systems don't approach the flexibility and convenience of motoring about in an automobile, the private car will not be supplanted by public transportation (Burkhardt, 2000; Mollenkopf, 2003). Thanks to new intelligent systems, it will become even easier to traverse both small and great distances quickly and efficiently (Hanowski & Dingus, 2000; Küting, 1999), changing the very definition of what is "near" or "far."

For dealing with various limitations to mobility, which range from the vague insecurity some elders feel when walking to the case of total immobility, various technical solutions, such as different types of rollators, stair lifts, elevators, and wheelchairs for every type of function loss, have been developed. These can improve, or at least facilitate, mobility inside and outside one's home. These advances have made it possible to provide an appropriate aid for every type of handicap. Examples of developments in mobility aids that can offer fascinating possibilities for compensating for sensory or physical impairment include travel guides that are based on *geographical information systems* (GIS) and *global positioning systems* (GPS), enabling users to plan their travel and providing them with orientation and navigation assistance during journeys (Strothotte, Johnson, Petrie, & Douglas, 1998; Rafik & Wright, 1999). Personal adaptive mobility aids guide the sensory or physically impaired users with the help of a robot-based walking frame, or rollator, with a handle and joystick user interface while at the same time giving them physical support as they walk (O'Neill, Petrie, Gallagher, et al., 1999; Hine & Nooralahiyan, 1998). Portable video magnifiers are ready to be connected to a TV or PC, so the World Wide Web (WWW) is getting accessible for the visually impaired, et cetera (Duchateau, Archambault, & Burger, 1999; Emiliani & Stephanidis, 1999).

ASSISTIVE DEVICES AND MEDICAL TECHNOLOGIES

With regards to health, medical interventions, patient care, and early detection and prevention, a great variety of assistive devices have been developed to address the impairments faced by handicapped persons and frail elders. The progress in the development of medical interventions with respect to replacement and/or repair of limbs, joints, and organs has had a profound effect on the life expectancy and usually the quality of life of older persons. Developments in the technology of the chronic administration of medicines and nutrients are relatively newer but equally impressive. Medical technologies and auxiliary devices such as special bathroom technology, nursing beds, and lifters help provide care for those with health impairments (Bühler & Knops, 1999; Tamura, Togawa, Ogawa, & Yamakoshi, 1998). Technological improvements in lighting and programmable hearing aids are steadily decreasing the adverse effects of age-associated declines in vision and hearing (Fozard, 2001; Fozard & Gordon-Salant, 2001). A randomized clinical trial indicated that providing assistive technology and environmental modifications can improve functional performance in older persons with severe physical and sensory impairment, slow down the rate of decline, and reduce the costs of institution-based health care (Mann, Ottenbacher, Fraas, et al., 1999).

Computer-supported training programs are suited to prevent the loss of physical and mental competence through disuse. Medical screening and routine check-ups increasingly become automatic, allowing the medical practitioner to make an early diagnosis without a personal consultation (Mix, Borchelt, Nieczaj, et al., 2000).

In view of the growing longevity and number of old persons, and the increasing prevalence of health impairments that go along with old age, both traditional forms of family care and professional care services will come up against limiting factors. In this regard, video- and computer-based tele-care and tele-rehabilitation systems are seen as a significant contribution toward dealing with future tasks and problems. An example for research in this domain is the "TeleReha" study, run between 1996 and 1998 at the Humboldt University, Berlin (Nieczaj, Trilhof, Mix, et al., 1999). The goal of this exploratory study was to evaluate to what degree mobility-impaired elderly people and their family caregivers can and will make use of video-supported communication and electronic information systems and whether this can contribute to improving their situation. The centre provided a variety of services such as professional onscreen-counseling, video-supported communication, and an electronic multimedia-information service. During the test period, frequencies of contact increased considerably, indicating that the system was well adapted to the needs of both the elderly and their caregivers. However, intensive training of all participants and permanent professional attendance was necessary in order to achieve successful use. Requests of several participants led to further improvements in the PC user interface. Orientation within the menus and navigation had to be facilitated. Furthermore, the estimation that one might get answers to questions of everyday life via computers or that videophones would facilitate striking up new contacts decreased during the test phase. This means, for future application, that first, technical systems have to meet the abilities and requirements of both elderly and caregivers if they are to be readily put to use in the geriatric-rehabilitative environment, and second, that their use can only be successful when based upon a concept comprising intensive training of all participants and permanent professional attendance (cf. also Schulz, Lustig, Handler, & Martire, 2002; Rubert, Czaja, & Walsh, 2002).

Over the next few years, significant advances can be expected in the use of technology in early detection and intervention in age-related diseases and functional decline. Many assessments for risk of cardiovascular disease, osteoporosis, and pulmonary disease have relatively high false alarm rates, even though they may have good sensitivity. Some of these difficulties could be overcome with more frequent, reliable measurements on the same individuals over time. The miniaturization of recording and data analysis equipment makes it possible to monitor physiological and behavioral functions unobtrusively in the same person over time, thereby improving the sensitivity and false alarm rates of the measure of risk and providing reliable longitudinal information that has been shown to improve early detection of disabilities in some areas (see Fozard, 1998, for a review). For example, longitudinal analyses of the relationship between elevated blood pressure and hearing loss was established through longitudinal studies (Brant, Gordon-Salant, Pearson, et al., 1996). In addition to impaired cardiovascular function as a cause of age-associated hearing loss, noise has been proposed as a competing risk factor for age as a contributor to hearing loss (Fozard & Gordon-Salant, 2001). Accordingly, Fozard (2001) has proposed using modern hearing aid technology to establish the relationship between long-term exposure to noise and age-associated hearing loss and the use of the same technology to reduce the impact of noise exposure on hearing loss.

SMART-HOME TECHNOLOGIES

The enormous potential of new "intelligent" or "smart" home technologies could also prove particularly useful with regards to aging individuals. They afford nearly unlimited possibilities by the integration of systems and the process of automation (see, e.g., Cooper & Ferreira, 1998). "Smart Home" or "home automation" refers to safety and security issues, living comfort, and technologies that, via internal computer networking, allow one to control several home appliances. In addition, external networking technologies in the field of ICT can offer the aging user a great variety of potential services, e.g., telemedicine, telecare, teleshopping, video on demand, home consulting via monitor, and education or entertainment services.

A recent consumer survey (Meyer, Schulze, Helten, & Fischer, 2001) focused on attitudes toward smart technologies and areas in which the usage of smart technologies is preferred. Data were obtained from standardized questionnaires administered to 423 individuals aged 16 to 83. When comparing younger and older (16 to 52 years and 53 to 83 years old, men/women 50:50) people's view of Smart Home, only small differences were found. Older persons tended to expect more from this kind of technology than younger persons did, which was a rather surprising find. Older people imagined that the Smart Home would simplify their everyday lives, would improve and expand their access to information and communication resources, and make their home environments more fun. These expectations could be the result of a greater need for such assistance, but might also arise from their relative inexperience with modern ICT—a situation that might change with future cohorts of older people.

Younger and older people differ also very little in their responses with respect to desired areas of Smart Home applications. The greatest differences are their interests in technological assistance found in the areas of security, health, and education. The desire for assistance in the health area is clearly stronger among older people. For older persons, technological assistance with health is just as important as help with housework and organizing everyday life. Security is the only area where the interests of older people in Smart Home applications outstrip that of health and household support. Older people also have a greater desire for Smart Home assistance in the area of education, whereas only small age differences were found in the organization of everyday living and housework, as well as in leisure and entertainment activities. Among the negative attributes attached to Smart Home, older people tend to emphasize that the technology will be too complicated. A larger number of younger people mention that Smart Home creates anxiety. Younger persons tend to express greater acceptance of comfort-related functions, whereas older persons, for their part, are more interested in energy-saving and security functions. Thus, older people have high expectations regarding Smart Home applications, but they also feel that this technology could be too complicated for them (Meyer & Mollenkopf, 2003; see also van Berlo, 2002).

The role of technology to enhance the quality of life of older persons in artistic self-expression, education, and leisure has received little research attention, a situation that should change over the next few years. Technology-based software for altering and creating visual and auditory images is widely available, but at least in the case of the music software, the learning needed to use the equipment is high. The growing popularity of Seniornet and similar organizations attests to the interests of older persons in using the computer for a variety of personal pursuits. Human factors studies are currently finding ways to facilitate use of the Internet by older persons (e.g., Ownby & Czaja, 2002; Pak, Rogers, & Fisk, 2002). Bouma and Harrington (2000) describe a technology-supported system to allow several persons to work on painting or creating an image. The potential of virtual reality for enhancing the endeavors of older persons has not yet received significant research and development efforts.

THE CHALLENGES OF TECHNOLOGY

The application of technology in everyday life reduces physical hardship, provides practical solutions to the daily grind, and frees the individual from unpleasant tasks. However, despite attempts of developers and manufacturers of technical devices and systems to make products as user-friendly as possible, including universal design guidelines (Coleman & Myerson, 2001), technological devices or particular features are not adequate for the needs and abilities of older people, and the increasing pace of proliferation of technological applications may even create new constraints.

ACCESSIBILITY

Many single devices are troublesome for a large proportion of elderly people. This has been confirmed, for example, through a study conducted in Germany with a sample of 1,417 persons aged 55 years or older (Mollenkopf, Meyer, Schulze, et al., 2000). Bad experiences with household appliances were reported by about 10 percent of the owners of a microwave oven, a pressure cooker, and a stove. Fears exist mostly among the owners of a pressure cooker (14 percent) and a nonelectric device, the ladder (11 percent). The need for simplification of use was expressed most often with regards to the microwave (11 percent), the washing machine (11 percent), and again the pressure cooker (9 percent).

Compared to these relatively low figures related to household technology, electronic communication, information, and entertainment devices obviously raise much more problems to their users. Among the 15 appliances that have been included in the survey, 9 are incriminated with bad experiences by their users, such as 10 percent (cordless phone) to 23 percent (video recorder). The computer is terrifying for every fifth older owner of such a device, and the need for simplification of use was expressed with respect to 7 of the questioned 15 ICT technologies. The most difficult device to handle seems to be the video recorder (33 percent cited a need for simplification). Bad experiences are reported in both technology domains to a similar extent by all age groups. Fears are more frequent among women in the domestic domain, but no significant gender differences were found with regards to ICT. In this domain, the frequency of bad experiences, fears, and the need of simplification is almost identical among men and women and among the different age groups (Mollenkopf & Kaspar, 2002).

Thus, the need for simplification does not depend on particular groups of the population but seems to be universal. More than 50 percent of the constraints encountered on daily living tasks are considered to be remediable by a combination of redesign and the provision of some training in the task (Rogers, Meyer, Walker, & Fisk, 1998, p. 121). The data make clear that a lot of work still has to be done to shape even widespread technologies such as the washing machine or the video recorder in a more user-friendly way in order to make these products accessible to, and usable and affordable by, all older people who might profit from them.

Problems of accessibility emerge especially when habitual behaviors have to be changed or when it requires courses of action that are totally new for the elderly and thus connected with a fear of failure, as is the case with the layered user interfaces of new electronic communication aids. When handling such software-style interfaces, older men and women who grew up with the electro-mechanical interaction style of consumer devices experience more difficulties than the "software generation" (born in the 1960s or later) (Docampo Rama, de Ridder, & Bouma, 2001). As this example illustrates, the shortcomings and deficits inherent to certain technologies can be falsely interpreted as an aging problem.

One proposal has been made for using smart technology to improve the usability of technical devices by older users. The idea is to devise self-adapting control devices that are sensitive to the preferences and usual uses of individual users, such as temperature and lighting controls in houses equipped with smart technology. The concept has not yet received systematic study in relation to aging. However, technology is commercially available for voice recognition of spoken commands to computers and stored telephone numbers in cellular telephones.

A number of positive developments have taken place in the area of assistive technologies (see, e.g., Bühler & Knops, 1999; Fernie, 1997; Mann et al., 1999; Placencia Porrero & Ballabio, 1998; Watzke, 2002), but despite the general assumption that older people benefit from whatever type of assistive device is made available to them, and despite the obvious changes that the availability and use of technology can bring to their everyday lives, surprisingly little systematic research has been done on the effectiveness and impact of those technologies (McWilliam, Diehl-Jones, Jutai, & Tadrissi, 2000).

PERSONAL, SOCIO-STRUCTURAL, AND ETHICAL CHALLENGES

A multitude of studies have shown that older adults are able to learn new skills—but that we also have to accept the reality of wide individual differences in the timing and rate of abilities and of age-related decline in cognitive abilities (e.g., Craik & Salthouse, 1992; Lindenberger & Baltes, 1997; Mayer, P. B. Baltes, M. M. Baltes, et al., 1999; Willis & Schaie, 1986). In any case, more time, training, and cognitive support are needed with increasing age when learning new skills is needed to optimize the use of devices. To merely provide a technical product or aid does not suffice; elderly people need encouragement and time to become familiar with it (Mann et al., 1999; Mollenkopf, 1994; Nieczaj, Trilhof, Mix, et al., 1999).

Training seems to hold promise for improving the competence of older adults with regard to their use of the Internet and personal computers (Czaja & Lee, 2001). The rapid pace and proliferation of technological development, in particular in the ICT domain, requires various new skills and abilities. The elderly of tomorrow will have had tremendous exposure to computer applications, even if they have not been formally educated in their proper use. In all likelihood, this will lead to a growing openness and increasing competencies with respect to using technological advances. One should note, however, that these new competencies could, under certain circumstances, lead to experiences of deficiency and feelings of being obsolete among the elderly. In the future, one may feel "old" when one can no longer use a computer mouse or interpret commands in the status bar of a software program. Similarly, frustration and despair can result when one lacks the fine motor skills necessary to manipulate miniaturized devices (e.g., changing the batteries in hearing aids). Moreover, not all older people will be able, or get the chance, to take advantage of such types of experiences. As a result, elderly nonusers run the risk of being labeled technologically illiterate and/or may be excluded from important social domains. Just as new social inequalities can come about through different socio-structural conditions, so can they result from technological surges, which are experienced by individual age generations in different phases and situations of life and hence are appropriated in different ways (Fozard, 1997; Sackmann & Weymann, 1994). Thus, in the future, the demarcation between the haves and the have-nots, that is, those who have technological means at their disposal, and those who do not or cannot use the latest technology, will probably continue to exist. Technology may well create even larger rifts between the rich and the poor, the young and the old. Therefore, it will not only be crucial to improve the design of systems and devices, but to identify necessary accompanying measures in order to avoid a "digital divide" (Brink, 2001; Mollenkopf, 2001; Schauer & Radermacher, 2001).

Thus, functional effectiveness is not everything. Older persons' equipment and use of domestic appliances, modern information, and communications technologies depend strongly on aspects of social structure as well as on individual attitudes and lifelong habits. Data from the interdisciplinary *sentha*-project (Mollenkopf et al., 2000) indicate that among sociostructural variables, age was found to be most important (negative) impact, followed by household composition, income, and parenthood. Negative attitudes towards technology, in fact domain-specific as well as general ones, were significant (negative) predictors, too: Persons who always have preferred to minimize the use of household technologies and/or ICT during their life course, those who think that it is not worth buying new products anymore, and those whose perceived obsolescence is generally high are more likely to be sparsely equipped in old age than those who express more positive attitudes. In the domain of ICT, a high level of education and the experience with technology ("I always had a lot to do with technology in my life") turned out to be significant positive predictors. Surprisingly, gender has no impact on the equipment and use of this type of appliances, whereas it is a strong predictor with respect to household technology (Mollenkopf & Kaspar, 2002).

Even more difficult ethical questions must be raised concerning the application of computerized devices for assisting persons with cognitive impairments (Marshall, 1996). Many new systems in the home, such as monitoring devices, will maximize access to the elderly individual's behavior and enable the identification of potential dangers in the interests of improving the supervision of the mentally ill and ensuring their safety, while at the same time involving both environmental and personal intrusion (the "virtual" presence of others; Severs, 1999). To some extent, such measures may lead to unjustified restriction and control, as, for instance, the infringement of the patient's rights of privacy and self-determination. Therefore, when considering the application of technological products to assist people with dementia, it is crucial to take into account the extent to which they are able to control the equipment.

The impact of technology's ever-widening use in society, such as the need for product standardization and supportive infrastructure, the automation of services, and the increase in motorized traffic, limits autonomous action to some degree and sometimes makes it difficult for elderly people to maintain their autonomy and social life outside the home (Ball, Wadley, & Edwards, 2002; Marcellini, Mollenkopf, Spazzafumo, & Ruoppila, 2000; Owsley, 2002; Rogers, Cabrera, Walker, et al., 1996; Smither & Braun, 1994). Information about many different spheres of life is increasingly offered in electronic form instead of printed media, and in a multitude of public domains, persons and services are being replaced by automatic devices.This means that technology takes on the role of social partner in once-human interactions (such as automatic ticket dispensers instead of train conductors, automatic teller machines instead of bank tellers, Internet information services and telecare instead of personal consultants and care providers). The mass of information can also increase stress such as the fear of not being up-to-date, and older persons, in particular, may feel lost in the flood of information provided by the World Wide Web. Therefore, a major challenge of, for example, adult education is to enable older persons to transform available information into knowledge that is meaningful to them.

ACCEPTABILITY

Technological products are socio-culturally shaped artifacts (e.g., MacKenzie & Wajcman, 1999) and, therefore, access to technical devices is not only made difficult through the fact that they often are too complicated and difficult to use, but also because they may be associated with aspects that are societally undesirable and thus not well accepted. Besides individual necessities and financial resources, the acceptance of technology is a crucial precondition for the acquisition and use of appliances (Blaich, 1992; Mollenkopf, 1994; Stewart, 1992; Zimmer & Chappell, 1999). This is particularly salient with respect to assistive devices, which may be perceived as a clear indication of old age and frailty. Awkward mobility aids, for exampe, although useful, may be felt to be embarrassing and jeopardize a person's self-awareness when used in public. This may, however, change with the implementation of modern electronic devices, which are connected with the image of modernity and efficiency.

Bouwhuis and Melenhorst (2001) provide some evidence that the willingness of older persons to utilize new technology depends on a subjective evaluation of the trade-off between the effort required to master the use of the technology against its value to the person. They argue that such willingness depends on the similarities and differences between the new technology and that which characterized the "technology generation" to which they belong (Docampo Rama, de Ridder, & Bouma, 2001).

In order to achieve a proper balance between the relentless development of technology and the interests of aging, the consumer, or end user, should be involved in all phases of the development, distribution, and dispersal of technologically based products, environments, and services. This proposal goes considerably beyond the use of consumer panels to choose colors or compare alternative prototypes, although this is part of the process. A basic tenet of gerontechnology is that consumer involvement in the development of a product means significant involvement in the decisions to develop a product or environment in the first place, as well as input into and evaluation of the product under development (Becker & Mollenkopf, 2002; Fozard et al., 1997). The argument is that the developing and marketing of new products should not be left completely to the imagination of designers or marketers. With respect to distribution, consumer input means input into and evaluation of consumer education about the products, ease of use of the product, and evaluation of marketing. With respect to technology dispersal, consumer input helps define the boundaries or range of application of particular technologies.

The idea of involving the end user of technology in design and distribution processes is somewhat different from the approaches used in other broad applications of technology to topics such as medical technology and environmental technology (Fozard, et al., 1997). In the former case, physicians and medical scientists provide advocacy and knowledge needed to guide technology development and use. In the latter, legal experts and engineers serve as the advocates and expert goal setters for environmental cleaning and greening approaches to environmental controls. In the case of gerontechnology, the roles of advocate and expert must be fulfilled more directly by the aging user of the technology. The variety of technological advances covers a wide range of products and services, of which only some are of interest to particular subgroups of aging individuals. Hence, implementing the concept of user involvement in technology in different areas of application takes considerable ingenuity and commitment-significant challenges in most areas of application that do not involve specific efforts in assistive technology for specific disabilities.

The fear of stigmatization aside, attitudes of elderly people toward domain-specific technologies are very positive. To 72 percent of the older adults in Germany, household technology means a major support of independence. About two-thirds (67.4 percent) of them feel the same with regards to ICT. At the same time, up to 1 in 5 persons expresses fears toward such appliances: 19 percent agree to the statement "Household technology is connected with a high risk," and hardly 15 percent feel this in view of ICT (Mollenkopf & Kaspar, 2002). In general, older adults are neither "enemies" of technology nor uncritical users of technological innovations. Instead, research revealed that four types of older people's relation to technology can be distinguished, namely the positive advocates of technology, the rationally adapting, the skeptical and ambivalent, and those critical and reserved with respect to technology (Wahl & Mollenkopf, in press). The most positively accepting respondents constitute the largest group (28.5 percent). Within the four types no significant gender differences exist. Among the positive advocates, the share of the "younger old" is significantly higher than the share of the older and "old-old," and the critical consist mainly of men and women aged 65 and older. Persons of higher education can be found significantly more often among the positive advocates of technology and persons of lower education most often are rationally adapting.

On the basis of the studies presented, we can conclude that both the objective and subjective preconditions for actively shaping one's environment by means of technical products are not equally distributed among older persons. Aspects of social structure as well as individual attitudes and lifelong habits constitute important preconditions for the equipment with, and use of, technical devices. Therefore, objective technical and financial, as well as cognitive and subjective emotional, barriers have to be minimized. The everyday needs and requirements of older people must be considered more seriously in future research and development, and technologies themselves must be optimized in a manner that does not create new barriers to the application of technologies designed for maintaining independence and enhancing the social participation of older persons.

TECHNOLOGY CHANGE AND HUMAN AGING— NEEDS FOR A COMPREHENSIVE CONCEPTUAL FRAMEWORK FOR PERSON-ENVIRONMENT INTERACTIONS

A systems, or transactional, view of P-E relationships is widely used in gerontology to analyze how the supports and demands provided by the environment for a particular behavior are different for older and younger persons (see Lawton & Nahemow, 1973; Lawton, 1998). Adding a temporal dimension to the systems view provides a way to describe the ever-changing dynamics of P-E relationships associated with secular changes in the environment and the human aging that occurs in it. The ideas are represented graphically in Figure 10.1 (adapted from Fozard, 2002).

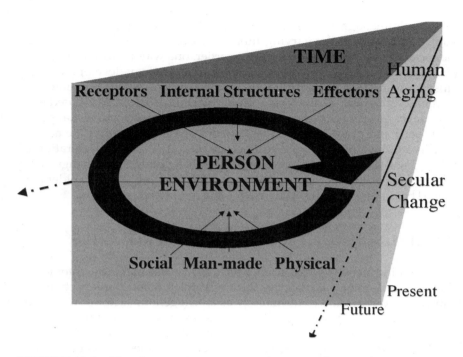

FIGURE 10.1   The changes in person-environment interactions over time.

The front surface of the figure represents the interface of the person (top half) and the environment (lower half). The third dimension of the figure represents time ranging from the past (back of figure) to the present (front plane of figure) to the future (dotted arrow in front of the figure). The upper half of the time dimension is labeled "human aging" to correspond with the person side of the interaction and the lower half is labeled "secular change" to represent changes in the environment side of the interaction over time. It is immediately apparent that secular changes will interact with aging in complex ways depending on the rate and amount of change in the environment. The circular arrow surrounding person and environment in the diagram depicts the continuous flow of information from the environment to the person and the response of the person—either reactive or proactive —to the information. The flow of information from the environment comes from three components: the social environment, the man-made or built environment, and the natural physical environment. The human response involves the receptors, internal states, and the effectors. All three components on both the human and environmental side change with time.

The figure suggests first that considerable planning should be carried out to understand the varying human responses to technology change associated with aging. As discussed earlier, one way to achieve this is to involve users in the development phases of technology development, not just its evaluation. It also suggests that the dynamics of P-E interactions depend on environmental factors other than those directly associated with the development of the technology itself—concurrent secular changes in the social and physical aspects of the environment will affect the acceptability and usefulness of the technology as well. A full consideration of changing P-E interactions goes beyond the observation that a change in the technological environment will affect a child differently than an older person. These points will be elaborated in the following discussion.

SOCIAL SCIENCE TECHNOLOGY APPROACHES

The genuine focus of social science technology research is the interaction between technology and society. Such research has been largely confined, however, to the study of technology as an exogenous factor of change in the process and organization of work and to the theoretical treatment of technology as artifacts that either rationalize human action or give it new latitude (see, e.g., Joerges, 1988). The discussion of the process of technology's pervasion of private daily life, outside the context of gainful employment and of the concomitant changes, was initially framed by the scientific paradigm of technological determinism. According to this view, modern industrialized societies are undergoing a profound change in all social domains because of an inherent logic of modern technology, making it the prime mover of socioeconomic change and social modernization. For example, Ogburn (1972) saw technical development as the engine of social change to which such institutions as the family can only adapt. Freyer (1960) stated that technological categories are becoming dominant in the life world of industrialized society, and Ellul (1954) concluded that the automatic nature and universality of that process is inescapable.

Beginning in the mid-1970s, an opposing view of technology as a social construct increasingly emerged. It was no longer held that technology permeates and changes human actions with its own rationale, but that humans develop, shape, and use technology according to their abilities and interests. However, this new phase of technology research on everyday existence has yet to leave much of a mark on studies about the elderly person's everyday technological reality. Instead, attention has been veering from the question of technology's use in everyday settings to the conditions governing technology's inception and the actors involved in that process (Dierkes & Hoffmann, 1992). In this socio-constructivist perspective, technology is seen as a product of social processes in the course of which the social environment, manifested as social groups and systems, influences the process by which technological artifacts are created by defining problems and driving technical developments forward amid different interests and orientations (Pinch & Bijker, 1987). No technology is of a purely technical nature but rather is always also social, and everything social is simultaneously also technical (Bijker & Law, 1992).

This theoretical approach, the social shaping of technology, also expands the perspective of research on technology in everyday settings. The users of everyday technology are an integral part of the process governing technology's increasing use. The integration of technological artifacts in daily patterns of action can give rise to new routines that open new latitude for action or can create new constraints and dependencies because the continual escalation of technology's dissemination and use perpetuates new technological development and broadens infrastructure systems and standardization (Braun, 1993). As for the daily life world of old people, the progressively wider use of technology in modern industrialized societies consequently means increasing breadth in the freedom of action and problem-solving alternatives in everyday practice. But the structuring, standardization, and anonymization of sequences of action that accompany old people's greater use of these alternatives are precisely what also restrict their self-determined action and direct experience. In this regard, social institutions such as welfare associations, as well as the legally mandated regulation of insurance benefits, are important for the use of technical aids in old age. Street traffic as a field of action shaped by society and technology alike illustrates especially well that technical developments can contain ways to expand one's scope of action as well as risks that constrict one's life space. The growing ability of elderly people to travel and the increasing ownership of cars among members of age cohorts below 65 years of age are contributing to a definite increase in individual mobility. But whether on the road as pedestrians, car drivers, users of local public transport, or bicyclists, elderly people also suffer from ever heavier and more aggressive street traffic and the danger of being injured or killed in a traffic accident (Mollenkopf, 2003).

Similarly, new electronic devices and systems offer considerable benefits, especially with regard to aging individuals and to people with physical disabilities, and they might also be capable of improving the quality of life of people with cognitive impairments. At the same time, their application clearly increases a new reliance—and by this, dependency—upon technology and the dangers of isolation and supervision. Therefore, to ensure that the elderly will be able to use the positive opportunities of technical products, and at the same time retain control over their destiny, it is necessary to take the social embeddedness of aging and technology into account.

ENVIRONMENTAL GERONTOLOGY APPROACHES

Environmental gerontology approaches that relate the social and physical environment provide a theoretical perspective to human aging that can integrate social aspects of aging as well as spatial and technical aspects of the environment. According to these models, the aging organism and its capacity for adaptation are vulnerable to environmental overdemands ("press") as well as underdemands; misfits between behavioral competence, personal needs, and environmental conditions might undermine life quality (Carp & Carp, 1984; Lawton & Nahemow, 1973). For instance, functional disabilities that might develop have far less impact under favorable environmental conditions and with appropriate technological products than under conditions that restrict the living space of elderly people and fail to meet their needs.

THE SYMBOLIC MEANING OF TECHNOLOGICAL PRODUCTS

In an ecologically oriented sociology of technology or in environmental gerontology, oriented primarily to technology, one must also consider the symbolic content that objects, in this case mostly technical artifacts, have as part of the environment for their owners and users. For example, technical aids that can make environmental demands easier to deal with for elderly people whose strength or physical competence is declining are frequently rejected because their very shape evokes associations of handicap and disease, stigmatizing the user and undermining self-esteem. In phenomenological approaches, the aspect of meaning is stressed, especially in relation to self-concept and identity (Boesch, 1976). In sociological theories, by contrast, the social inequalities precipitated by the differentiating character of things are highlighted (Bourdieu, 1988).

This raises the question of the way in which technological products and systems contribute to both the construction of identity and the differentiation meant by Bourdieu. In the future, technology seems likely to lose much of its prosthetic nature; it will no longer be viewed as a replacement for a missing body part or a means of compensation for a particular deficiency. Rather, the distinction between "natural" and "technological" will become blurred, as will the distinctions between "health" and "illness," between the individual as subject, with his or her own body and identity, and technology as an object separate from the individual.

COMPLEMENTING MICRO AND MACRO PERSPECTIVES OF PERSON-TECHNOLOGY INTERACTIONS

Consequently, a comprehensive and dynamic framework for P-E interactions should include at least four perspectives (see also Wahl & Mollenkopf, in press):

1. The *microperspective of individual aging processes*, including age-related decrements in perception, attention, memory, and (fluid) intelligence (e.g., Howard & Howard, 1997); personal attitudes; and symbolic meanings attributed to environmental (including technical) features. Within this perspective, mostly combined with a strong research orientation, three models have been used in the recent literature on aging and technology. First, human factors models draw from the in-depth knowledge of man-machine interactions. Charness and Bosman have shown already, in 1990, how much empirically based quantitative material is available with respect to light and auditory environments and their interaction with aging individuals (see also Fisk & Rogers, 1997). Secondly, the information-processing view on age and technology interactions has substantial overlap with the human factors approach. A third family of models, just summarized as ecological models, focuses on the aging-technology relation at the microlevel and points to age-related changes in the role of the environment (e.g., Fozard & Popkin, 1978; Scheidt & Windley, 1998; Wahl, 2001).

2. Within the second, *application-oriented microperspective*, extensive knowledge and data are available with regard to design directives and home adaptation guidelines based on practical planning experience and intervention (see Regnier & Pynoos, 1987, for a classic volume in this regard). Such knowledge can be of great benefit for adapting technical products to the needs and abilities of the aging and the aged, but often is applied with no consideration for their emotional sensitivity.

Both of these perspectives neglect, however, the macro conditions of the reciprocal aging-technology relationship. Human factors approaches, as well as microlevel perspectives in general, must always be framed within historical contexts and consider the socio-structural conditions and policy background of technology development, deployment, acquisition, and use.

3. From a macrolevel perspective, the already-mentioned historical relativity of aging and technology has to be considered first. For instance, in modern industrialized countries with highly differentiated sections of society, heterogeneous life courses, and singularized ways of living, communication and mobility become increasingly important to each individual to secure active participation in society. Thus, the social integration of elderly

people is not only made difficult through the loss of function of the senses or age-related illness, but also through the societal processes of differentiation and pluralization (Mollenkopf, 1996). Moreover, future cohorts of older technology users will continue to have their special "technology biography" that will be different from earlier cohorts, respectively.

Secondly, the social and structural forces that determine access to education and income—and thus to technology-relevant competencies and devices—have to be taken into account. Future generations of older men and women will experience the industrialization and mechanization of working life and the penetration of almost all private domains by technology. However, not all of them will be able to acquire the new skills and competencies necessary to cope with the growing pace of technological changes, and not all of them will afford the necessary economic resources for purchasing the requisite technological products. In the near future, a bridging of the divide between the "haves" and the "have-nots" does not come into sight. Rather, it will persist into the remote future (Mollenkopf, 2001).

4. There is a further macro perspective when it comes to the planning of social policy and legislative regulations (Mayer, Baltes, Gerok, et al., 1992). They directly impact the application of technological products and technology-related interventions such as programs for prevention, training, or rehabilitation (Mollenkopf, 1994; Watzke, 2002).

Therefore, microlevel perspectives need to be strongly amplified by macrolevel perspectives. This wider theoretical approach also implies a stronger collaboration between researchers and professionals from a variety of disciplines, such as psychologists, human factors researchers, designers, and architects, as well as between sociologists, anthropologists, and social policy researchers.

Finally, and summing up, it should be emphasized that how individual persons age depends not only on their personal resources and attitudes, but also on the historical time, society, and (technological) environment he or she lives in, all of which influence each other in complex interactive processes. Therefore, there is a strong need to counteract the existing tendency in research to attend predominantly to the micro level and to neglect other levels of analysis or available knowledge when targeting the relation of aging and technology.

CONCLUSIONS

For decades, modern societies have become societies not the least characterized by the high degree to which technology is used in them. There are few domains that in some respect would even have been possible without technology. These developments may have divergent influences on future aging —depending on the traditions, the level of mechanization, and the economic resources of the countries in which the older person lives. However, the basic trends discussed here can be observed all over the world.

The meaning that technology's progressive infiltration of the environment has for people in old age hardly needs to be emphasized. Modern gerontologists agree that aging processes and outcomes depend not only on biological, but also on contextual influences. In western industrial societies, this means that technology is becoming an ever more crucial "environment" for aging and the aged.

Beyond the issue of direct everyday relevance, society in general—and the aging population in particular—are confronted by far more encompassing changes that coincide with processes of technology's proliferation. Just as new social inequalities can come about through different sociostructural conditions, so also can they result from technological surges, which are experienced by individual age generations in different phases and situations of life and hence are appropriated in different ways. In the future, the demarcation between the haves and the have-nots, that is, those who have technological means at their disposal, and those who do not or cannot use the latest technology, will probably continue to exist. Thus, technology may well create even larger rifts between the rich and the poor, the young and the old.

To avoid, or at least mitigate, new social inequalities or discrimination, the conditions for older individuals to profit from the opportunities offered by the broad range of old and new technological products, they have to be improved substantially. Such improvements comprise, first of all, the design of devices. The design of technologies that might contribute to enhancing autonomy and social participation of older persons leaves much to be desired. For this reason, the developers and suppliers of such technologies and programs need to take the interests, needs, and possibilities of older people into greater consideration.

But to ensure that elderly people will use technology's positive opportunities, it will not only be crucial to improve their design, but to identify necessary accompanying measures. To merely provide a technical device does not suffice; elderly people need encouragement and time to become familiar with the rapid pace and proliferation of technological innovations. In addition, to preserve the quality of life in old age, it is necessary that these devices also fulfill the criteria of social functionality. This would allow people of all ages to resort to technical aids at the proper time and without fear of discrimination.

From a theoretical perspective, there is a strong need for better integrated micro and macro perspectives as well as research- and application-oriented approaches in order to take into account the complex interchange processes between individuals and their technological environments in an appropriate manner. Both aging individuals and the technological products and systems they can or cannot use are embedded in societal and technological modernization processes. The dynamic aging and technology interaction does not least depend on the socio-structural and legislative conditions and the stocks of technological artifacts and knowledge prevailing in a particular society at a historical time.

REFERENCES

Ball, K. K., Wadley, V. G., & Edwards, J. D. (2002). Advances in technology used to assess and retrain older drivers. *Gerontechnology, 1(4)*, 251-261.

Becker, S., & Mollenkopf, H. (2002). Guidelines for senior friendly product development. *Gerontechnology, 2(1)*, 109.

Bijker, W. E., & Law, J. (Eds.). (1992). *Shaping technology/building society. Studies in sociotechnical change.* Cambridge/London: MIT Press.

Blaich, R. I. (1992). Taming technology for the benefit of the aging—and everyone else. In H. Bouma & J. A. M. Graafmans (Eds.), *Gerontechnology* (pp. 7-14). Amsterdam: IOS Press.

Boesch, E. E. (1976). *Psychopathologie des Alltags* [Psycho-pathology of everyday life]. Bern, Germany: Huber.

Bonner, S. (1998). AID HOUSE. Edinvar housing association smart technology demonstrator and evaluation site. In I. Placencia Porrero & E. Ballabio (Eds.), *Improving the quality of life for the European citizen* (pp. 396-400). Amsterdam: IOS Press.

Bouma, H., & Graafmans, J. A. M. (Eds.). (1992). *Gerontechnology.* Amsterdam: IOS Press.

Bouma, H., & Harrington, T. L. (2000). Information and communication. In T. L. Harrington & M. K. Harrington (Eds.), *Gerontechnology—why and how* (pp. 139-164). Maastricht, NL: Shaker.

Bourdieu, P. (1988). *Die feinen Unterschiede.* Frankfurt: Suhrkamp (original: La distinction. Critique sociale du jugement. Paris: Les éditions de minuit, 1979).

Bouwhuis, D. G., & Melenhorst, A. S. (2001). Perceived cost-benefit ratios of using interactive communication equipment. In K. Sagawa & H. Bouma (Eds.), *Proceedings of the International Workshop on Gerontechnology* (pp. 75-78). Tsukuba, Japan: National Institute of Bioscience and Human-Technology.

Brant, L. J., Gordon-Salant, S., Pearson, J. D., Klein, L. L., Morrell, C. H., Metter, E. J., et al. (1996). Risk factors related to age-associated hearing loss in the speech frequencies. *Journal for the American Academy of Audiology, 7*, 152-160.

Braun, I. (1993). *Technik-Spiralen. Vergleichende Studien zur Technik im Alltag* [Technology spirals. Comparative studies on technology in everyday life]. Berlin, Germany: edition sigma.

Brink, S. (2001). Digital divide or digital dividend? Ensuring benefits to seniors from information technology. In National Advisory Council on Aging (Ed.), *Writings in gerontology: Seniors and technology* (Vol. 17, pp. 19-32). Ottawa, Canada: Minister of Public Works and Government Services, Canada.

Bühler, C., & Knops, H. (Eds.). (1999). *Assistive technology on the threshold of the new millennium*. Amsterdam: IOS Press.

Burkhardt, J. E. (2000). Limitations of mass transportation and individual vehicle systems for older persons. In K. W. Schaie & M. Pietrucha (Eds.), *Mobility and transportation in the elderly* (pp. 97-123). New York: Springer.

Campbell, T., Dries, J., & Gilligan, R. (1999). *The older generation and the European information society: Access to the information society* (Final project report). Düsseldorf, Germany: European Institute for the Media.

Carp, F. M., & Carp, A. (1984). A complementary/congruence model of well-being or mental health for the community elderly. In I. Altman, M. P. Lawton, & J. F. Wohlwill (Eds.), *Human behavior and environment* (Vol. 7, pp. 279-336). New York: Plenum Press.

Charness, N., & Bosman, E. A. (1990). Human factors and design for older adults. In J. E. Birren & K.W. Schaie (Eds.), *Handbook of the psychology of aging* (3rd ed., pp. 446-464). New York: Academic Press.

Charness, N., Czaja, S., Fisk, A. D., & Rogers, W. (2001). Why Gerontechnology? *Gerontechnology, 1*(2), 85-87.

Charness, N., Park, C., & Sabel, A. (Eds.). (2001). *Communication, technology and aging. Opportunities and challenges for the future.* New York: Springer.

Coleman, R. (1998). Improving the quality of life for older people by design. In J. Graafmans, V. Taipale, & N. Charness (Eds.), *Gerontechnology: A sustainable investment in the future* (pp. 74-83). Amsterdam: IOS Press.

Coleman, R., & Myerson, J. (2001). Improving life quality by countering design exclusion. *Gerontechnology, 1*(2), 88-102.

Cooper, M., & Ferreira, J. (1998). Home networks for independent living, support and care services: Issues impinging on the successful introduction of products and services. In I. Placencia Porrero & E. Ballabio (Eds.), *Improving the quality of life for the European citizen* (pp. 359-363). Amsterdam: IOS Press.

Craik, F. I. M., & Salthouse, T. E. (Eds.). (1992). *The handbook of aging and cognition*. Hillsdale, NJ: Erlbaum.

Czaja, S. J. (1996). Aging and the acquisition of computer skills. In W. A. Rogers, A. D. Fisk, & N. Walker (Eds.), *Aging and skilled performance: Advances in theory and application* (pp. 201-220). San Diego: Academic Press.

Czaja, S. J. (1997). Using technologies to aid the performance of home tasks. In A. D. Fisk & W. A. Rogers (Eds.), *Handbook of human factors and the older adult* (pp. 311-334). San Diego: Academic Press.

Czaja, S. J., & Lee, C. C. (2001). The Internet and older adults: Design challenges and opportunities. In N. Charness, D. C. Park, & B. A. Sabel (Eds.), *Communication, technology and aging: Opportunities and challenges for the future* (pp. 60-80). New York: Springer.

Czaja, S. J., & Sharit, J. (1998). Age differences in attitudes toward computers. *Journal of Geronotology: Psychological Sciences, 53B*(5), P329-P340.

Dierkes, M., & Hoffmann, U. (Eds.) (1992). *New technology at the outset—social forces in the shaping of technological innovations*. Frankfurt, Germany: Campus.

Docampo Rama, M., de Ridder, H., & Bouma, H. (2001). Technology generation and age in using layered interfaces. *Gerontechnology, 1*, 25-40.

Duchateau, S., Archambault, D., & Burger, D. (1999). The accessibility of the World Wide Web for visually impaired people. In C. Bühler & H. Knops (Eds.),

Assistive technology on the threshold of the new millennium (pp. 34-38). Amsterdam: IOS Press.

Ellul, J. (1954). *La technique ou l'enjeu du siècle.* Paris: Librairie Armand Colin [The Technological Society. New York: Knopf, 1964. Rev. ed.: New York: Knopf/Vintage, 1967].

Emiliani, P. L., & Stephanidis, C. (1999). Accessing the information society. In C. Bühler & H. Knops (Eds.), *Assistive technology on the threshold of the new millennium* (pp. 28-33). Amsterdam: IOS Press.

Fabris, N., Marcellini, F., & Brizioli, E. (1996). Gerontechnology: From simple aids to domotica. In H. Mollenkopf (Ed.), *Elderly people in industrialised societies: Social integration in old age by or despite technology?* (pp. 195-205). Berlin, Germany: edition sigma.

Fernie, G. (1997). Assistive devices. In A. D. Fisk & W. A. Rogers (Eds.), *Handbook of human factors and the older adult* (pp. 289-310). San Diego, CA: Academic Press.

Festervand, T. A., & Wylde, M. A. (1988). The marketing of technology to older adults. *International Journal of Technology and Aging, 1*(2), 156–162.

Fisk, A. D., & Rogers, W. A. (Eds.). (1997). *Handbook of human factors and the older adults.* San Diego, CA: Academic Press.

Fisk, A. D., & Rogers, W. A. (2002). Psychology and aging: Enhancing the lives of an aging population. *Current directions in psychological science, 11*, 107-110.

Fozard, J. L. (1997). Aging and technology: A developmental view. In W. A. Rogers (Ed.), *Designing for an aging population: Ten years of human factors and ergonomics research* (pp. 164-166). Santa Monica, CA: Human Factors and Ergonomics Society.

Fozard, J. L. (1998). Contributions of longitudinal studies to epidemiology and disease prevention: An overview. *Australasian Journal on Ageing, 17* (1), 22-24.

Fozard, J. L. (2001). Gerontechnology and perceptual-motor function: New opportunities for prevention, compensation, and enhancement. *Gerontechnology, 1*, 5-24.

Fozard, J. L. (2002). Gerontechnology—Beyond ergonomics and universal design. *Gerontechnology, 1(3)*, 137-139.

Fozard, J. L., & Gordon-Salant, S. (2001). Changes in vision and hearing with aging. In J. E. Birren & K. W. Schaie (Eds.), *Handbook of the psychology of aging* (5th ed., pp. 241-266). San Diego, CA: Academic Press.

Fozard, J. L., Graafmans, J. A. M., Rietsema, J., van Berlo, G. M. W., & Bouma, H. (1997). Gerontechnology: Technology to improve health, functioning and quality of life for aging and aged adults. *Korean Journal of Gerontology, 7*(1), 229-255.

Fozard, J. L., & Popkin, S. J. (1978). Optimizing adult development. Ends and means of an applied psychology of aging. *American Psychologist, 33*, 975-989.

Fozard, J. L., Rietsema, J., Bouma, H., & Graafmans, J. A. M. (2000). Gerontechnology: Creating enabling environments for the challenges and opportunities of aging. *Educational Gerontology, 26*, 331-344.

Freudenthal, A. (1998). Transgenerational design of "Smart Products," a checklist of guidelines. In J. A. M. Graafmans, V. Taipale, & N. Charness (Eds.), *Gerontechnology. A sustainable investment in the future* (pp. 406-410). Amsterdam: IOS Press.

Freyer, H. (1960). Über das Dominantwerden technischer Kategorien in der Lebenswelt der industriellen Gesellschaft [On the advancing dominance of technical categories in the everyday world of industrialized societies]. In Akademie der Wissenschaften und der Literatur (Ed.), *Abhandlungen der Geistes- und Sozialwissenschaftlichen Klasse, 7* (pp. 539-551). Mainz, Germany: Akademie der Wissenschaften und der Literatur.

Glatzer, W., Fleischmann, G., Heimer, T., Hartmann, D. M., Rauschenberg, R. H., Schmenau, S., et al. (1998). *Revolution in der Haushaltstechnologie. Die Entstehung des Intelligent Home.* Frankfurt, Germany: Campus.

Graafmans, J., Taipale, V., & Charness, N. (Ed.). (1998). *Gerontechnology. A sustainable investment in the future.* Amsterdam: IOS Press.

Haber, P. A. L. (1986). Technology and aging. *Gerontologist, 26,* 350-357.

Hanowski, R. J., & Dingus, T. A. (2000). Will intelligent transportation systems improve older driver mobility? In K. W. Schaie & M. Pietrucha (Eds.), *Mobility and transportation in the elderly* (pp. 279-298). New York: Springer.

Harrington, T. L., & Harrington, M. K. (2000). *Gerontechnology: Why and how.* Maastricht, The Netherlands: Shaker.

Hine, J., & Nooralahiyan, A. (1998). Improving mobility and independence for elderly, blind and visually impaired people. In I. Placencia Porrero & E. Ballabio (Eds.), *Improving the quality of life for the European citizen* (pp. 283-287). Amsterdam: IOS Press.

Hjortol, R., & Sagberg, F. (2000). Changes in elderly persons' modes of travel. In European Conference of Ministers of Transport (ECMT) (Ed.), *Transport and aging of the population. Report of the 112th round table on transport economics* (pp. 177-209). Paris Cedex, France: OECD Publications.

Howard, J. H., & Howard, D. V. (1997). Learning and memory. In A. D. Fisk & W. A. Rogers (Eds.), *Handbook of human factors and the older adults* (pp. 7-26). San Diego, CA: Academic Press.

Joerges, B. (1988). *Technik im Alltag* [Technology in everyday life]. Frankfurt, Germany: Suhrkamp.

Kruse, A. (1992). Altersfreundliche Umwelten: Der Beitrag der Technik [Age-friendly environments. The contribution of technology]. In P. B. Baltes & J. Mittelstrass (Eds.), *Zukunft des Alterns und gesellschaftliche Entwicklung. Akademie der Wissenschaften zu Berlin* (Vol. 5: Forschungsbericht, pp. 668-694). Berlin, Germany: De Gruyter.

Küting, H. J. (1999). Supporting mobility of the elderly by means of safe and comfortable cars. In M. Tacken, F. Marcellini, H. Mollenkopf, & I. Ruoppila (Eds.), *Keeping the elderly mobile. Outdoor mobility of the elderly: Problems and solutions* (pp. 293-299). Delft, The Netherlands: Delft University Press.

Lawton, M. P. (1998). Environment and aging: Theory revisited. In R. J. Scheidt & P. G. Windley (Eds.), *Environment and aging theory. A focus on housing* (pp. 1-31). Westport, CT: Greenwood Press.

Lawton, M. P., & Nahemow, L. (1973). Ecology and the aging process. In C. Eisdorfer & M. P. Lawton (Eds.), *The psychology of adult development and aging* (pp. 619-674). Washington, DC: American Psychological Association.

Lesnoff-Caravaglia, G. (Ed.). (1988). *Aging in a technological society.* New York: Human Sciences Press.

Lindenberger, U., & Baltes, P. B. (1997). Intellectual functioning in old and very old age: Cross-sectional results from the Berlin Aging Study. *Psychology and Aging, 12*, 410-432.

MacKenzie, D., & Wajcman, J. (Eds.) (1999). *The social shaping of technology* (2nd ed.). Buckingham, Philadelphia: Open University Press.

Mann, W. C., Ottenbacher, K. J., Fraas, L., Tomita, M., & Granger, C. V. (1999). Effectiveness of assistive technology and environmental interventions in maintaining independence and reducing home care costs for the frail elderly: A randomized controlled trial. *Archives of Family Medicine, 8*(3), 210-217.

Marcellini, F., Mollenkopf, H., Spazzafumo, L., & Ruoppila, I. (2000). Acceptance and use of technological solutions by the elderly in the outdoor environment: Findings from a European survey. *Zeitschrift für Gerontologie und Geriatrie, 33*(3), 169-177.

Marshall, M. (1996). Dementia and technology: Some ethical considerations. In H. Mollenkopf (Ed.), *Elderly people in industrialised societies. Social integration in old age by or despite technology?* (pp. 207-215). Berlin, Germany: edition sigma.

Mayer, K. U., Baltes, P. B., Baltes, M. M., Borchelt, M., Delius, J., Helmchen, H., et al. (1999). What do we know about old age and aging? Conclusions from the Berlin Aging Study. In P. B. Baltes & K. U. Mayer (Eds.), *The Berlin Aging Study. Aging from 70 to 100* (pp. 475-519). Cambridge, UK: Cambridge University Press.

Mayer, K. U., Baltes, P. B., Gerok, W., Häfner, H., Helmchen, H., Kruse, A., et al. (1992). Gesellschaft, Politik und Altern [Society, Politics, and Aging]. In P. B. Baltes & J. Mittelstrass (eds.), *Zukunft des Alterns und gesellschaftliche Entwicklung* [The future of aging and societal development] (pp. 721-757). Berlin/New York: de Gruyter.

McWilliam, C. L., Diehl-Jones, W. L., Jutai, J., & Tadrissi, S. (2000). Care delivery approaches and seniors' independence. *Canadian Journal on Aging / La Revue canadienne du vieillissement, 19*(suppl. 1), 101-124.

Meyer, S., & Mollenkopf, H. (2003). Home technology, smart home, and the aging user. In K. W. Schaie, H. W. Wahl, H. Mollenkopf, & F. Oswald (Eds.), *Aging Independently: Living arrangements and mobility* (pp. 148-161). New York: Springer.

Meyer, S., Schulze, E., Helten, F., & Fischer, B. (2001). *Vernetztes Wohnen. Die Informatisierung des Alltagslebens* [Networked housing. The informatization of everyday life]. Berlin, Germany: edition sigma.

Mix, S., Borchelt, M., Nieczaj, R., Trilhof, G., & Steinhagen-Thiessen, E. (2000). Telematik in der Geriatrie—Potentiale, Probleme und Anwendungserfahrungen [Telematics in geriatrics—potentials, limitations, and experience]. *Zeitschrift für Gerontologie und Geriatrie, 33*(3), 195-204.

Mollenkopf, H. (1994). Technical aids in old age—Between acceptance and rejection. In C. Wild & A. Kirschner (Eds.), *Technology for the elderly: Safety-alarm systems, technical aids and smart homes* (pp. 81-100). Knegsel, The Netherlands: Akontes.

Mollenkopf, H. (1996). Social integration of elderly people in industrialised societies: An introduction. In H. Mollenkopf (Ed.), *Elderly people in industrialised societies: Social integration in old age by or despite technology?* (pp. 13-22). Berlin, Germany: Edition sigma.

Mollenkopf, H. (2001). Technik—ein "knappes Gut?" Neue soziale Ungleichheit im Alter durch unterschiedliche Zugangs und Nutzungschancen [Technology—a "scarce good?" New social inequalities in old age through unequal chances of access and usage]. In G. Backes, W. Clemens, & K. R. Schroeter (Eds.), *Zur Konstruktion sozialer Ordnungen des Alter(n)s* (pp. 223-238). Opladen, Germany: Leske + Budrich.

Mollenkopf, H. (2003). Impact of transportation systems on mobility of elderly persons in Germany. In K. W. Schaie, H. W. Wahl, H. Mollenkopf, & F. Oswald (Eds.), *Aging independently: Living arrangements and mobility* (pp. 177-191). New York: Springer.

Mollenkopf, H., & Kaspar, R. (2002). Attitudes to technology in old age as preconditions for acceptance or rejection. In A. Guerci & S. Consigliere (Eds.), *Vivere la vecchiaia / Living in old age: Western world and modernization* (Vol. 2, pp. 134-144). Genova, Italy: Erga edizioni.

Mollenkopf, H., Marcellini, F., Ruoppila, I., Széman, Z., Tacken, M., & Wahl, H. W. (2002). The role of driving in maintaining mobility in later life: A European view. *Gerontechnology, 1*(4), 231-250.

Mollenkopf, H., Meyer, S., Schulze, E., Wurm, S., & Friesdorf, W. (2000). Technik im Haushalt zur Unterstützung einer selbstbestimmten Lebensführung im Alter. Das Forschungsprojekt "sentha" und erste Ergebnisse des sozialwissenschaftlichen Teilprojekts [Everyday Technologies for Senior Households: The project "sentha" and first results of its social science part]. *Zeitschrift für Gerontologie und Geriatrie, 33*(3), 155-168.

Mynatt, E. J., & Rogers, W. A. (in press). Learning to use a home medical device: Mediating age-related differences with training. *Human Factors.*

Nieczaj, R., Trilhof, G., Mix, S., Kwon, S., Borchelt, M., & Steinhagen-Thiessen, E. (1999). Telematikeinsatz in der geriatrischen Rehabilitation und Pflege—Die TeleReha-Studie [Telematics applications in geriatric rehabilitation and care—the TeleReha study]. *Geriatrie Forschung, 9*(1), 21-30.

Ogburn, W .F. (1972). Die Theorie des "Cultural Lag" [Cultural lag as theory]. In H.P. Dreitzel (Ed.), *Sozialer Wandel* (pp. 328-338). Neuwied, Germany: Luchterhand.

O'Neill, A. M., Petrie, H., Gallagher, B., Hunter, H., Lacey, G., & Kavetas, N. (1999). Initial evaluations of a robot mobility aid for frail and elderly visually impaired persons. In C. Bühler & H. Knops (Eds.), *Assistive technology on the threshold of the new millenium* (pp. 352-356). Amsterdam: IOS Press.

OTA—Office of Technology Assessment. (1984). *Technology and aging in America* (Vol. OTA-BA-265). Washington, DC: U.S. Congress, Office of Technology Assessment.

Ownby, R., & Czaja, S. (2002). Problems with web page design for the elderly. *Gerontechnology, 2*(1), 101.

Owsley, C. (2002). Driving mobility, older adults, and quality of life. *Gerontechnology, 1*(4), 220-230.

Oxley, R. R. (2000). Introductory report (United Kingdom). In European Conference of Ministers of Transport (ECMT) (Ed.), *Transport and aging of the population: Report of the 112th round table on transport economics* (pp. 211-241). Paris Cedex, France: OECD Publications.

Pak, R., Rogers, W. A., & Fisk, A. D. (2002). An investigation of the relationship between spatial abilities and hypertext navigation: It's not as simple as it seems! *Gerontechnology, 2(1)*, 100.

Pieper, R., Vaarama, M., & Fozard, J. L. (Eds.). (2002). *Gerontechnology: Technology and aging starting into the third millennium*. Aachen, Germany: Shaker.

Pinch, T. J., & Bijker, W. E. (1987). The social construction of facts and artefacts: Or how the sociology of science and the sociology of technology might benefit each other. In W. E. Bijker, T. P. Hughes, & T. J. Pinch (Eds.), *The social construction of technological systems* (pp. 17-50). Cambridge/London: MIT Press.

Placencia Porrero, I., & Ballabio, E. (Eds.). (1998). *Improving the quality of life for the European citizen*. Amsterdam: IOS Press.

PROMISE Consortium (Ed.). (1998). *The promise of the information society: Good practice in using the information society for the benefit of older people and disabled people*. Helsinki, Finland: STAKES National Research and Development Centre for Welfare and Health.

Rafik, T. A., & Wright, D. K. (1999). Advanced electronic mobility aids for visually impaired people. In C. Bühler & H. Knops (Eds.), *Assistive technology on the threshold of the new millennium* (pp. 609-613). Amsterdam: IOS Press.

Reents, H. (1996). *Handbuch der Gerontotechnik: interdisziplinäre Forschung.* [Handbook gerontechnology: interdisciplinary research] Landsberg, Germany: ecomed.

Regnier, V., & Pynoos, J. (1987). *Housing the aged: Design directives and policy considerations*. New York: Elsevier.

Rogers, W. A., Cabrera, E. F., Walker, N., Gilbert, D. K., & Fisk, A. D. (1996). A survey of automatic teller machines usage across the adult life span. *Human Factors, 38*, 156-166.

Rogers, W. A., Meyer, B., Walker, N., & Fisk, A. D. (1998). Functional limitations to daily living tasks in the aged: A focus group analysis. *Human factors, 40*, 111-125.

Rosenbloom, S. (2000). Report by the chairperson (United States). In European Conference of Ministers of Transport (ECMT) (Ed.), *Transport and aging of the population: Report of the 112th round table on transport economics* (pp. 7-42). Paris Cedex, France: OECD Publications.

Rubert, M., Czaja, S., & Walsh, S. (2002). Tele-care: Helping caregivers cope with cancer. *Gerontechnology, 2(1)*, 144.

Rudinger, G. (1996). Alter und Technik [Old age and technology]. *Zeitschrift für Gerontologie und Geriatrie, 29(4)*, 246-256.

Sackmann, A., & Weymann, A. (1994). *Die Technisierung des Alltags. Generationen und technische Innovationen* [The technization of everyday life. Generations and technical innovations]. Frankfurt, Germany: Campus.

Schauer, T., & Radermacher, F. J. (Eds.). (2001). *The challenge of the digital divide. Promoting a global society dialogue*. Ulm, Germany: Universitätsverlag.

Scheidt, R. J., & Windley, P. G. (Eds.). (1998). *Environment and aging theory: A focus on housing*. Westport, CT: Greenwood Press.

Schulz, R., Lustig, A., Handler, L. M., & Martire, L. M. (2002). Technology-based caregiver intervention research: Current status and future directions. *Gerontechnology, 2(1)*, 15-47.

Severs, M. (1999). Will the information technology revolution improve services to elderly people in the new millennium? *Age and Aging, 28,* 5-9.

Smith, M. W., Czaja, S. J., & Sharit, J. (1999). Aging, motor control and the performance of computer mouse task. *Human Factors, 41,* 389-397.

Smither, J. A., & Braun, C. C. (1994). Technology and older adults: Factors affecting the adoption of automatic teller machines. *Journal of General Psychology, 121*(4), 381-390.

Stewart, T. (1992). Physical interfaces or "obviously it's for the elderly, it's grey, boring and dull!" In H. Bouma & J. A. M. Graafmans (Eds.), *Gerontechnology* (pp. 197-208). Amsterdam: IOS Press.

Strothotte, T., Johnson, V., Petrie, H., & Douglas, G. (1998). Evaluation of an orientation and navigation aid for visually impaired travellers. In I. Placencia Porrero & E. Ballabio (Eds.), *Improving the quality of life for the European citizen* (pp. 279-282). Amsterdam: IOS Press.

Tamura, T., Togawa, T., Ogawa, M., & Yamakoshi, K. (1998). Fully automated health monitoring at home. In J. A. M. Graafmans, V. Taipale, & N. Charness (Eds.), *Gerontechnology. A sustainable investment in the future* (pp. 280-284). Amsterdam: IOS Press.

TNO Institute for Strategy Technology and Policy. (1998). *Telematics applications programme "Design for All" for an inclusive information society* (TNO-report-98-70). Delft, The Netherlands: TNO.

van Berlo, A. (2002). Smart home technology: Have older people paved the way? *Gerontechnology, 2*(1), 77-87.

van Berlo, A., Bouma, H., Ekberg, J., Graafmans, J., Huf, F. A., Koster, W. G., et al. (1997). Gerontechnology. In R. Dulbecco (Ed.), *Encyclopedia of human biology* (2nd ed., Vol. 4, pp. 305-311). San Diego, CA: Academic Press.

Wahl, H. W. (2001). Environmental influences on aging and behavior. In J. E. Birren & K. W. Schaie (Eds.), *Handbook of the psychology of aging* (5th ed., pp. 215-237). San Diego, CA: Academic Press.

Wahl, H. W., & Mollenkopf, H. (in press). Impact of everyday technology in the home environment on older adults' quality of life. In K. W. Schaie & N. Charness (Eds.), *Impact of technology on successful aging.* New York: Springer.

Watzke, J. (2002). Assistive Technology for Older Adults: Challenges of Product Development and Evaluation. *Gerontechnology, 2*(1), 68-76.

Willis, S. L., & Schaie, K. W. (1986). Practical intelligence in later adulthood. In R. J. Sternberg & R .K. Wagner (Eds.), *Practical intelligence: Nature and origins of competence in the everyday world* (pp. 236-268). Cambridge, UK: Cambridge University Press.

Zimmer, Z., & Chappell, N. L. (1999). Receptivity to new technology among older adults. *Disability and Rehabilitation 2,* 222-230.

CHAPTER 11

The Urban-Rural Distinction in Gerontology: An Update of Research

STEPHEN M. GOLANT
DEPARTMENT OF GEOGRAPHY, UNIVERSITY OF FLORIDA

This review examines a large, and mostly U.S., literature to assess whether the distinctive environments found in the urban and rural settings of older persons influence their personal well-being or quality of life. Although these studies are rarely framed in the language of Lawton's, "Ecological Theory of Aging" (Lawton, 1998), their empirical findings can potentially shed light on three theoretical inquiries relevant to environmental gerontology. First, does the "environmental press" of urban and rural places—the real and perceived content of a setting that evokes the behaviors and responses of older persons—offer different opportunities or constraints for older residents to satisfy their health care, supportive service, and long-term care needs, and does it influence their personal well-being? Second, are older persons in rural or urban settings less competent or more vulnerable—as indicated by their poorer health, ability to perform everyday activities, less education, lower economic status, and their living alone? And third, do the facilitating and inhibiting influences of a rural setting make a greater difference in the lives of its more vulnerable older residents? Altogether, this literature holds promise of elucidating a fundamental issue in environmental gerontology: Does the place one grows old matter and does it matter more for some groups of older persons than for others (Golant, 1984)?

This chapter reviews the generalizations offered by this literature and the conceptual and methodological challenges of interpreting its findings. Though focused on U.S. settlements, its questions and issues are relevant to rural areas in developed and developing countries alike. The author initially examined over 500 publications written after 1990 cited in four major databases, PUBMED, AGELINE, SOCIAL SCIENCES CITATION INDEX, and SCIENCE CITATION INDEX.

RURAL AND URBAN CONTEXTS: CONCEPTUAL CHALLENGES

The Ecological Diversity of Urban and Rural Settlements in the United States

Just under a quarter of the U.S. population age 65 and over lived in rural America in the year 2000. This vast area represents 83 percent of the land area of the United States and consists of almost 2,300 counties. It is comprised of an extraordinarily diverse array of settlements. It is not hyperbole that "endangered and dying small towns" (Norris-Baker & Scheidt, 1991, p. 342) are worlds apart from the fast growing nonmetropolitan counties that are the destinations of higher income retirees. It is similarly true that metropolitan areas consist of a complex mosaic of central business districts, inner cities, gentrified neighborhoods, and older and newer suburbs. Thus, an analysis of residential analytical aggregations can easily smooth over sharp disparities both within and between these urban and rural contexts (Wallace & Wallace, 1998).

Researchers have relied on only a few classifications to describe these urban and rural contexts and have distinguished them by a relatively few ecological attributes: size, density, population heterogeneity, and remoteness (implying large traveling distances). Although sharing more similarities than differences, these typologies rely on different measures to establish their settlement boundaries, use different data collection units, and specify different numbers of urban-rural categorical gradations. They include urban (urbanized areas) and nonurban typologies from the U.S. Census Bureau, metropolitan-nonmetropolitan dichotomies of the Office of Management and Budget, the nine Urban Influence code categories of the Economic Research Service of the U.S. Department of Agriculture (Figure 11.1), the 10-category Beales or Rural-Urban Continuum code categories, and the "frontier areas" of the Department of Health and Human Services, distinguished by their sparsely populated areas with 6 to 10 persons per square mile (Ricketts, Johnson-Webb, & Taylor, 1998). Specific U.S. government programs have relied on variants of these typologies including the 1977 legislation that created Rural Health Clinics (to provide primary care services in rural underserved areas) and the zip code zones of the U.S. Administration of Aging and its 1992 Amendments to the Older Americans Act (Ricketts, Johnson-Webb, & Taylor, 1998).

The *U.S. Department of Agriculture* (USDA) *Economic Research Service* (ERS) focuses on a very different set of ecological categories, the diverse economic landscapes of rural America. It classifies nonmetropolitan

Code	County Definitions
1	Large—Central and fringe counties of large metropolitan areas of 1 million or more
2	Small—Counties in small metropolitan areas of fewer than 1 million population
3	Adjacent to a large metropolitan area with a city of 10,000 or more
4	Adjacent to a large metropolitan area without a city of at least 10,000
5	Adjacent to a small metropolitan area with a city of 10,000 or more
6	Adjacent to a small metropolitan area without a city of 10,000 or more
7	Not adjacent to a metropolitan area and with a city of 10,000 or more
8	Not adjacent to a metropolitan area and with a city of 2,500 to 9,999 population
9	Not adjacent to a metropolitan area and with no city or a city with a population less than 2,500

Source: Ricketts, T. C., Johnson-Webb, K. D., & Taylor, P. (1998). *Definitions of rural: A handbook for health policy makers and researchers.* Chapel Hill, NC: Cecil G. Sheps Center for Health Services Research, University of North Carolina at Chapel Hill.

FIGURE 11.1   United States Department of Agriculture Urban Influence Codes

counties into six nonoverlapping economic types: farming-dependent, mining-dependent, manufacturing-dependent, government-dependent, services-dependent, and nonspecialized counties (Cook & Mizer, 1994). A related typology classifies counties into five overlapping categories likely to inform public policy: retirement-destination counties, federal lands counties, commuting counties, persistent poverty counties, and (government) transfers-dependent counties. There are many obvious reasons to expect that these economic- and public-policy based approaches would capture the diversity of rural America, but except for the research of the ERS, studies have rarely incorporated these frameworks (Cook & Mizer, 1994).

   When research analyses rely on different settlement classifications to evaluate how urban and rural settings differ, it becomes more difficult to compare their findings and to make generalizations. A greater risk exists that the documented variations simply reflect methodological decisions regarding the categorization of the places and groups of people included in rural and urban America. Even when researchers use the same typology, findings may be difficult to interpret, because for statistical reasons, they collapse or combine their urban and rural settlement categories differently. Omission is no less a problem. Research analyses that fail to distinguish the "economic" or "public policy" types of their settings risk making generalizations that are not representative of the mosaic of landscapes found in rural America. Studies will be especially biased if, by chance or design, they focus on rural areas that only belong to a single classification category —such as "persistent poverty" counties.

The urban-rural typologies used in past research suffer from yet another potential methodological weakness. They fail to recognize that the urban-rural continuum is but one dimension of a "multidimensional hierarchical system" comprised of causally linked settlement components (Wachs, 1999, p. 359). Operationally, this is reflected by research investigations that fail to examine how the regional context of their urban and rural settlements influences their findings. Most studies, of course, will identify the regional location of their study or will report on regional differences (Rogers, 1999). Few will assess whether their documented urban-rural differences are spurious because they can be mainly attributed to a regional context effect.

Studies that assess the variation in the housing quality of urban and rural older residents in the United States illustrate how ignoring such hierarchical influences easily leads to misleading findings. Housing quality analyses always show that elderly homeowners living in rural areas are more likely than those in urban areas to be occupying dwellings in poor physical condition (Housing Assistance Council, 2000). Further analysis shows, however, that this generalization applies primarily to the dwellings occupied by older households in the U.S. South. In each of the other three U.S. Census regions (West, Midwest, and Northeast), the older homeowners in nonmetropolitan locations are equally or less likely than those in the central cities or the suburbs of metropolitan areas to occupy physically deficient dwellings (Golant, 2002).

Altogether, these alternative ways to classify urban and rural locales offer another unfortunate example of how researchers inconsistently classify older people's environments (Weisman, Chaudhury, & Moore, 2000).

A BROADER ECOLOGICAL CONCEPTUALIZATION OF URBAN AND RURAL CONTEXTS

Past research has infrequently conceptualized urban and rural contexts in a manner that is consistent with the "ecology of aging" literature (Lawton, 1998; Moos & Lemke, 1996; Scheidt & Windley, 1985). This broader perspective would distinguish at least three additional environmental categories.

The first would distinguish urban and rural contexts according to the strength of their "personal environments" (Lawton, 1998), that is, the emotional and material supports provided by family members to help frail older persons cope better with their impairments and help them to age in place. The long-term care literature has often speculated about how older persons and their family members trade off formal and informal sources of care. Nonetheless, most research from the United States and the United

Kingdom reports that rural and urban families do not assist their older members any differently (Coward & Dwyer, 1991; Glasgow, 2000). Compared with other inquiries, however, this is an underdeveloped area of research.

The second category would distinguish urban and rural contexts by the ecological characteristics of their built or natural environments (Lawton, 1998), encompassing human-made or physically modified environmental features and their natural settings. Studies often identify the harsh living conditions of rural America—difficult to transverse terrains, inadequate roads, poor quality bridges and highways, and weather extremes—or the transportation disadvantages for its elderly occupants (Ricketts, Johnson-Webb, & Randolph, 1999). Urban-rural comparisons, however, infrequently rely on these distinctions.

The third category would distinguish what Lawton (1998) referred to as the "social environment." This includes the programmatic, regulatory, and social institutional features that differentiate U.S. urban and rural areas. This is also an underdeveloped area of research, but the following examples suggest another basis for an urban-rural typology:

• Managed health care coverage is less available in rural than urban areas, though recent changes in the Balanced Budget Act of 1997 may make it more feasible to develop such plans in rural areas (Schoenman, 1999).

• Government-funded programs offer lower reimbursement payments to health care providers in rural than urban areas, making it difficult for them to attract high quality labor (Medicare, Payment Advisory Commission, 2001).

• Fewer health networks in rural than urban areas organizationally integrate the services provided by physicians, hospitals, and other health care providers (Medicare, Payment Advisory Commission, 2001; Schlenker & Shaughnessy, 1996).

• Rural health care providers have a less adequate information system infrastructure than their counterparts in urban areas (Medicare, Payment Advisory Commission, 2001).

DISTINGUISHING THE TEMPORAL PROPERTIES OF URBAN AND RURAL CONTEXTS

Temporal influences play a key role in how studies interpret differences between urban and rural contexts (Golant, 2003). Profound changes have occurred in the demographic, social, political, cultural, and economic characteristics of rural America (Fuguitt, Beale, & Tordella, 2002; Rogers, 1999). Traditionally, for example, rural America was thought to have an informal social support network built around the assumption of "a community

space and culture that involves shared assumptions, expectations, obligations, and codes of conduct regarding the appropriate way to interact with
older people" (Rowles, 1998, p. 111). This was a view of rural America in
which family and neighbors offered reliable assistance to their older residents. This generalization is now difficult if not impossible to make
(Rowles, 1998; Scheidt & Windley, 1987). Other key indicators of rurality,
access or remoteness, can also change relatively quickly. Over a relatively
short, five-year span (from 1993 to 1998), there was a substantial increase
in the availability and costs of rural public transportation services in the
United States: a 10 percent increase in the number of rural public transportation systems, a 79 percent increase in trips on these systems, and a 10
percent increase in the average cost per trip (Burkhardt, 2001). Similarly,
future assessments of rural access must increasingly consider the effects of
changes in telecommunications, digital communications, and specifically,
in telemedicine technologies (Redford & Whitten, 1997). Thus, studies conducted even a decade ago may offer invalid generalizations. The reporting
of outdated findings is extraordinarily pervasive in the rural gerontology
literature. Repeated referencing often elevates a study's credibility far
beyond its methodology would justify.

The timing of historical events will also influence urban-rural differences. Although one would expect to find health care facilities in more
accessible counties, many hospitals were initially built in nonmetropolitan
counties without interstate connections and they "have more hospitals and
beds per resident than do nonmetropolitan counties with interstates, as
well as metropolitan counties" (Ricketts, Johnson-Webb, & Randolph,
1999, p. 10). Urban and rural places also will adapt differently to health
care delivery regulations. Rural areas, for example, were slower to adopt
organizational and financial changes required by federal health care policies (Mueller, Coburn, Cordes, Crittenden, et al., 1999).

Interpreting the significance of temporal influences is complicated for
at least two reasons. First, rural America is not changing uniformly (Cook
& Mizer, 1994; Fuguitt, Beale, & Tordella, 2002). Thus, there is a danger of
under- or overstating the significance of demographic and economic transitions in particular locations. Second, most studies do not control for the
length of time that older persons have lived in their current locations or
have not documented their migration histories (Scheidt, 1998). Older rural
women, for example, who have recently migrated from urban places, are
more likely to be married and have higher income and education levels
than their traditional rural female neighbors. Yet, even as rural women
who are long-time occupants are socioeconomically more disadvantaged,
they may cope more successfully with the "barriers to economic well-
being, health care, transportation, and other needs" because they have
"inherited a sense of permanence and worth of rural life from their early
farm forebears" (McCulloch & Kivett, 1998, p. 151).

A less known methodological artifact can influence generalizations about how urban and rural settings differ. Over time, the population density of a rural county often increases or more of its workers commute to a neighboring urban county. These changes may trigger its reclassification as an urban county. Data sets, however, may not automatically change their urban and rural county designations. To insure a consistent comparison of the same set of rural (or urban) counties between 1990 and 2000, for example, 1990 urban-rural boundary definitions may be used. This is the case even though a significant number of the rural-defined counties of 1990 are officially a part of urban America in the year 2000. Although this "apples to apples" comparison may appear reasonable, it can yield very misleading findings.

An analysis that compared the physical conditions of the dwellings occupied by older persons in urban and rural contexts offers a revealing example. The 1999 *American Housing Survey* (AHS)—a data set usually relied on when making public policies regarding the unmet housing needs of older (and younger) Americans—defines metropolitan and nonmetropolitan areas based on a constant set of 1983 boundaries (Commission on Affordable Housing and Health Facility Needs for Seniors in the 21st Century, 2002; Golant, 2002). Thus, its findings are based on an urban-rural county classification that is 16 years out of date. Two inevitable results: first, the *prevalence* of rural older households living in housing in poor physical condition will be understated because many of the so-called 1983 rural counties are now the suburban counties of metropolitan areas. Relatively large shares of their housing stock will be new and in good physical condition. Thus, the inclusion of these counties in rural America dilutes the percentage share of dwellings deemed in poor condition. Second, the *number* of rural dwellings in poor physical condition that is occupied by older households will be inflated, because dwellings are counted in so-called 1983 rural counties that by 1999 have become reclassified as urban. The unreasonableness of relying on such historically dated urban and rural boundaries is demonstrated when a researcher selects a sample of rural counties to study. Would such a sample include counties that are *now* "rural" or *were* "rural" 16 years earlier?

THE POPULATION COMPOSITION ATTRIBUTES OF RURAL AND URBAN CONTEXTS

Defining and Justifying Indicators

Composition attributes generally refer to the socio-demographic characteristics of older persons, such as age, income, family/household types, education, and race. Conceptually, most analyses treat these attributes as indicators of the vulnerability of older persons. Two rationales exist for focusing on how the composition attributes of urban and rural elderly populations differ.

First, this category of constructs is specifically incorporated in Lawton's (1998), "Ecological Theory on Aging" that was designed to explain why environment press of a given magnitude would differently influence older people's adaptive behavior or psychological well-being. The model's, "environmental docility hypothesis" predicts that seniors who are less competent or more vulnerable will be more susceptible to the vagaries of their environment. Thus, in a remote rural community, older persons who are less educated or lived alone would be predicted to have more difficulty securing needed health care than better-educated and married couples (Calsyn & Winter, 1999). Unfortunately, studies have not tested the validity of the proposition by comparing the adaptive responses of more and less vulnerable elderly groups in equally adverse rural settings.

There is a second and equally important rationale to study such differences. Government programs must allocate scarce fiscal resources to older persons with the greatest unmet needs. At issue is whether it is informative to distinguish their residential contexts. One group of researchers argues that once taking into consideration the differences in the composition of an older population, residential category membership is a poor predictor of unmet need or, at worse, obfuscating. This group argues that unmet needs attributed to ecological context differences only persist when a study inaccurately takes into account how elderly populations differ. They point to studies that fail to control statistically for the share of rural seniors who are very old. Thus, when rural areas are more top-heavy with age 75 and over seniors than urban areas, they will appear as having worse quality of life outcomes (Wallace & Wallace, 1998).

Two research analyses inspired by the need to inform public policy specifically focused on this question. Under the Older Americans Act, many states maintain an Intrastate Funding Formula designed to target planning and service areas occupied by seniors with the greatest economic and social needs (Coward, Vogel, Duncan, & Uttaro, 1995). Composition features, such as educational status, race, poverty, family size, and age, distinguish at-risk populations. At issue is whether empirically documented differences in the unmet needs of urban and rural elders would persist even after accounting for their population composition differences. One analysis concluded that not only is it uninformative to differentiate older persons by their residential context, it is also inequitable. That is, the "inclusion of rural weighting may divert already scarce fiscal resources away from urban areas where greater levels of need can be demonstrated"

(Harlow, 1993, p. 440). A second analysis disagreed and showed that "residing in a nonmetropolitan area increases the likelihood of poor health and higher levels of physical cognitive impairments and the need for services after controlling for age, income, and race" (Coward, Vogel, Duncan, & Uttaro, 1995, p. 24).

These contradictory findings argue for caution when drawing generalizations from this literature. The findings of the second study emphasize that the urban-rural differences in the well-being of older rural dwellers cannot be simply reduced to the effects of their composition differences. On the other hand, the findings of the first study emphasize the need for careful statistical analysis before a researcher concludes that urban-rural quality of life differences can be attributed to their ecological context variations.

URBAN-RURAL VARIATIONS IN INDICATORS OF POPULATION COMPOSITION

The early literature often portrayed rural or nonmetropolitan areas in the United States as the homes of more vulnerable older persons (Glasgow, 1988). A consideration of the most frequently identified composition indicators reveals a less clear-cut contemporary locational pattern.

Sociodemographic Structure

Just under 15 percent of the population in U.S. nonmetropolitan or rural areas but less than 12 percent of the population in metropolitan or urban areas were age 65 and over in the year 2000 (Table 11.1). Both metropolitan and nonmetropolitan areas, however, had about the same share of the age 65 and over population that was in the oldest age groups (age 75 and over; Table 11.2). Predictably, the age 65 and over population with the smallest share of age 75 plus persons lived in the suburbs (outside the central cities of metropolitan areas).

Similar percentages of the older population occupying metropolitan and nonmetropolitan areas were women and lived alone, though there were slightly smaller percentages of younger (age 65 to 74) nonmetropolitan elderly living alone, and slightly higher shares of older (age 85 and over) nonmetropolitan elderly who were women and living alone (USDA, ERS, 2002).

Much higher percentages of the nonmetropolitan older population had less than a high school education. This metro-nonmetro gap was the greatest for the age 85 and over population (Rogers, 1999). Rural America was also disproportionately occupied by Nonhispanic, white older persons and had underrepresentations of Black, Hispanic, and Asian populations. This generalization was less true for certain regions than for others.

TABLE 11.1 Relative Size of the Older Population in Metropolitan and Nonmetropolitan Locations, 2000

Location	Size of Total Population	Total Population	Percent of Total Population in Older Age Groups					
			60-64	65-74	75-84	85+	65+	75+
United States	281,421,906	100.0	3.8	6.5	4.4	1.5	12.4	5.9
Metropolitan Areas	225,981,679	100.0	3.7	6.2	4.2	1.4	11.9	5.6
Inside Central Cities	85,401,127	100.0	3.4	5.9	4.2	1.5	11.5	5.7
Outside Central Cities	140,580,552	100.0	3.9	6.5	4.2	1.4	12.1	5.6
Nonmetropolitan Areas	55,440,227	100.0	4.5	7.7	5.1	1.8	14.7	6.9

Source: U.S. Census Bureau. (2001). Profiles of general demographic characteristics, 2000 Census of Population and Housing, United States. Washington, DC: U.S. Government Printing Office.

TABLE 11.2 Age Distribution of the Elderly Population in Metropolitan and Nonmetropolitan Locations, 2000

Location	Size of Age 65 and Over Population	Percent of Age 65 and Over Population in Older Age Groups					
		65+	65-74	75-84	85+	75+	
United States	34,991,753	100.0	52.6	35.3	12.1	47.4	
Metropolitan Areas	26,858,060	100.0	52.5	35.5	12.0	47.5	
Inside Central Cities	9,856,307	100.0	50.9	36.1	13.0	49.1	
Outside Central Cities	17,001,753	100.0	53.5	35.1	11.4	46.5	
Nonmetropolitan Areas	8,133,693	100.0	52.7	34.8	12.6	47.3	

Source: U.S. Census Bureau. (2001). Profiles of general demographic characteristics, 2000 Census of Population and Housing, United States. Washington, DC: U.S. Government Printing Office.

Economic Status

The incomes of older persons are lower in rural than urban areas (U.S. Bureau of the Census, 2001). As of 2000, 13.2 percent of the age 65 and over nonmetropolitan area population had incomes below the 100 percent poverty level. This compared with elderly poverty rates of 7.5 percent in the suburbs, and 12.4 percent in the central cities. The metropolitan-non-metropolitan poverty rate gap was larger for the age 85 and over population than for the younger elderly groups and especially large for older persons living alone (USDA, ERS, 2002).

Elderly poverty rates in nonmetropolitan areas varied substantially by U.S. Census region in the year 2000: 16.4 percent in the South, 11.7 percent in the Midwest, 9.3 percent in the West, and 9.7 percent in the Northeast (U.S. Bureau of the Census, 2001). In 1999, 83 percent of the country's "persistent poverty" counties were located in the U.S. South even though only 44 percent of U.S. nonmetropolitan counties overall were located in this region (Cook & Mizer, 1994). The most rural counties (the most remote, with the smallest populations) had the highest poverty rates (USDA, ERS, 2002).

The nonmetropolitan older population will spend more years in poverty and is less likely than the metropolitan older population to escape from their poverty status. This generalization persists even after controlling for other population composition differences (Jensen & McLaughlin, 1997). Elders in nonmetropolitan areas also have lower lifetime earnings, fewer income generating assets, lower Social Security and pension benefits, and they are less likely to hold skilled professional, managerial, or technical jobs (Glasgow & Brown, 1998).

This pattern of income inequality results partly from the selective migration patterns of older and younger persons. Younger populations often relocated from counties in regions dependent on farming and mining leaving behind economically disadvantaged older persons who did not have the means or motivation to move elsewhere (Fuguitt, Beale, & Tordella, 2002; Rogers, 1999). In contrast, nonmetropolitan counties receiving wealthier retiree in-migrants have lower elderly poverty rates (Longino, 1990; Serow, 2001).

A reliance only on poverty rate indicators without considering cost of living differences may misleadingly overstate the number of rural elders experiencing economic difficulties. The Department of Housing and Urban Development expresses the incomes of households as a ratio of their metropolitan area's or nonmetropolitan county's area median income (adjusted for household size). This agency often designates households as poor if they are living in areas where their incomes are 50 percent or less of their area's median income. By this standard, 47 percent of nonmetropolitan older households compared with 53 percent of central city and 49 percent of the suburban elderly are poor (Golant, 2002).

It is also important to consider other sources of wealth besides income. The owned dwelling is the single most important asset of older Americans. Older households in nonmetropolitan areas are more likely to be home-owners and to occupy paid-up dwellings or hold very small mortgages (Rogers, 1999). Offsetting this advantage is the generally lower values of the dwellings owned by rural elders (Housing Assistance Council, 2000). Overall, however, rural older homeowners have lower housing costs than do their urban counterparts.

INDICATORS OF BOTH VULNERABILITY AND WELL-BEING

Defining and Justifying Indicators

A second set of indicators describes the physical, functional, and mental health status of older persons. These can be conceptually interpreted in at least four distinctive ways. First, they are constructs depicting the vulner-ability of individuals or populations. Second, models predicting the well being or quality of life of individuals or populations often propose them as antecedents. Third, analyses treat them as distinctive quality of life or well-being constructs. And, fourth, they are defined as outcome constructs that inform about the success or failure of social or economic programs for-mulated to alleviate the unmet needs of older persons.

Physical Health

Nonmetropolitan elders in the United States overall, and specifically in the most remote rural counties, were more likely than metropolitan elders to assess their own health as poor or fair (Rogers, 1999). Studies reporting this difference, however, have not controlled for the possible spurious effects of population composition differences (Coburn & Bolda, 1999). On the other hand, a Florida-based study reported that low-income and less educated older persons did not report significantly poorer self-health and did not have more physician-diagnosed medical conditions than a comparable urban older population sample (Ranelli & Coward, 1996).

An analysis of a large 1993 Medicare Current Beneficiary sample also showed that rural older persons did not have a higher prevalence of chronic health problems (Call, Casey, & Radcliff, 2000). Several other U.S. studies have similarly found few such differences (Dwyer, Folts, &

Rosenberg, 1994; Rogers, 1999). A British review reached a similar conclusion (Wenger, 2001). Older and rural seniors have also not been found to differ significantly with respect to smoking or drinking heavily, eating healthful diets, or being overweight (Van Nostrand, Furner, Brunelle, & Cohen, 1993). One study was especially unequivocal:

> The results question blanket assertions about population density and health status. It is concluded that analyzing population data as an urban/rural dichotomy may bias understanding and misguide health policy. It is recommended that health policy initiatives require community based studies to establish medical care needs. (Gillanders, Buss, & Hofstetter, 1996, p, 7)

When studies focus on particular health problems, they are more likely to report that the health status of urban and rural elders differs. A Geneva, Switzerland study found that age 65 and over urban residents had a 31 percent higher incidence of hip fractures than older rural residents after controlling for age, class, gender, and home vs. institutional occupancy (Chevalle, Herman, Delmi, Stern, et al., 2002). In the U.S., the rate of edentulism (loss of natural teeth) for the overall age 65 and over population and for the low-income group particularly is higher in nonmetropolitan counties and this difference persists in all regions except the Midwest (Eberhardt, Ingram, & Makuc, 2001). Lower-income rural older adults were also significantly more likely to have root caries (Ringelberg, Gilbert, Antonson, Dolan, et al., 1996).

Functional Health

Functional health status, the capability of older persons to perform their everyday activities without assistance, is the most important basis by which families, professionals, and programs judge older people's need for more supportive housing and long-term care accommodations. *Instrumental Activities of Daily Living* (IADLs) typically include preparing meals, doing light housework, taking the right amount of medicine, keeping track of money or bills, and going outside the home. *Activities of Daily Living* (ADLs) typically include getting in and out of bed or a chair, taking a bath or shower, dressing, walking, eating, and using or getting to a toilet.

Prior to 1990, studies in the U.S. routinely concluded that functional limitations were more prevalent among rural than urban elders (Dwyer, Lee, & Coward, 1990). More recent studies offer inconsistent findings. A national study (not controlling for variation in population composition effects) found that a slightly greater proportion of rural elders suffered from five to six ADL impairments, but higher proportions of elders in small cities and other urban areas had IADL limitations, or had one to four ADL impairments (Dwyer, Barton, & Vogel, 1994). A national survey of older persons not living in institutions found that after controlling for population composition effects, nonmetropolitan elders were actually *more* functionally able (Rabiner, Konrad, DeFriese, Kincade, et al., 1997). A small study of centenarians found that urban elders had higher levels (but not significantly) of functional health after controlling for race and gender. Explanations for why rural elders would have better functional health focus on their lower life-style expectations and strong self-reliance. That is, they judge their inabilities less harshly or compensate for their lost abilities by using assistive devices or modifying their behaviors (Clayton, Dudley, Patterson, Lawhorn, et al., 1994; Rabiner, Konrad, DeFriese, Kincade, et al., 1997). A methodological artifact, however, may be at work. Community-based studies typically exclude the institutionalized population, and thus they undercount the impaired seniors in rural areas who are disproportionately more likely to occupy nursing homes than their urban counterparts (Wallace & Wallace, 1998).

Mental Health

Findings on how the mental health of rural and urban seniors differs are difficult to interpret for several reasons. First, analyses focus on different mental health constructs, including psychological well-being (e.g., happiness, life satisfaction, and morale) and cognitive disorders (e.g., anxiety, depression, agitation, and dementias; Scheidt, 1998). Second, they are based only on regional or local samples. Third, they may not carefully control for urban-rural variations in chronological age, even as cognitive impairment rates are higher for persons who are age 85 and older (Chumbler, Cody, Booth, & Beck, 2001).

Several studies in the United States and in other countries found that some dementing illnesses are more common in rural than in urban elderly populations. Current screening instruments, however, may misclassify rural elders as "false positive" dementia cases (Keefover, Rankin, Keyl, Wells, et al., 1996). The largest U.S. psychiatric epidemiological study (*Epidemiological Catchment Area* [ECA] collaborative program) found only a weak residential category influence on mental disorders such as depression, cognitive impairments, or the lifetime prevalence of any psychiatric disorder. Regional effects were stronger (Robins & Regier, 1991). The researchers link the lower self-reported mental illness rates of rural elders to the stronger stigma against admitting to mental illness (Lawrence & McCulloch, 2001).

In the above ECA study, subjective well-being also did not simply vary by residential context, though urban dwellers had more daytime sleepiness and nighttime sleep complaints (Hays, Blazer, & Foley, 1996). A large national study also found that nonmetropolitan older residents had more positive perceptions of well-being (Mookherjee, 1998). A small study additionally found that urban older women reported higher levels of stress (Gale, 1993). In contrast, a 1986 Nebraskan study of depressive symptoms among older women (Warheit Depression Scale) found no significant differences by community type (Craft, Johnson, & Ortega, 1998). The authors conclude that a convergence in rural and urban lifestyles explains the lack of significant mental health differences. Inconsistently, a 1992 telephone survey of U.S. rural older subjects (without controlling for composition differences) found that they had significantly more suicide attempts over a one-year period (Rost, Zhang, Fortney, Smith, et al., 1998).

Empirical research on the mental health problems of ethnic minorities in rural areas is sparse, inconsistent, and controversial. A small study of black older persons in western Tennessee, found that depressive symptoms were more likely among urban dwellers reflecting the rural residents' stronger and more extensive social support network of family, friends, and neighbors (Okwumabua, Baker, Wong, & Pilgrim, 1997). Nonetheless, Scheidt (2001) argues that researchers may be underestimating or misdiagnosing the mental health problems of elderly African Americans and Hispanics because of deficient methodologies and a misunderstanding of the links between culture and mental health.

UNEQUAL QUALITY OF LIFE OUTCOMES IN URBAN AND RURAL AMERICA

Four Quality of Life Categories and the "Urban" Standard

This section reviews evidence that the variation in the older population's quality of life outcomes or personal well-being can be attributed to their urban and rural ecological contexts. Urban-rural comparisons will be made for four quality of life categories:

1. mortality rates
2. the availability, use, and accessibility of community-based health care and other supportive services
3. the availability and use of home health care services
4. the availability and use of nursing homes

Most of the studies implicitly assume that an urban way of life is the more desirable or strived for societal standard. The following review also follows this convention though it may not be justifiable for two reasons. First, the conditions found in urban America are not necessarily more desirable. Rural and urban crime rates may be similar, but both may be intolerably high. Second, not all urban activities, features, or attributes will be appropriate or desirable in rural contexts. As one example, the introduction of conventional buses may not be the best solution to serve the transportation needs of rural elders, but the increased availability of demand-responsive transit options offering flexible door-to-door transportation may greatly improve their mobility (Burkhardt, 2001).

Mortality Rates as an Indicator of Urban-Rural Differences in Quality of Life

The most important causes of death among older persons are heart disease, cancer, stroke, chronic obstructive pulmonary disease, and pneumonia (Eberhardt, Ingram, & Makuc, 2001). Several studies have linked the variation in the mortality rates of older adults to the unequal health risks found in their urban and rural contexts. Over the period of 1996-1998, the national age-adjusted death rate for age 65 and over men or women was higher in nonmetropolitan counties and was the lowest in larger metropolitan counties. These mortality rate differentials, however, were not consistently found in all regions and they did not generally apply to black elders. In the Midwest and Western regions of the country, for example, the age-adjusted death rate of age 65 and over blacks was the *lowest* in the nonmetropolitan counties (Eberhardt, Ingram, & Makuc, 2001).

One study also reported relatively lower rural mortality rates when it controlled for the sociodemographic differences among urban and rural elders (Smith, Anderson, Bradham, & Longino, 1995). This longevity advantage, however, was only conferred on age 55 to 64 and 65 to 74 cohorts, and not on persons age 75 and over. Moreover, another study suggested that the additional years of life experienced by rural older adults might have downsides, because they were sometimes entirely spent in poor health and inactivity (Geronimus, Bound, Waidmann, Colen, et al., 2001). The conclusion is that once considering other risk factors, only a small and unpredictable amount of variation in the mortality rates of older persons is explained by their different urban and rural locations (Wallace & Wallace, 1998). Nonetheless, the higher elderly death rates in some parts of rural America mean that there will be "more actual end-of-life-related need for health services" (Ricketts, Johnson-Webb, & Randolph, 1999, p. 19).

Generalizations are also difficult to make about the risk of accidental causes of death in urban and rural places. Death rates of older persons (age 65 and over) due to motor vehicle crashes were higher in counties with lower population density. In contrast, elderly persons were more involved in fatal crashes at intersections, but these occurred at higher population densities (Clark, 2001). Older occupants of nonmetropolitan areas were more likely to die from excessive heat or cold. It is possible, however, that the variation primarily reflected the lower incomes of the rural elders (Macey & Schneider, 1993).

The Availability, Use, and Accessibility of Physicians, Health Care Clinics, Hospitals, Pharmacies, and Other Supportive Services

Rural America is fundamentally disadvantaged because its health and human service programs cater to smaller and more geographically spread-out markets. Thus, its programs have more difficulty achieving the beneficial economies of scale enjoyed by urban areas and as a result, they incur more expensive capital and operating costs (Medicare, Payment Advisory Commission, 2001). The physical remoteness of parts of rural America similarly results in programs having higher transportation costs (Burkhardt, 2001).

On a per capita basis, physicians are overall less available in rural than in urban areas. This disparity, however, primarily results from the higher concentration of specialists in urban areas who "require a large population base, sophisticated hospitals and laboratories, and specialty colleagues . . ." (Rosenblatt & Hart, 1999, p. 41). In contrast, except in the more remote rural areas, family or primary care physicians are just as available in rural areas (Medicare, Payment Advisory Commission, 2001). Moreover, the supply of rural physicians has also steadily increased over the past 20 years, especially in larger communities near metropolitan areas (Rosenblatt & Hart, 1999). The federal government has also increased its assistance (e.g., Medicare bonus reimbursement payments) to underserved rural areas with very low physician to population ratios. These *health professional shortage areas* (HPSAs) typically have small populations, poor physical and cultural amenities, extreme poverty, and high concentrations of minorities (Rosenblatt & Hart, 1999). During the 1990s, the growth of rural health clinics also offered a substitute for physician office visits (Medicare, Payment Advisory Commission, 2001). The above trends suggest that rural pockets still exist where there is a strong unmet need for physicians, but that this inequality is not readily revealed by making urban comparisons (Rosenblatt & Hart, 1999).

Studies do not agree on whether older Medicare beneficiaries receive less physician care in rural than urban areas (Chumbler, Cody, Beck, & Booth, 2000; Coburn & Bolda, 1999; Himes & Rutrough, 1994; McConnel & Zetzman, 1993). Dansky, Brannon, Shea, Vasey, et al. (1998) argue that it is misleading in any case to rely only on physician visits overall as a single indicator. They found that rural elders see general practitioners more frequently, but internal medicine and other specialty physicians less frequently than do urban elders. The locational variations in physician use rates are also difficult to interpret because studies inconsistently control for differences in the physical, functional, or mental health needs of patients. Thus, even when urban and rural seniors have equivalent physician use rates, rural seniors may be receiving inappropriate care if they have more serious health problems (Medicare, Payment Advisory Commission, 2001).

The number of hospitals in rural America has dropped sharply over the past 20 years because of a declining demand for in-patient services. To increase market share, hospitals have become more diversified and are more likely to offer long-term care services (swing beds, nursing facility, and home health) than urban hospitals (Medicare, Payment Advisory Commission, 2001; Schlenker & Shaughnessy, 1996).

Urban hospitals are used more for specialized surgical care, such as cardiovascular procedures, whereas rural hospitals are used more for routine procedures (Buczko, 2001). Studies disagree, however, about the hospital utilization rate differences of the urban and rural elderly. A recent analysis found that nonfarm rural elders have more hospital inpatient stays per beneficiary (Medicare, Payment Advisory Commission, 2001). Yet other investigations find few residential differences in the number of short-term hospital stays or in the number of days of bed disability (Blazer, Landerman, Fillenbaum, & Horner, 1995; Coburn & Bolda, 1999; Himes & Rutrough, 1994; McConnel & Zetzman, 1993).

Older rural Medicare beneficiaries must endure longer travel times to obtain medical care, but they are as satisfied as older urban beneficiaries with their access to and quality of medical care. Only older Medicare beneficiaries in the most rural locations are somewhat less satisfied with the ease of getting to a doctor (Medicare, Payment Advisory Commission, 2001). Older beneficiaries in the rural counties adjacent to a metropolitan area actually reported higher satisfaction levels than those in urban counties (Stearns, Slifkin, & Edin, 2000). Other research argues that it is the low income rather than urban or rural residential category that is the more important influence of self-reported access difficulties and satisfaction level (Stearns, Slifkin, & Edin, 2000). Similarly, it is the type of health insurance held by older persons and their ability to afford medical costs that are more important than physician access (Blazer, Landerman, Fillenbaum, & Horner, 1995; Seccombe, 1995; Stearns, Slifkin, & Edin, 2000).

Residential location differences inconsistently explain whether older persons are receiving needed medical care. Only older persons in the most rural locations (particularly in HPSAs) are less likely to receive needed care, particularly electrocardiograms, timely follow-up after hospital discharge, mammograms, and dental care (Medicare, Payment Advisory Commission, 2001; Stearns, Slifkin, & Edin, 2000). Rural diabetic elderly patients receiving office-based care in three states also were less likely to receive appropriate services (Weiner, Parente, Garnick, Fowles, et al., 1995).

Emergency response time to rural patients also was longer than for urban patients, partly because of less available ambulance service (Medicare, Payment Advisory Commission, 2001). On the other hand, medical care outcomes for older persons hospitalized for community-acquired pneumonia were unrelated to residential context (Whittle, Lin, Lave, Fine, et al., 1998). Similarly, discharged rural cardiac patients had better outcomes (Dellasega, Orwig, Ahern, & Lenz, 1999). In a small study (Maine, New Hampshire, and Vermont during 1989), the likelihood of hospitalization for older persons at risk did not differ by distance (Goodman, Fisher, Stukel, & Chang, 1997).

Prescription drug use in Pennsylvania also did not substantially differ by residential location (Lago, Stuart, & Ahern, 1993). A possible explanation is that rural seniors have more personal, medication-related discussions with their pharmacists than their urban counterparts (Ranelli & Coward, 1996). Additionally, in Minnesota, North Dakota, and South Dakota, most rural residents (of all ages) lived within 20 miles of a pharmacy. Rural establishments may also be more accessible because they were open during evenings and weekends, had pharmacists on-call after hours, and delivered prescriptions to private homes. Rural elders reported that the cost of pharmacy services was a more serious concern (Casey, Klinger, & Moscovice, 2002).

Older adults in rural areas have available to them a smaller and less diverse array of community-based supportive services, although the urban-rural gap has become smaller (Coward, Duncan, & Freudenberger, 1994). Rural-based *Area Agencies on Aging* (AAA) have smaller budgets and fewer volunteer and paid staff than urban AAAs (Krout, 1998). One study found, however, that a national sample of disabled nonmetropolitan older respondents had a greater volume of AAA-sponsored services available per capita than their metropolitan area counterparts (Clark, 1993). Such contradictory findings can be explained by the variation in the availability of supportive services for older persons found throughout rural America (Krout, 1998). The use of services by older Americans, however, may not be simply related to their availability. Krout (1998) reports that older rural elders attend their AAAs less frequently than do older urban elders. Availability of services and the frequency older people use them may also be unrelated to their unmet needs. No residential differences in unmet ADL and IADL needs for care were found for a large national sample of older persons after controlling for variations in population composition effects (Clark, 1992). This finding was partly explained by the rural elderly sample receiving more person days of informal assistance with IADL activities. Another study of urban and rural senior center attendees in Pennsylvania found that even when older persons in rural areas had more health complaints, they did not use more services or report more unmet needs. This discrepancy was explained by the greater self-reliance of rural seniors in health care matters (Clark & Dellasega, 1998).

The Availability and Use of Home Health Care Services

Understanding the unequal availability of home health care services (mostly provided under the Medicare home health benefit) in urban and rural areas is important for several reasons. First, if these services are less available in rural areas, older persons may be at greater risk of prematurely entering nursing homes. Second, hospitals are motivated under current Medicare reimbursement patterns to discharge older persons faster than in the past, and thus these elders often need posthospital care. Third, if rural home health care services are in shorter supply, it is important to understand why. It may reflect the inadequate supply of nurses and therapists in rural areas, possibly because of the lower wages offered to these workers, in turn a result of lower Health Care Financing Administration rates for Medicare reimbursements (Cheh & Phillips, 1993).

Research examining how home health care use patterns of Medicare beneficiaries differ in urban and rural areas offers contradictory findings. Home health care use rates are also difficult to interpret because it is unclear whether seniors are receiving appropriate care without controlling for their health conditions and their treatment outcomes (Medicare, Payment Advisory Commission, 2001).

Several studies found that rural older Medicare beneficiaries were less likely to be home health care clients (Clark, 1992; Nyman, Sen, Chan, & Commins, 1991). They also showed that rural home health care agencies were more likely to be addressing post-acute than long-term or chronic care needs. A recent analysis (in 28 states) reported that for the period 1995-1996, "similar elderly home health patients (controlling for case mix) served by similar agencies will receive somewhat fewer services, particularly on a per-day basis, if they are in rural rather than urban areas" (Schlenker, Powell, & Goodrich, 2002, p. 367). It also found that patient outcomes after discharge were less favorable for rural home health clients. Another study found that rural older Medicare beneficiaries using home health care were less likely to receive the number of physical therapy visits specified in the guidelines. To compensate, home health agencies substituted skilled nursing services for physical therapy services (Cheh & Phillips, 1993).

Other studies have reached very different conclusions. Two investigations found no significant differences in the use of formal home care by urban and rural elders (Netzer, Coward, Peek, Henretta, et al., 1997; Rabiner, 1995). Another study found that older residents in the most rural areas received significantly more Medicare reimbursed home health care visits than in the more urbanized rural counties. The authors speculated that home health care visits were substituting for physician visits and community-based services (Dansky, Brannon, Shea, Vasey, et al., 1998). This pattern of home care use was particularly applicable to older people with diabetes (Dansky, Brannon, Shea, Vasey, et al., 1998). Kenney's (1993) frequently cited study shows why it is difficult to draw conclusions. It reported that home health use rates by older Medicare beneficiaries (in 1987) were 14 percent higher in urban than in rural areas. Two other findings, however, are infrequently reported. First, when the rural beneficiaries did receive home care, they had three more visits on average than did urban users. Second, the home health use rates in urban areas were higher in only 58 percent of the states, but in 42 percent of the states, the rural use rates were higher, particularly in the East South Central and Middle Atlantic regions (Kenney, 1993). Overall, the current literature suggests that the availability and use of home health care services varies more *among* rural counties than *between* urban and rural areas (Salmon, Nelson, & Rous, 1993).

The Availability and Use of Nursing Homes

A key question is whether rural elders are prematurely more at risk of entering nursing homes than urban elders because they have less available alternative long-term care options, including family assistance, home care, community-based services, or noninstitutional accommodations, such as assisted living facilities (Krout, 1998). If impaired rural elders must enter a nursing home to receive needed personal and health care assistance, environmental theories argue that they may experience maladaptive behaviors and negative affect because they are unnecessarily receiving too much environmental support (Lawton, 1998).

Nonmetropolitan counties have a larger supply of nursing homes per capita than metropolitan counties. This is partly because of the Medicare swing-bed program, whereby a high percentage of nursing homes in rural areas—especially in the more remote counties—are hospital-based (Coburn & Bolda, 1999; Dubay, 1993). Rural nursing homes, however, are less likely to offer certified skilled nursing beds or special care units and are more likely to offer only a custodial level of care. Thus, rural elders may have more difficulty finding heavier skilled nursing care (Coburn & Bolda, 1999).

Older persons in rural areas had a higher nursing home admission rate (Coward, Netzer, & Mullens, 1996; Dubay, 1993). The admission rates of Medicare enrollees in 1987 ranged from 8.8 admissions per 1,000 enrollees in urbanized counties adjacent to a metropolitan area, to 14.5 admissions per 1,000 enrollees in the more remote and thinly populated counties not adjacent to a metropolitan area.

Accounting for this higher rate of rural institutionalization is not straightforward. Rural elders admitted to nursing homes are not necessarily younger or healthier than their urban counterparts (Duncan, Coward, & Gilbert, 1997). That is, they were not at higher risk of being admitted to nursing homes at lower levels of functional disability (Penrod, 2001). Moreover, rural elders do not display a greater *need* for skilled nursing care, as measured by sociodemographic, health, or living alone risk factors. Higher admission rates may simply reflect the greater availability of nursing homes in rural areas. Alternatively, physicians in rural areas may be more likely to refer older persons to nursing homes. Others have theorized that rural elders hold more positive attitudes toward the nursing home, believing it to be integral to their community (Rowles, Concotelli, & High, 1996). Other research, however, shows that rural residents entering nursing homes were more likely than their urban counterparts to report needing services (after controlling for variations in their health) that were unavailable in their communities (Coward, Duncan, & Freudenberger, 1994). Another study found that nursing home admissions of urban elders were more likely a result of a serious injury from a fall or an acute illness than from a chronic illness. In contrast, rural elders were more likely to report that changing and unfavorable family circumstances were responsible for their nursing home occupancy, implying that they could not rely on home-based informal assistance to address their chronic health problems (Jett, Coward, Schoenberg, Duncan, et al., 1996).

TRANSACTIONAL AND ETHNOGRAPHIC PERSPECTIVES ON THE RURAL ELDERLY

A significant category of studies is less interested in whether rural or urban older adults are more vulnerable or in how their ecological contexts systematically differ. Rather, this research seeks to understand how rural dwellers materially, emotionally, and symbolically use, interpret, experience, and adapt to their settings (Rowles, 1998; Scheidt, 1998). These studies are inspired by the transactional research paradigm and its focus on events and phenomena involving the confluence of people, space, and time (Altman & Rogoff, 1987). "Rural" for these inquiries is nothing less than a holistic and undifferentiated amalgam of ecological and composition attributes and quality of life outcomes subjectively interpreted through both historical and contemporaneous lens. Seeking causal explanations, artificially separating individuals from their environmental con-

text or environmental components from each other, demarcating the objective and subjective worlds of older adults, establishing urban-rural boundaries, or sorting environmental attributes into specific construct categories,
are considered artificial and contrived tasks (Rowles & Johansson, 1993;
Scheidt & Norris-Baker, 1993).

Several empirical studies offer examples. One investigation of the food
sharing practices of persons age 70 plus in two rural counties in central
North Carolina emphasized that food intake was not merely a source of
nutrition, but was inseparably joined with older participants' sense of community and the availability of emotional and instrumental supports
(Quandt, Arcury, Bell, McDonald, et al., 2001). A second study of small and
economically depressed communities (Norris-Baker & Scheidt, 1991)
showed how older residents were willing to volunteer unselfishly to maintain the operations of their declining community and by so doing felt more
hopeful and in control. Another study emphasized that assessments of the
health care needs of older rural residents and effective programmatic
responses must be "grounded within a total community context" (Rowles,
1991, p. 383) that recognizes the interacting influences of family, neighbors,
and clergy and thus requires that "practitioners . . . become integrated
within the community rather than remain aloof" (Rowles, 1991, p. 384).

These transactional inquiries enrich our understanding of the basis for
older people's quality of life, but it is often difficult to judge if their insights
are unique to rural America. First, it is often unclear whether the rurality
of a setting has more to do with the composition of its occupants or its ecological features. These studies often offer incomplete information about
their ecological contexts and their role in shaping the experiences of their
older occupants. Second, researchers have carried out these case studies in
only a very few states, mostly in North Carolina, Kentucky, Florida,
Kansas, and Minnesota, and their interpretations are necessarily regionally
biased. Third, researchers conduct these investigations in a very narrow set
of economic contexts. Thus, there are various qualitative examinations of
persistent poverty or economically deprived areas of West Virginia and
Kansas (Norris-Baker & Scheidt, 1991; Rowles, 1991; Rowles & Johansson,
1993; Scheidt & Norris-Baker, 1993), but few examinations of the settings
that belong to the other economic/public policy categories of rural
America. Fourth, the older samples are often studied because they are predefined as "problem groups," that are impoverished, lonely, isolated,
impaired, abused, or suffer from nutritional disorders (Longres, 1994;
Quandt, Arcury, Bell, McDonald, et al., 2001). The prevalence or perva-
siveness of the problem is usually not a focus of these studies nor is the
question of whether it is unique to rural America. Altogether, these issues
make it difficult to make generalizations from this category of studies.

CONCLUSIONS

Rural America consists of an ecological mosaic of settlements that range from remote and very sparsely populated frontier counties to thriving towns and villages located adjacent to large sprawling metropolitan areas. Rural counties are found in stagnant and economically depressed regions but also in those that are rapidly growing and economically prosperous. Many rural counties are attracting younger, healthy, and active retirees as in-migrants, whereas very old, impaired, impoverished, and long-time elderly residents "left-behind" occupy others. Thus, it should not be surprising that this panoply of rural settlements should defy simple generalizations regarding the quality of life or well-being of its older occupants. Predictably, the large and primarily U.S. research literature does not yield simple conclusions about whether rural America is the home of more vulnerable older populations with poorer quality of life outcomes.

The determination of whether the quality of life outcomes of older persons with varying vulnerabilities are causally linked to their urban and rural environments will require especially sophisticated methodologies. Too often the case, however, the reported findings are based on oversimplified and incompatible settlement and regional classifications that treat quality of life outcomes as unidimensional constructs, that ignore confounding temporal influences, and that fail to control statistically for variations in the composition and vulnerability status of their urban and rural seniors. It is thus difficult to conclude with any confidence that the environmental press of the rural context is more harmful or less facilitative. An unfortunate byproduct of this ambiguity is that rural advocates are less able to convey a clear and compelling message when they seek to inform and change public policy.

These qualifications aside, some studies offer convincing evidence that selected parts of rural America are more likely to be occupied by vulnerable older persons in environmentally challenged settings. Their ecological features—remoteness, low density, and sparse populations—and their depressed economies undoubtedly help explain their less favorable quality of life outcomes. The contrarian's view, however, is that urban America is as likely to contain comparable pockets of deprivation and that in both urban and rural America, the root of the problem may have more to do with the low incomes and poor educational attainment of older persons than with the attributes of their ecological context. Rural America after all does not have a monopoly on human vulnerability and deprivation. Cynics will also argue that until we more carefully isolate the demographic, economic, and cultural influences of the regional context, we must table simple generalizations about how the quality of life of older people differs in these residential categories. Furthermore, the mere documentation of adverse environments and vulnerable seniors does not always result in an older rural population that is objectively or subjectively worse off. Federal and state governments currently offer a variety of program benefits to compensate for these disparities (Reeder & Calhoun, 2002). Disentangling how the population composition and vulnerability makeup of older persons combine with ecologically diverse urban and rural contexts to produce different quality of life outcomes is a fruitful area of future research.

Qualitative studies by transactionalists attempt to deal with the multiple personalities of rural America by largely avoiding them. They have presented vivid vignettes of the ways of life of disadvantaged rural elderly populations but have largely failed to paint like portraitures of advantaged rural dwellers. Faithful to the integrated and holistic focus of their paradigm, they do not address whether their findings are unique to rural places. On the other hand, proponents of the transactionalist research paradigm appropriately challenge the unrealistic assumptions made by the "ecological theory on aging" scientific model. They justifiably question if the composition and vulnerability status of older rural adults and the features of their ecological contexts can be surgically separated into discrete constructs with measurable structural relationships. It is not always easy to challenge their assertion that a vulnerable older population transacting materially and emotionally with an economically and a physically challenging environment is in fact the essence of a rural place—what it means to be "rural." Despite the absence of transactionalist inquiries into amenity-rich rural counties dominated by wealthy and active retirees, it is likely that these places could be interpreted similarly as "rural" environments. Thus, the transactionalists can reasonably argue that the "rural" or the "urban" cannot be conceptualized merely as a geographic location associated with objective but crudely conceptualized ecological and population attributes. The very difficult question, however, is how these qualitative portrayals can achieve the same respectability as scientific investigations, and this certainly is a fruitful direction of future research.

Even as some of the studies considered in this review offered rigorous conceptualizations of individual and environmental constructs and have carefully examined the dynamics of the individual-environment interface, their formulations did not address the third theoretical inquiry of environmental gerontology—earlier identified as the "environmental docility hypothesis." These research efforts have not disentangled the complex linkages that bind rural older occupants with their settings. They have not investigated whether incompetent or more vulnerable older groups who live in socially and economically adverse and resource-deficient rural environments display more maladaptive behaviors, or experience more negative quality of life outcomes than do their more competent or less vulnerable counterparts. This too would be a fruitful future area of research.

What is beyond debate is that rural America is a moving target comprised of older occupants and environments that are continually changing. The reality of these settlement dynamics will require that future studies give greater priority to the role of the temporal dimension as a central research inquiry (Golant, 2003). A failure to do so will yield quickly false and transient conclusions. The future scenario of settlement change in the United States will probably be best characterized as urban-rural convergence rather than urban-rural divergence. In such a future world where settlement differences have melted away, researchers and policy makers will be tempted to do away with urban and rural constructs and focus their efforts on understanding how individual or population differences explain quality of life variations. Exploring these changing and blurring urban and rural boundaries is also a fruitful area of research, especially for those concerned that without such a dichotomy the quality of life choices of older persons will be forever narrowed.

REFERENCES

Altman, I., & Rogoff, B. (1987). World views in psychology: trait, interactional, organismic, and transactional perspectives. In D. Stokols & I. Altman (Eds.), *Handbook of environmental psychology* (Vol. 1, pp. 7-40). New York: John Wiley.

Blazer, D. G., Landerman, L. R., Fillenbaum, G., & Horner, R. (1995). Health services access and use among older adults in North Carolina: urban vs. rural residents. *American Journal of Public Health, 85,* 1384-90.

Buczko, W. (2001). Rural Medicare beneficiaries' use of rural and urban hospitals. *The Journal of Rural Health, 17,* 53-8.

Burkhardt, J. E. (2001). Transportation support for healthy aging among the rural elderly. In U.S. Special Committee on Aging, United States Senate (Ed.), *Healthy aging in rural America.* (pp. 5-29). Washington, DC: U.S. Government Printing Office.

Call, K. T., Casey, M. M., & Radcliff, T. (2000). Rural beneficiaries with chronic conditions: Does prevalence pose a risk to Medicare managed care? *Managed Care Quarterly, 8,* 48-57.

Calsyn, R. J., & Winter, J. P. (1999). Predicting specific service awareness dimensions. *Research on Aging, 21,* 762-780.

Casey, M. M., Klinger, J., & Moscovice, I. (2002). Pharmacy services in rural areas: Is the problem geographic access or financial access? *The Journal of Rural Health, 18,* 467-477.

Cheh, V., & Phillips, B. (1993). Adequate access to posthospital home health services: Differences between urban and rural areas. *The Journal of Rural Health, 9,* 262-269.

Chevalle, T., Herman, F. R., Delmi, M., Stern, R., Hoffmeyer, P., Rapin, C. H., et al. (2002). Evaluation of the age-adjusted incidence of hip fractures between urban and rural areas: The difference is not related to the prevalence of institutions for the elderly. *Osteoporosis International, 13,* 113-8.

Chumbler, N. R., Cody, M., Beck, C. K., & Booth, B. M. (2000). Older adults use of primary care physicians for memory related problems. In J. J. Kronenfeld (Ed.), *Health care providers, institutions, and patients: Changing patterns of care provision and care delivery* (pp. 31-44). Stamford, CN: JAI Press.

Chumbler, N. R., Cody, M., Booth, B. M., & Beck, C. K. (2001). Rural urban differences in service use for memory-related problems in older adults. *Journal of Behavioral Health Services and Research, 28,* 212-221.

Clark, D., & Dellasega, C. (1998). Unmet health care needs: Comparison of rural and urban senior center attendees. *Journal of Gerontological Nursing, 24,* 24-33.

Clark, D. E. (2001). Motor vehicle crash fatalities in the elderly: Rural versus urban. *The Journal of Trauma, 51,* 896-900.

Clark, D. O. (1992). Residence differences in formal and informal long-term care. *Gerontologist, 32,* 227-233.

Clark, D. O. (1993). Volume and distribution of AAA-sponsored services and service use by disabled older adults. *Home Health Care Services Quarterly, 14,* 175-198.

Clayton, G. M., Dudley, W. N., Patterson, W. D., Lawhorn, L. A., & Poon, L. W. (1994). Influence of rural/urban residence on health in the oldest old. *International Journal of Aging and Human Development, 38,* 65-89.

Coburn, A. F., & Bolda, E. J. (1999). The rural elderly and long-term care. In T.C. Ricketts (Ed.), *Rural health in the United States* (pp. 179-189). New York: Oxford University Press.

Commission on Affordable Housing and Health Facility Needs for Seniors in the 21st Century. (2002). *A quiet crisis in America: A Report to Congress.* Washington, DC : U.S. Government Printing Office.

Cook, P. J., & Mizer, K. L. (1994). *The revised ERS county typology: An overview.* Washington, DC: U.S. Dept. of Agriculture, Economic Research Service.

Coward, R. T., Vogel, W. B., Duncan, R. P., & Uttaro, R. (1995). Should Intrastate Funding Formulas for the Older Americans Act Include a Rural Factor. *Gerontologist, 35,* 24-34.

Coward, R. T., Duncan, R. P., & Freudenberger, K. M. (1994). Residential differences in the use of formal services prior to entering a nursing home. *Gerontologist, 34,* 44-49.

Coward, R. T., & Dwyer, J. W. (1991). Longitudinal study of residential differences in the composition of the helping networks of impaired elders. *Journal of Aging Studies, 5,* 391-407.

Coward, R. T., Netzer, J. K., & Mullens, R. A. (1996). Residential differences in the incidence of nursing home admissions across a six-year period. *Journals of Gerontology: Series B: Psychological Sciences and Social Sciences, 51B,* S258-S267.

Craft, B. J., Johnson, D. R., & Ortega, S. T. (1998). Rural-urban women's experience of symptoms of depression related to economic hardship. *Journal of Women and Aging, 10,* 3-18.

Dansky, K. H., Brannon, D., Shea, D. G., Vasey, J., & Dirani, R. (1998). Profiles of hospital, physician, and home health service use by older persons in rural areas. *Gerontologist, 38,* 320-330.

Dellasega, C., Orwig, D., Ahern, F., & Lenz, E. (1999). Postdischarge medication use of elderly cardiac patients from urban and rural locations. *The Journals of Gerontology. Series A, Biological Sciences and Medical Sciences, 54,* M514-20.

Dubay, L. C. (1993). Comparison of rural and urban skilled nursing facility benefit use. *Health Care Financing Review, 14,* 25-37.

Duncan, R. P., Coward, R. T., & Gilbert, G. H. (1997). Rural-urban comparisons of age and health at the time of nursing home admission. *The Journal of Rural Health, 13,* 118-25.

Dwyer, J. W., Barton, A. J., & Vogel, W. B. (1994). Area of residence and the risk of institutionalization. *Journals of Gerontology: Social Sciences, 49,* S75-S84.

Dwyer, J. W., Folts, W. E., & Rosenberg, E. (1994). Caregiving in social context. *Educational Gerontology, 20,* 615-631.

Dwyer, J. W., Lee, G. R., & Coward, R. T. (1990). The health status, health services utilization, and support networks of the rural elderly: a decade review. *The Journal of Rural Health, 6,* 379-98.

Eberhardt, M. S., Ingram, D. D., & Makuc, D. M. (2001). *Health, United States, 2001: Urban and rural chart health chartbook.* Hyattsville, MD: National Center for Health Statistics.

Fuguitt, G. V., Beale, C. L., & Tordella, S. J. (2002). Recent trends in older population change and migration for nonmetro areas, 1970-2000. *Rural America, 17,* 11-19.

Gale, B. J. (1993). Psychosocial health needs of older women: Urban versus rural comparisons. *Archives of Psychiatric Nursing, 7,* 99-105.

Geronimus, A. T., Bound, J., Waidmann, T. A., Colen, C. G., & Steffick, D. (2001). Inequality in life expectancy, functional status, and active life expectancy across selected black and white populations in the United States. *Demography, 38,* 227-251.

Gillanders, W. R., Buss, T. F., & Hofstetter, C. R. (1996). Urban/rural elderly health status differences: The dichotomy reexamined. *Journal of Aging and Social Policy, 8,* 7-24.

Glasgow, N. (1988). *The nonmetro elderly.* Washington, DC: U.S. Department of Agriculture, Economic Research Service.

Glasgow, N. (2000). Rural/urban patterns of aging and caregiving in the United States . *Journal of Family Issues, 21,* 611-631.

Glasgow, N., & Brown, D. L. (1998). Older, rural, and poor. In R. T. Coward & J. A. Krout (Eds.), *Aging in rural settings: Life circumstances and distinctive features* (pp. 187-207). New York: Springer.

Golant, S. (1984). *A place to grow old: The Meaning of environment in old age.* New York: Columbia University Press.

Golant, S. M. (2002). The housing problems of the future elderly population, Appendix G-1. In Commission on Affordable Housing and Health Facility Needs for Seniors in the 21st Century (Ed.), *A quiet crisis in America: A report to Congress* (pp. 189-370). Washington, DC: U.S. Government Printing Office.

Golant, S. M. (2003). Conceptualizing time and behavior: Promising pathways in environmental gerontology. *The Gerontologist, 43, 18-28.*

Goodman, D. C., Fisher, E., Stukel, T. A., & Chang, C. (1997). The distance to community medical care and the likelihood of hospitalization: Is closer always better? *American Journal of Public Health, 87,* 1144-1150.

Harlow, K. S. (1993). Proxy measures, formula funding, and location—Implications for delivery of services for the aging. *Journal of Urban Affairs, 15,* 427-444.

Hays, J. C., Blazer, D. G., & Foley, D. J. (1996). Risk of napping: Excessive daytime sleepiness and mortality in an older community population. *Journal of the American Geriatrics Society, 44,* 693-698.

Himes, C. L., & Rutrough, T. S. (1994). Differences in the use of health services by metropolitan and nonmetropolitan elderly. *The Journal of Rural Health, 10,* 80-88.

Housing Assistance Council. (2000). *Why housing matters: HAC's 2000 Report on the state of the nation's rural housing.* Washington, DC: Housing Assistance Council.

Jensen, L., & McLaughlin, D. K. (1997). The escape from poverty among rural and urban elders. *Gerontologist, 37,* 462-8.

Jett, K. M. F., Coward, R. T., Schoenberg, N. E., Duncan, R. P., & Dwyer, J. W. (1996). Influence of community context on the decision to enter a nursing home. *Journal of Aging Studies, 10,* 237-254.

Keefover, R. W., Rankin, E. D., Keyl, P. M., Wells, J. C., Martin, J., & Shaw, J. (1996). Dementing Illnesses in Rural Populations: The Need for Research and Challenges Confronting Investigators. *Journal of Rural Health, 12,* 178-187.

Kenney, G. M. (1993). Rural and urban differentials in Medicare home health use. *Health Care Financing Review, 14,* 39-57.

Krout, J. A. (1998). Services and service delivery in rural environments. In R. T. Coward & J. A. Krout (Eds.), *Aging in rural settings: Life circumstances and distinctive features* (pp. 247-266). New York: Springer.

Lago, D., Stuart, B., & Ahern, F. (1993). Rurality and prescription drug utilization among the elderly: an archival study. *The Journal of Rural Health, 9,* 6-16.

Lawrence, S. A., & McCulloch, B. J. (2001). Rural mental health and elders: Historical inequities. *Journal of Applied Gerontology, 20,* 144-169.

Lawton, M. P. (1998). Environment and aging: Theory revisited. In R. J. Scheidt & P. G. Windley (Eds.), *Environment and aging theory: A focus on housing* (pp. 1-31). Westport, CN: Greenwood Press.

Lawton, M. P., & Lawrence, R. H. (1994). Assessing health. In M. P. Lawton & J. Teresi (Eds.), *Annual review of gerontology and geriatrics* (pp. 23-56). New York: Springer.

Longino, C. F., Jr. (1990). Geographical mobility and family caregiving in nonmetropolitan America: Three decade evidence from the U.S. Census. *Family Relations, 39,* 38-43.

Longres, J. F. (1994). Self-neglect and social control: A modest test of an issue. *Journal of Gerontological Social Work, 33,* 3-20.

Macey, S. M., & Schneider, D. F. (1993). Deaths from excessive heat and excessive cold among the elderly. *Gerontologist, 33,* 497-500.

McConnel, C. E., & Zetzman, M. R. (1993). Urban/rural differences in health service utilization by elderly persons in the United States. *The Journal of Rural Health, 9,* 270-280.

McCulloch, B. J., & Kivett, V. R. (1998). Older rural women: Aging in historical and current contexts. In R. T. Coward & J. A. Krout (Eds.), *Aging in rural settings: Life circumstances and distinctive features* (pp. 149-166). New York: Springer.

Medicare, Payment Advisory Commission. (2001). *Report to the Congress: Medicare in rural America.* Washington, DC: Medicare Payment Advisory Commission.

Mookherjee, H. N. (1998). Perceptions of well-being among the older metropolitan and nonmetropolitan populations in the United States. *Journal of Social Psychology, 138,* 72-82.

Moos, R. H., & Lemke, S. (1996). *Evaluating residential facilities.* Thousand Oaks, CA: Sage.

Mueller, K. J., Coburn, A., Cordes, S., Crittenden, R., Hart, J. P., McBride, T., et al. (1999). The changing landscape of health care financing and delivery: How are rural communities and providers responding? *Milbank Quarterly, 77,* 485-510, ii.

Netzer, J. K., Coward, R. T., Peek, C. W., Henretta, J. C., Duncan, R. P., & Dougherty, M. C. (1997). Race and residence differences in the use of formal services by older adults. *Research on Aging, 19,* 300-332.

Norris-Baker, C., & Scheidt, R. J. (1991). A contextual approach to serving older residents of economically threatened small towns. *Journal of Aging Studies, 5,* 333-346.

Nyman, J. A., Sen, A., Chan, B. Y., & Commins, P. P. (1991). Urban/rural differences in home health patients and services. *Gerontologist, 31,* 457-466.

Okwumabua, J. O., Baker, F. M., Wong, S. P., & Pilgrim, B. O. (1997). Characteristics of depressive symptoms in elderly urban and rural African Americans. *Journals of Gerontology: Series A: Biological Sciences and Medical Sciences, 52A,* M241-M246.

Penrod, J. D. (2001). Functional disability at nursing home admission: A comparison of urban and rural admission cohorts. *The Journal of Rural Health, 17,* 229-238.

Quandt, S. A., Arcury, T. A., Bell, R. A., McDonald, J., & Vitolins, M. Z. (2001). The social and nutritional meaning of food sharing among older rural adults. *Journal of Aging Studies, 15,* 145-162.

Rabiner, D. J. (1995). Patterns and predictors of noninstitutional health care utilization by older adults in rural and urban America. *The Journal of Rural Health, 11,* 259-273.

Rabiner, D. J., Konrad, T. R., DeFriese, G. H., Kincade, J., Bernard, S. L., Woomert, et al. (1997). Metropolitan versus nonmetropolitan differences in functional status and self-care practice: Findings from a national sample of community dwelling older adults. *Journal of Rural Health, 13,* 14-27.

Ranelli, P. L., & Coward, R. T. (1996). Residential differences in the use of pharmacies by older adults and their communication experiences with pharmacists. *Journal of Rural Health, 12,* 19-32.

Redford, L. J., & Whitten, P. (1997). Ensuring access to care in rural areas: The role of communication technology. *Generations, 21,* 19-23.

Reeder, R. J., & Calhoun, S. D. (2002). Federal funding in nonmetro elderly counties. *Rural America, 17,* 20-27.

Ricketts, T. C., Johnson-Webb, K. D., & Randolph, R. K. (1999). Populations and places in rural America. In T. C. Ricketts III (Ed.), *Rural health in the United States* (pp. 7-24). New York: Oxford University Press.

Ricketts, T. C., Johnson-Webb, K. D., & Taylor, P. (1998). *Definitions of rural: A handbook for health policy makers and researchers.* Chapel Hill: Cecil G. Sheps Center for Health Services Research, University of North Carolina at Chapel Hill.

Ringelberg, M. L., Gilbert, G. H., Antonson, D. E., Dolan, T. A., Legler, D. W., Foerster, U., et al. (1996). Root caries and root defects in urban and rural adults: The Florida dental care study. *The Journal of the American Dental Association, 127,* 885-891.

Robins, L., & Regier, D. (1991). *Psychiatric disorders in America: The empidemiologic catchment area study.* New York: Free Press.

Rogers, C. C. (1999). *Changes in the older population and implications for rural areas.* Washington, DC: U.S. Department of Agriculture, Economic Research Service.

Rosenblatt, R. A., & Hart, G. L. (1999). Physicians and rural America. In T. C. Ricketts III (Ed.), *Rural health in the United States* (pp. 38-51). New York: Oxford University Press.

Rost, K., Zhang, M., Fortney, J., Smith, J., & Smith, G. R., Jr. (1998). Rural-urban differences in depression treatment and suicidality. *Medical Care, 36,* 1098-1107.

Rowles, G. D. (1991). Changing health culture in rural Appalachia: Implications for serving the elderly. *Journal of Aging Studies, 5,* 375-389.

Rowles, G. D. (1998). Community and the local environment. In R. T. Coward & J. A. Krout (Eds.), *Aging in rural settings: Life circumstances and distinctive features* (pp. 105-125). New York: Springer.

Rowles, G. D., Concotelli, J. A., & High, D. M. (1996). Community integration of a rural nursing home. *Journal of Applied Gerontology, 15,* 188-201.

Rowles, G. D., & Johansson, H. K. (1993). Persistent elderly poverty in rural Appalachia. *Journal of Applied Gerontology, 12,* 349-367.

Salmon, M., Nelson, G. M., & Rous, S. G. (1993). Continuum of care revisited: A rural perspective. *Gerontologist, 33,* 658-666.

Scheidt, R. J. (1998). The mental health of the elderly in rural environments. In R. T. Coward & J. A. Krout (Eds.), *Aging in rural settings: Life circumstances and distinctive features* (pp. 85-103). New York: Springer.

Scheidt, R. J. (2001). Individual-cultural transactions: Implications for the mental health of rural elders. *Journal of Applied Gerontology, 20,* 195-213.

Scheidt, R. J., & Norris-Baker, C. (1993). The environmental context of poverty among older residens of economically endangered Kansas towns. *Journal of Applied Gerontology, 12,* 335-348.

Scheidt, R. J., & Windley, P. G. (1985). The ecology of aging. In J. E. Birren & K. W. Schaie (Eds.), *Handbook of the psychology of aging* (pp. 245-258). New York: Van Nostrand Reinhold.

Scheidt, R. J., & Windley, P. (1987). Environmental perceptions and patterns of well-being among older Americans in small rural towns. *Comprehensive Gerontology, 1,* 24-29.

Schlenker, R. E., Powell, M. C., & Goodrich, G. K. (2002). Rural-urban home health care differences before the Balanced Budget Act of 1997. *The Journal of Rural Health, 18,* 359-372.

Schlenker, R. E., & Shaughnessy, P. W. (1996). The role of the rural hospital in long-term care. In G. Rowles, J. E. Beaulieu, & W. W. Myers (Eds.), *Long-term care for the rural elderly* (pp. 132-155). New York: Springer.

Schoenman, J. A. (1999). Impact of the BBA on Medicare HMO payments for rural areas. *Health Affairs, 18,* 244-254.

Seccombe, K. (1995). Health insurance coverage and use of services among low-income elders: Does residence influence the relationship? *The Journal of Rural Health, 11,* 86-97.

Serow, W. J. (2001). Retirement migration counties in the southeastern United States: Geographic, demographic, and economic correlates. *The Gerontologist, 41,* 220-227.

Smith, M. H., Anderson, R. T., Bradham, D. D., & Longino, C. F., Jr. (1995). Rural and urban differences in mortality among Americans 55 years and older: Analysis of the National Longitudinal Mortality Study. *The Journal of Rural Health, 11,* 274-85.

Stearns, S. C., Slifkin, R. T., & Edin, H. M. (2000). Access to care for rural Medicare beneficiaries. *Journal of Rural Health, 16,* 31-42.

U.S. Bureau of the Census. (2001). *Annual demographic survey, March supplement, poverty status of people in 2000.* Washington, DC: U.S. Government Printing Office.

U.S. Department of Agriculture, Economic Research Service. (2002). *Briefing room: Rural population and migration: Rural Elderly.* Washington, DC: U.S. Department of Agriculture, Economic Research Service.

Van Nostrand, J. F., Furner, S. E., Brunelle, J. A. , & Cohen, R. A. (1993). Health. In J.F. Van Nostrand (Ed.), *Common beliefs about the rural elderly: What do national data tell us?* (pp. 51-62). Washington, DC: U.S. Dept. of Health and Human Services, National Center for Health Statistics.

Wachs, T. D. (1999). Celebrating complexity: Conceptualization and assessment of the environment. In S. L. Friedman & T. D. Wachs (Eds.), *Measuring environment across the life span: Emerging methods and concepts* (pp. 357-292). Washington, DC: American Psychological Association.

Wallace, R. E., & Wallace, R. B. (1998). Rural-urban contrasts in elder health status: Methodologic issues and findings. In R. T. Coward & J. A. Krout (Eds.), *Aging in rural settings: Life circumstances and distinctive features* (pp. 67-83). New York: Springer.

Weiner, J. P., Parente, S. T., Garnick, D. W., Fowles, J., Lawthers, A. G., & Palmer, R. H. (1995). Variation in office-based quality. A claims-based profile of care provided to Medicare patients with diabetes. *JAMA, 273,* 1503-1508.

Weisman, G., Chaudhury, H., & Moore, K. D. (2000). Theory and practice of place: Toward an integrative model. In R. L. Rubinstein, M. Moss, & M. H. Kleban (Eds.), *The many dimensions of aging* (pp. 3-21). New York: Springer.

Wenger, G. C. (2001). Myths and realities of ageing in rural Britain. *Ageing and Society, 21,* 117-130.

Whittle, J., Lin, C. J., Lave, J. R., Fine, M. J., Delaney, K. M., Joyce, D. Z., et al. (1998). Relationship of provider characteristics to outcomes, process, and costs of care for community acquired pneumonia. *Medical Care, 36,* 977-987.

CHAPTER 12

Kinship and Supportive Environments of Aging

CHRISTINE L. FRY
LOYOLA UNIVERSITY CHICAGO

"Aging is a family affair." This often quoted statement in the practical literature on caregiving highlights the moral obligations of kin to support their older, frail, and often disabled members. A frail older person enters a short or protracted period of dependency and altered relationships with his or her spouse, if surviving, and his or her children, if available. Caregiving has its rewards, but it is the challenges and stresses of caring for another who is unable to fulfill the requirements for daily living that have received the most attention. Consequently, caregiving has become a major, if not the most central topic in gerontology.

Caregiving takes place in a context. Sociocultural factors fill that environment with meaning. Individuals are linked in meaningful ways to one another. Relationships are defined. How families respond in looking after their members is conditioned by expectations. What constitutes support? Who is available to do the work of care? The focus is on families, kin networks, and older people. Although kinship is primarily a cultural matter, the resultant social arrangements can profoundly shape the environmental context of growing old. Our intent is to examine diversity in kinship and the ways in which support is provided. To do this we must place the experience of caregiving in the industrialized urban societies of Europe and North America in a much broader perspective. The work of kinship and care can best be understood through cross-cultural comparisons. Our goal is to understand the workings of kinship and caregiving in industrial societies in light of a fuller range of variation.

Our initial sentence, "Aging is a family affair," contains two issues universal to the experience of being human: age and family. First, aging is universal since human lives take place through time. Humans are conceived and born, then they grow up, and eventually die. What happens across the course of any human life is a complex interplay of cultural expectations, individual volition, and historical circumstance. This interplay is represented by theories about the life course in gerontology (Settersten, 1999, 2003) and in anthropology on comparative age structure (Kertzer, 1989; Fry, 2003). Secondly, every human is born into some kind of a family and will, across his or her life course, interact with a class of people identified as relatives. Although families, in their variability, defy simple definition, the study of kinship is well developed in social anthropology. The reason for this is that kinship is the primary institution organizing the lives of people in small-scale cultures. Also, as a multiple functioned institution, kinship is adaptable to a myriad of circumstances. How does kinship shape the ordinary daily environment of older adults? Five topics structure our inquiry:

1. The work of kinship
2. The life course and the developmental cycle of domestic groups
3. Kinship and social support in domestic scaled societies
4. Kinship and social support in large scaled industrialized societies
5. Kinship as an environmental contingency

THE WORK OF KINSHIP

Why do all cultures have families in one form or another? Families structure interdependency between members of a society who live together and interact on a daily basis. All animals living in social groups, including humans, do so because there are advantages in being interdependent. The rewards are quite diverse, including such issues as defense of territory, protection from predation, access to mates, or to ensure success in reproduction and nurturing infants into adulthood. In comparison to most primate and other mammalian societies, human families are quite distinctive. Given the immaturity and helplessness of human infants and the length of time it takes for them to mature, coordinated efforts of a number of adults are needed (Lovejoy, 1988; Foley, 1992). Adult humans provision their offspring and each other. Men provide their wives, children, and other related adults with food they have tracked, killed, and butchered. Women provide their husbands, children, and other related adults with food they have gathered. Provisioning behavior is not unique to humans, but long-term provisioning is quite distinctive.

Caregiving is more than simply feeding another. Care is one of the basic tasks of kinship. Within a framework of individuals who consider themselves to be related, support is extended to those who need it. The kind of support we refer to as caregiving extends beyond the generalized reciprocity and domestic divisions of labor that characterize the daily operation of households. Caregiving involves dependency on the part of individuals who are unable to perform the tasks of adults. This includes children who either lack the physical skills or cultural competence to care for themselves or others. Also included are the ill and chronically disabled, who are often older adults. Thus, kinship is the care network through which one gives and receives varying forms of care across a lifetime.

Kin networks are cultural constructions. The ideology of kinship is a contingency shaping the social environment and arrangements in the material environment. On the one hand, the rules of descent and marriage define who is a relative and their roles in the network. At some point, the rules of relatedness set the boundaries between who is, and who is not a relative. As a result the social world is divided into relatives, distant relatives, other families, and other people. On the other hand, kinship exists in a broader cultural context and is shaped by economic and political factors. We first address the issue of variability in defining relatives and then examine the larger contexts in which families function.

WHO IS A RELATIVE?

Beyond maternal and matrifocal connections, kinship linkages are by no means obvious simply because of the length of gestation. Humans solve this problem by devising cultural maps of who is a relative and who is not related. A near universal incest taboo creates the boundaries. On one side are consanguineal or blood relatives. Sexual relations are prohibited within this class of people, especially among an ego, parents, siblings, and children. On the other side are a class of people from whom one can select sexual partners. If stable longer-term relationships are established between an ego and one or more of these people, he or she becomes a spouse and an affinal relative. Marriage connects the consanguineal kin of man and wife into an allied set of relatives called affines. For example, on marriage a woman acquires her husband's consanguineal kin as her affines or in-laws.

Ever since the pioneering work of Lewis Henry Morgan (1871), anthropologists have scrutinized and dissected kinship systems from all over the world (see Parkin, 1997, for a review). What is clear from our accumulated knowledge is that the definition of who is a relative is specific to a cultural context. A major division is found in rules of descent. We find cultures that place equal emphasis on both maternal and paternal linkages. In comparison there are cultures that place emphasis on either maternal or paternal linkages but not both. We identify these principles of descent respectively as 1) bilateral and 2) unilineal (see Table 12.1). At issue are the ways in which descent rules shape environments of aging.

TABLE 12.1   Type of Descent and the Prevalent Rules of Residence

Type of Descent	Most Prevalent Residence Rule
Bilateral Descent Bilateral descent is also called cognatic descent. In bilateral descent there are no preferences or emphasis on the linkages within the kinship network. Relatives are reckoned through all linkages – male and female and ascending and descending generations. An ego in bilateral descent is the center of a kindred organized around a core of lineal kin and bounded by degrees of collaterality.	**Neolocal: 40%** Residence of a newly married couple is the formation of a new household. **Bilocal: 56%** Bilocal residence is also called ambilocal residence. A newly married couple is affiliated with the household of one of the parental households. No preference is made as to the bride's or groom's parents. Choices are influenced by economic opportunities, prestige, or personal choice.
Unilineal Descent: Unilineal descent is unilateral with emphasis being placed on kin linkages of one gender. Relatives are reckoned through a constricted network of male or female links. Although egos are sometimes used, they are not necessary since the resulting kin groups, lineages and clans, are bounded by a core a people linked by descent through a male or female line.	
Patrilineal: Emphasis is placed on descent through a male line.	**Patrilocal: 95%** Residence of a newly married couple is with the groom's family. The new family becomes a part of and is allied with the family of the groom's father.
Matrilineal: Emphasis is placed on descent through a female line.	**Matrilocal: 42%** Residence of a newly married couple is with the bride's family. The new family becomes a part of and is allied with the family of the bride's mother. **Avunculocal: 28%** Residence of a newly married couple is with the groom's maternal uncle (mother's brother). The new family becomes a part of and is allied with that of a uncle forming a core of males who are linked through matrilineal descent. **Patrilocal: 23%**

BILATERAL DESCENT

Descent is inherently bilateral or cognatic. With the exception of medical-ized reproductive technology, it takes a male and a female to conceive a child. They, in turn have parents, who also have parents. From the per-spective of any ego, in every generation they see a bifurcation (two par-ents, four grandparents, eight great-grandparents, etc.) These systems of descent are organized around a set of a person's lineal kin who are linked through descent. In the ascending generations these are parents, grand-parents, and degrees of great-grandparents. In descending generations, these are children, grandchildren, and degrees of great-grandchildren. Around this core of lineal kin are assorted collateral relatives connected by sharing lines of descent or siblings. Collaterals are not only siblings, but are siblings of parents (aunts and uncles) and their descendents (cousins). As one goes up and down generations, this class of relatives can become quite large. Bilateral descent is very flexible and fluid. It is all-inclusive and is limited only by the ability to keep track of relationships. Practically bilat-eral kin are bounded by degrees of collaterality and social distance. Usually individuals classified as a fifth cousin or greater are too socially distant to be considered a relative.

UNILINEAL DESCENT

Unlike bilateral descent, unilineal descent is more restrictive in the empha-sis on gender-specific linkages. Emphasis on female linkages results in matrilineal descent. Patrilineal descent is the emphasis on male linkages. We do not see the bifurcation in past generations. Instead the line is straight. If matrilineal, the line of descent is through mother, mother's mother, mother's mother's mother, and so on. Likewise, if patrilineal, the line is through father, father's father, father's father's father, and so on. Likewise, the emphasis on linkage through only one gender has profound consequences for the descending lineal relatives and collaterals. For a female in matrilineal descent, her sisters and female children will usually be the important kin linkages and will remain within the natal unit. Brothers and sons will marry out and their children will belong to the kin units of their wives. A male ego will maintain connections with his mother and sisters, but his children are descendants of his wife's family. The con-verse is true of patrilineal descent. Unilineal descent is anything but flexi-ble and fluid. It is exclusionary and restrictive. The resulting units are well bounded. Corporate groups are easy to create using unilineal descent because members are recruited through birth. The gender not emphasized is recruited into these units through marriage.

Beyond the symmetry or asymmetry of the linkages, what is the net difference between bilateral and unilineal descent? If kinship is one kind of interdependence, these rules of descent reflect different patterns of interdependence. Bilateral descent, by being inclusive and flexible, extends exchange beyond the lineal core, through ascending and descending generations and out all lines of collaterality. Unilineal descent, by being exclusive and bounded, restricts exchange within a part of the lineal core and the collaterals. The effects of these exchange boundaries are seen once we add a temporal dimension to the resulting social units as their members pass through their life courses. For older adults in need of more supportive environments, the interdependency within domestic units can be of profound importance. With extreme old age, one can face a danger of out surviving their relatives.

DESCENT, DOMESTIC ORGANIZATION, AND THE LIFE COURSE

When looking at the composition and configuration of descent groups, we tend to emphasize a static picture, anchored in the group, not individual egos. Individuals are recruited into these domestic groups by birth and pass through one or more of these groups as they mature and ultimately exit at death. At any one point in time the composition of households is conditioned by residence rules. These rules reflect the residence expectations for a newly married couple. Residential preferences place people in preexisting kin groups and alliances. Quite predictably, these residence rules are shaped by the prevailing principle of descent. On the basis of ethnographic data from 563 cultures around the globe (Murdock, 1981) we can statistically document these patterns.[1]

Bilateral descent is decidedly associated with neolocal and bilocal residence (Table 12.1). Of the cultures that are bilateral and for which we have information on the rule of residence, 56 percent are bilocal and 40 percent are neolocal. Bilocality of residents happens when the married couple selects either the husband's or the bride's family to live near. Their decision may be conditioned by the relative wealth of families and may shift over time. Neolocality means that a new residential unit is formed through marriage that is distinctive and not a part of either the bride's or groom's family of orientation. Less than five percent of cultures with unilineal

---

[1]Murdock spearheaded the creation of the Human Relations Areas Files in the 1930s and 1940s. These files organized ethnographic reports from around the world into a topical code book, *Outline of Cultural Materials* (Murdock, 2000). An electronic version of this data set is available through the Microcase Corporation, 1301 120th Avenue, N.E., Bellevue, WA 98005 (Microcase 1994). The statistics presented in this section are from this data set.

descent are also bilocal or neolocal. Neolocality does not mean isolation. Quite to the contrary, most of these families are extended families either matrilateraly or patrilateraly, especially in the case of bilocal residence. Neolocality and bilocality is what we would expect with cognatic descent because of the flexibility it accords. Alliances and exchanges with other domestic units are not predetermined. The bifurcation of bilateral descent casts a wide network of possibilities. These are potential relationships for interdependency and support.

Unilineal descent, on the other hand, is associated with other, very specific residence rules. Patrilineal descent is predominately patrilocal (95 percent). Patrilocal means that following marriage, the couple moves in with the groom's relatives. Matrilineal descent is less clearly linked to a specific residence rule. Of our matrilineal cultures, 23 percent are patrilocal, 42 percent matrilocal and 28 percent avunculocal. Matrilocality means the new family resides with the bride's family whereas avunculocality means the couple lives with the groom's uncle (mother's brother). Patrilocal, matrilocal, and avunculocal residence is very different from neolocal and bilocal. Individuals, as they become adults at marriage, have little choice with whom they are going to live and with whom they are going to work. Here we see little flexibility because groups are fairly rigidly defined in long-term membership. Instead of a network of possibilities, we see a network of certainties. Corporate groups and unilineal descent seem to go hand in hand.

What are the implications of the ideology of descent for older people who in extreme old age could out survive their relatives? Figure 12.1 depicts the potential temporal dynamics of bilateral kindreds. Here we assume that at any one point in time, there are three living generations. Bilateral descent places a younger person (midlife) in the center of a kin network extending in all directions. In this case we would shift the ego to the G-1 generation. Lineal kin are of both older and younger generations and most are living. Collateral and affinal linkages (not depicted in the diagram) have individuals of older and younger generations and most of them are alive also. For an older person, especially one of advanced age, this picture changes considerably. In the figure, our reference point is an older ego (generation zero). For this individual, the lineal ascending generations are deceased (dashed lines). This person can only look down descending generations for living lineal relatives (children and grandchildren). Affinal and collateral linkages also will be affected by time and death. Spouses may die and the linkages to in-laws may become attenuated. Siblings may die, leaving the links to their descendants with possible abbreviation. The net effect of bilateral descent and aging is the shrinkage of kindreds to the lineal core and to a few other relatives.

Unilineal descent (Figure 12.2) presents a very different picture. First, egos are not depicted because the group is our point of reference. The

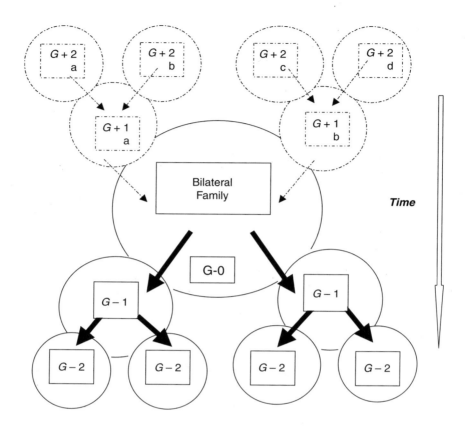

FIGURE 12.1   Bilateral descent from the perspective of an older ego. The bifurcation of lineal kin is displayed. Those families depicted in solid lines (G –1, G –2) descending from ego (G–0)are living. Those families depicted in dashed lines (G +1, G +2) are deceased. The implication is by the time one has reached an advanced age, a very significant part of the bilateral kindred has vanished through death, leaving linkages to the living network weakened.

descent group passes through time and changes through time. Members enter through birth or marriage. Members exit through death or marriage. Membership is determined by restriction in the gender of the kinship linkage. Individuals of any age are connected to the designated kin. All that happens to an older person is they rise to the apex of the genealogical pyramid and remain linked to the kin who make up the descent group. Thus, unilineal descent shields older people from the risks of survivorship.

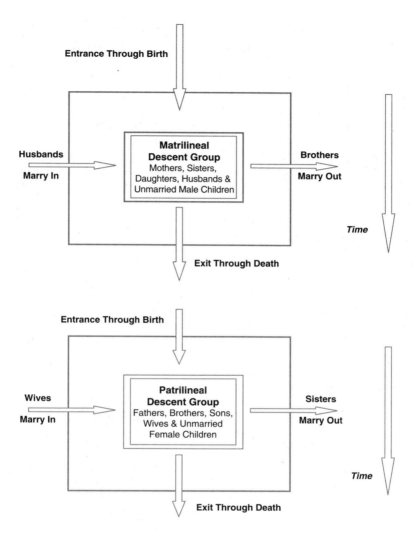

FIGURE 12.2   Unilineal descent groups. Groups are restricted and bounded in membership. The implication is for any ego reaching an advanced age, attrition through the death of ascending generations will have little impact on the kinship network.

Metaphorically, unilineal descent is like journeying through life in a boat. One may change boats at marriage, but one always has a boat. Bilateral descent is like climbing a tree. At the bottom the trunk and branches are thick. At the top, the branches are thin and the support can be shaky.

SOCIETAL SCALE AND THE CONSEQUENCES OF DOMESTIC ORGANIZATION FOR OLDER PEOPLE

One of the first questions asked in anthropology about old age concerned the experience of aging in simpler societies. Simpler societies provide sharp contrasts to the environments of aging in socially more complex societies. Also, the lack of technological buffering from the physical environment enables a more direct examination of the way the interdependency within social groups promotes the welfare of their members. In *The Role of the Aged in Primitive Society*, Simmons (1945) introduced the topic of the treatment of older adults to both comparative research and gerontology. He looked at old age in 71 societies around the world by statistically discovering relationships between 232 variables. The type of society identified as "primitive" in 1945 we now call "small scaled" or "domestic scaled." For example, peoples such as the !Kung of Southern Africa or the Iroquois of Northeastern North America are organized on the basis of a domestic economy. These societies are not industrialized. They are predominately egalitarian with only a limited political hierarchy and social stratification. Domestic units organize basic economic activities such as production, exchange, and consumption. It is societies such as these that we are most likely to see the interaction of descent and consequences in old age.

In his sample of 71 societies, Simmons discovered that in a third of these societies older adults were abandoned, killed, or in some way had their deaths hastened. Since the 1940s, the kind of comparative research Simmons began has been transformed by technology and methodological sophistication (Ember & Ember, 2001). Simmons was working with the then new *Human Relations Area Files* (HRAF). HRAF is a database organizing ethnographic reports from all over the globe by major topics and variables as outlined in *Outline of Cultural Materials* (Murdock, 2000). Since then these files have been expanded, probability samples developed, and the text converted from microfiche to electronic form known as e-HRAF.[2]

Of the many variables in Simmons' analysis, patrilineal and matrilineal descent are included. Bilateral descent is not. Although Simmons does not discuss these results in detail, it appears that unilineal descent, especially matrilineal descent, is not associated with the killing of older people.[3] On the other hand, older males in patrilineal societies are at a slightly greater risk of being killed. The later studies used HRAF to further understand the extent of nonsupportive treatment of older people and the reasons for mal-

---

[2]E-HRAF is available on the web at www.yale.edu.hraf or can be found in the library resources at member institutions.
[3]The data that Simmons utilizes is nominal data conceived as traits and recorded as present or absent with occasional notations for "strength." There are no tests of significance used.

treatment (Glascock, 1982; Glascock and Feinman, 1980, 1981; Maxwell & Maxwell, 1980; Silverman and Maxwell, 1987). Variables used in these studies are definitions of old, categories of older people, environment, subsistence, resource control, and the availability of kin. None systematically explores the issue of descent. Thus there are no comparative data for descent ideology and the treatment of older people.

A sample of societies to be found in e-HRAF was explored for this analysis by focusing on treatment of older adults, descent, and subsistence. The societies in the sample coded for evidence of supportive and nonsupportive treatment.[4] Nonsupport can range from dramatic forms of death hastening, which include gerontocide, abandonment, and encouraged suicide, to milder forms such as disrespect and inadequate food and shelter. In this data set, non-supportive treatment of older people is quite prevalent (43 percent).[5] Table 12.2 looks at the distribution of societies arranged by descent ideology (bilateral or unilineal) and by subsistence. In terms of descent ideology, bilateral societies tend to be evenly split on treatment of older adults. Unilineal societies tend to be more supportive with only about a third reported to be nonsupportive. Subsistence reveals another pattern. From past research it is clear that the factors predictive of nonsupportive treatment of older people is a combination of subsistence based on foraging that requires mobility and harsh environmental conditions. Indeed, that is exactly what we find in this sample. Seventy-two percent of societies reporting nonsupportive treatment are foragers (31 percent), horticulturists relying on foraging (38 percent), or pastoralists herding partially domesticated reindeer (6 percent).

Nearly 90 percent (seven out of eight) of the foragers who are bilateral are noted to have some form of nonsupportive treatment of older people. The highest percentage of unilineal societies with nonsupportive treatments is horticultural, but also relies on foraging (84 percent or 11 out of

---

[4]This coding follows Glascock and Wagner (1986) except where additional information is now available and with the addition of 15 societies that are not included in the probability sample. Treatment of elderly is a multiple coded variable ranging from fairly neutral behavior to abandonment and killing. Glascock and Fienman (1980) discovered that with multiple forms of treatment some societies are both supportive and nonsupportive of older people. The difference between support and nonsupport depends on the level of frailty and disablement. In this analysis, any evidence of nonsupport, even where there is evidence of support, is taken as evidence of nonsupport.

[5]Glascock reports that nonsupportive behavior is as high as 84 percent with the availability of data on treatment (Glascock & Fienman, 1981). In all probabilities it is even higher. HRAF data is secondary data derived from ethnographers who have studied and written about cultures around with work with very diverse sets of research issues. None of them set out to study treatment of older people. Certainly the maltreatment of a frail disabled person is likely to get the attention of most observers. If nonsupportive treatment is reported, it is reasonable to conclude that nonsupportive behavior toward older people is not rare within that society.

TABLE 12.2 Treatment of Older People as Shaped by Subsistence and Type of Descent

Subsistence	Bilateral Descent		Unilineal Descent	
Treatment of Old People	Non-supportive	Supportive	Non-supportive	Supportive
Foraging	7 (50%)	1 (7%)	3 (17%)	2 (7%)
Foraging/ Horticulture	1 (7%)	2 (13%)	11 (61%)	2 (7%)
Horticulture	0	4 (27%)	1 (6%)	3 (11%)
Pastoralism	2 (14%)	0	0	5 (18%)
Agriculture	4 (29%)	8 (53%)	3 (17%)	16 (57%)
	14 (100%)	15 (100%)	18 (100%)	28 (100%)
				75 Total

13). Likewise, pastoralists who rely on foraging are noted for nonsupportive treatment. In the Table 12.2, these are two bilateral pastoralists, the Chukchee and Saami who herd semi-domesticated reindeer in the Arctic of Asia and Europe respectively. With other forms of subsistence, horticulture, cattle pastoralism, and agriculture, supportive treatment prevails. It is noteworthy that a third (4 out of 12) of the bilateral societies that are also agricultural have nonsupportive treatment whereas only 16 percent of the unilineal and agricultural societies are noted for nonsupportive treatment. Again, this ranges from death hastening, to abuse, to ridicule, or milder forms of joking about infirmities.

Subsistence is most clearly related to the management of frail and disabled elderly. Foraging is difficult for older people because of the mobility required. The immediacy of the return in gathering and hunting places a premium on productivity and continuous production. Wealth is very difficult to accumulate because of a combination of the importance of mobility, portability of material culture, lack of storage technology, and the marginality of the habitat. Older people compensate for declining abilities by overproducing during seasons of abundance, adopting or fostering children as helpers, making fewer demands, working beyond their abilities, or requesting death (Guemple, 1969).

Bilateral descent is the descent rule of choice for foragers. In Murdock's large sample (1981), 64 percent of foraging societies are bilateral. This is not surprising. Bilateral descent, as we have seen above, is noted for its flexibility. Foraging requires fluidity. For foraging to work, people have to move to resources, collect, eat, and move again. To reduce unevenness in the luck of hunting or failures in collecting, people need to exchange resources through generalized reciprocity. Bilateral descent provides a network of possibilities. It is a kin network connecting in all sorts of genealogical directions and through many different kin types for sharing, residence, work efforts, and other forms of interdependence. Difficulties develop when that network shrinks, kin are not available, abilities to exchange decline, and resources become problematic.

Unilineal descent is the rule of choice for people whose subsistence is based on domestication. Some 68 percent of these societies are unilineal. Again, this is not surprising. Unilineal descent, by restricting the kin network, is not flexible. For subsistence based on domesticated plants and animals to work, people must be connected to those productive resources. Unlike foraging, the return on their labors is delayed. Labor has to be mobilized to prepare fields, plant, and maintain them through to harvest several months later. Because of the investment in land or animals, issues of ownership and property are important. Descent groups are most often corporate groups. With domestication, the premium on mobility vanishes. Groups become more sedentary, and it is possible to accumulate wealth. Both of these conditions should and do promote favorable treatment of older adults as members of a descent group. Yet, when entire villages have to move on seasonal food quests and warfare, resources, and technology are limited, we find frail adults left behind.

In spite of a focus on negative treatment of older people, supportive treatment is by far the most prevalent. There are very few societies that have evidence of only nonsupportive treatment. One extreme is the Chukchee who maintain an ideology that only a premature death will ensure one of better fortunes in the afterlife. One reason for this is a nearly invisible form of stratification inherent in kinship: the age hierarchy. Parents are always older than children and one generation above them. As one ascends generational levels with age, one also ascends the age hierarchy. Older people have more experience and accumulated knowledge than younger people. In societies without writing or the ability to store information in some form of written or visual media, this is very important. Older people become the keepers of tradition because they have a deep knowledge of a community because they have seen its members born and grow up in that social arena. Being at the apex of the age hierarchy will not guarantee a secure old age. It helps to also have a large family, property, wealth, and a number of other things that will reinforce that position.

KINSHIP AND SOCIAL SUPPORT IN LARGE-SCALE INDUSTRIALIZED SOCIETIES

Over the course of the last half of the twentieth century, capitalistic nation states have defined old age as a social problem (Katz, 1996). With apoplectic demographic projections and the increased medicalization of old age, most nations are afraid they cannot afford an aging population and the caregiving involved. How do the families in these societies compare with their counterparts in domestic scaled cultures? Popular images of families in these societies point to a transformation and decline of kinship. A very extensive literature documents an altered, but still important kinship system (Bengtson, Rosenthal, & Burton 1996; Blieszner & Bedford, 1996; Troll, 1986).

Kinship is bilateral in Europe and North America. Individuals are surrounded by a network of kin extending out to about the third or fourth degree of collaterality. Bilateral descent in a capitalistic society has superficial similarities with bilateral descent in smaller scaled societies. The one point of similarity is flexibility. Individuals are mobile as they seek opportunities in the labor market. They deactivate or attenuate part of their kindred when they physically move considerable distances (Climo, 1992). Like foragers in search of food opportunities, workers are on a quest for career opportunities. More importantly, there are major differences conditioned by the context in which people live. These are as follows:

• **Smaller families:**   Populations in most industrialized societies have experienced the demographic transition. Decreased mortality and fertility not only result in aging populations, but kindreds shrink in the size of their members. Families faced with the costs of rearing children and the necessity of two paycheck households, combined with reproductive technologies that permit the planning of offspring, simply have fewer children. The net result of lower fertility is a "bean pole family" (Bengston, Rosenthal, & Burton, 1990). These families are small and distinguished by marked generational differences because children have been born within a few years of each other.

• **Nuclear families:**   One major point of departure is that the families in industrialized societies are nuclear families. Bilateral descent is congruent with neolocal and bilocal residence, which we have seen in domestically organized cultures. However, the vast majority of those families, even if residentially distinct, are a part of an extended family. Nuclear families are not only residentially distinct, but manage separate domestic budgets. Wage labor and increased wealth have promoted neolocal residence and nuclear families (Gratton & Haber, 1993). With increases in wealth and social security for older adults, working and middle class families have consistently through time moved toward nuclear families of two and often single generations. More affluent families have usually maintained nuclear households. Nuclear families are diverse. Perhaps the modal form is parents and children. Other forms are single parent families, grandparents and grandchildren, even siblings (sisters) raising children together.

• **Economic functions of families:** Capitalistic economies are organized very differently than those of small-scaled cultures. Production shifts to units concerned with the creation of goods and services such as factories, corporations, firms, service agencies, and the like. Very few families remain as producing units. The division of labor changes from a domestic division of labor broadly based on gender to the true division of labor of specialized production. Families are interdependent with production units through wage labor to be able to purchase necessary goods and services on a market. Consequently, families have become units concerned with consumption. This places the small nuclear households in industrialized economies in sharp contrast to their counterparts in smaller-scaled economies.

INDIVIDUATION AND KINSHIP IDEOLOGY

The autonomous individual is a predominate theme in theories about people and personal developmental possibilities in an urban and industrialized world. Understandings of kinship has been transformed (Strathern, 1992). Kin, as defined by descent and marriage, the model used above, is largely the framework of earlier centuries codified by social anthropology in early to mid twentieth century. By late twentieth century, the meaning of kinship emphasizes diversity in forms and individualism. Individuals reproduce individuals who are nurtured and developed as individuals and less as kin. Developments in reproductive technologies further erode the meaning of descent. With frozen eggs, sperm, and embryos, along with test tube fertilization and surrogate mothers, a child no longer needs parents. All that is needed is a uterus in a living woman. Cloning will only further make descent a more questionable basis of connection to other individuals. The frequency of divorce also has altered the meaning of affinal connections. Broken links either bring attenuated bonds to affines or creates multiple sets of in-laws with ambiguous relationships.

Families in domestically organized societies are groups of people connected by genealogical links who have learned to live and work together. Kin, especially children, in the United States, are not seen as reservoirs of labor. They are individuals who have their own trajectories and whose accomplishments are to be enjoyed. Families are fun. Families and households should be the institution of intimacy in an otherwise predominately bureaucratic society (Bella, 1985).

FAMILIES AND CAREGIVING

Caregiving has different requirements in industrialized societies. First, older people do not face many of the hazards that must be dealt with in smaller scale cultures. Wealth can be and should be accumulated. Households need not be mobile on a seasonal basis. Technology has reduced the physical stamina needed to manage a household. Innovations such as central heating, indoor plumbing, stoves, refrigerators, washing machines, and vacuum cleaners are all labor saving devices designed to reduce the drudgery of home management to free up people for the labor force. These devices enable older people, even those living alone, to manage their homes for a long time with significant levels of disablement. Another feature of caregiving in industrialized societies is very distinctive of capitalism: markets. The service sector of this market has expanded throughout the twentieth century. If one cannot do a task, or chooses not to, he or she can purchase the service on the market. Services range from such things as tax preparation, lawn care, house painting, house cleaning, restaurants, car care, et cetera, including the entire range of the activities of daily living. Indeed, one of the first tasks of caregiving when an elder becomes frail is to figure out the services available in the eldercare market and the rules and regulations. Besides the market, there is growing evidence that non-kin get involved in supporting individuals they care about (Barker, 2002).

KINSHIP AS AN ENVIRONMENTAL CONTINGENCY

By being an integral part of the way humans relate to the natural world and to each other, culture is a set of contingencies. Cultural knowledge is conspecific knowledge about how the world works that has been worked out by individuals living together. This knowledge is negotiated, tested by experience, and shared with others comprising the sociocultural group. Kinship is a major domain of life, shaped by the rules and the work of kin. All humans spend significant parts of their lives from birth to death in some kind of domestic unit. Understandings about kin most clearly affect life with the more private household unit. Kinship also has its public side because families interact with each other and a larger community. What then are the contingencies of kinship that shape the environmental consequences for older people? We examine this issue by looking at contingencies of 1) Who can one count on? 2) Who lives with a person? and 3) Is blood really thicker than water?

WHO CAN I COUNT ON?

"Blood is thicker than water" is an aphorism highlighting inherent allegiances between a person and his or her kin as compared to other people. As we have seen above, who those relatives are is subject to culturally specific rules and circumstances. On a comparative basis, the major axis of variability is the rules of descent.

• **Contingencies of unilineal descent:**   Both matrilineal and patrilineal descent emphasize descent linkages and restrict those linkages to one gender only. The resulting kin groups tend to be corporate and well bounded. With a fixed pool of relatives combined with an age hierarchy, unilineal descent works well for older people. Inheritance rules often reinforce the certainties of who is responsible for a dependent older kinsperson. Unilineal descent, however, has its risks. An individual's welfare is dependent on the group's welfare. Lineages are very concerned with issues of continuity and successes. Reproductive failures, premature deaths, and economic setbacks can and do have disastrous effects on a family's fortunes. For older people, the risks of survivorship may be that their entire descent group declines. With an already restricted kin network, there may be even fewer kin to count on.

• **Contingencies of bilateral descent:**   Bilateral descent is far less restrictive in linkages than unilineal descent. Resultant kindreds are networks of potential kin limited only by the abilities to reckon relatedness, degrees of collaterality, and social distance. Adding to the flexibility of bilateral descent is that one's welfare is not entirely dependent on that of one's household. One can reach out to a related household in exchange, alliances, or just an extended visit to improve fortunes. For foragers, this effectively overcomes inequities of environmental productivity at any age. For older people, the risk of survivorship is that the network of potential kin linkages will shrink through the deaths of ascending kin as well as those of an ego's own generation.

WHO LIVES WITH ME?

Residence rules are the most obvious environmental contingency of kinship.These rules set preferences and often predetermine household composition and affiliation. The relatives with whom one lives and interacts with on a daily basis are "real" relatives. Because of the interdependency and generalized reciprocity that come with coresidence, these are the relatives one can count on.

• **Contingencies of patrilocal and matrilocal residence:**   The residence rules associated with unilineal descent result in fairly large extended families and a blurring of the boundaries between the coresident nuclear families. The resulting contingencies that work well for older people are twofold. First, generalized reciprocity is extended between coresident families. Consequently, the reversal of reciprocity caused by disability is not obvious and is absorbed in the lifetime of exchange. Secondly, pre-arranged residence has the advantage of shielding older people from the effects of a developmental cycle and differential survivorship.

• **Contingencies of neolocal residence:**   Neolocality is the residential choice of bilateral descent. Neolocality is also associated with productive activities that are individuated (i.e., wage labor) or involve short-term coordination (i.e., foraging). Advantages of residentially and economically distinct nuclear families are that the resulting unit directly benefits from the labors and fortunes of their adult members. Food and wealth do not have to be distributed to related households on a regular basis. Here, the costs for older adults whose incapacities undercut their abilities to maintain a separate household are obvious. Because of separate household economies or budgets, the need for assistance makes the exchange and shift in reciprocity toward dependency explicit to the kin involved. Also, as we have seen, older nuclear households can be at the risk of differential survivorship and shrinking kindreds. Resolution of problems associated with disability can, and often does, result in moving an older adult to be physically near the relatives who will look after him or her. That physical move may also involve incorporating the older person into an existing household of a younger person, thus creating an extended family. This is an alternative form of locality anchored in a descending generation (daughter, son, niece, and nephew) and not that of a parental generation.

IS BLOOD REALLY THICKER THAN WATER?

If kin are more likely to extend support, then we should examine some of the demands placed on relatives by economic and social factors. We also should look at the meaning of care and the activities required by caregiving. Support inherent in the interdependency of household members is not seen as problematic until it breaks down. When parents abuse children, when adult children abuse parents, their spouses, or try to hasten the deaths of any of their relatives, it is seen as problematic. The support extended to individuals in need of care because of immaturity or incapacity is different. It is different in that interdependency is transformed into dependency that may trigger kin units to confront other contingencies in their environment.

One factor, as we have seen, is mobility, especially mobility with limited technology. As we have seen above, when residence must be shifted on a periodic or seasonal basis, the result produces hardships for both children and elders. Foragers are known to space births through abortion, infanticide, or prolonged lactation to ensure the survival of existing children.

When a camp or even an entire village must move, frail older people are provisioned and sometimes left behind. Cross-cultural data suggests that bilateral descent is the most problematic for the support of frail older people in mobile foraging societies. Likewise, horticulturalists also relying on foraging are the unilineal societies that are reported as having nonsupportive treatment of their elders. It is among sedentary agriculturalists that we find older people experiencing the supportive benefits of unilineal descent.

Urban industrial societies present other conditions shaping kin and care. Mobility for job opportunities has different meanings as the problems of moving and distance are overcome technologically. Kin units respond to two markets. The first is the labor market where individuals work for wages. The second is a consumer market where goods and services are purchased. The care work of kin is contingent on these two markets. To participate in these markets, families have responded by having fewer children, by emphasizing bilateral descent with neolocal residence, and by transforming the meaning of kinship.

In the last half of the twentieth century, families have found it advantageous, if not necessary, to have more than one adult participating in the labor force. With women working, difficulties arise over schedules and the availability of caregivers. Solutions can be found in the service market. Parents, desiring two career families, will spend the equivalent of college tuition in day care for a child. Adult day care and other senior services are the parallels in the elder care market. With affluence, elders and their families may find supportive environments and care in a wide variety of alternative residential arrangements ranging from retirement communities with recreational amenities to assisted living and nursing homes.

The meaning of care is also transformed and shaped by the market. Caregiving is more than provisioning, clothing, sheltering, and generally looking after a person. With the medicalization of old age, caregiving involves appointments with medical personnel, supervision of drug regimes, physical therapy, coordinating services, and being an advocate and interpreter for an older person in need.

KINSHIP IS THE ENVIRONMENT OF AGING

We end with our opening statement; "Aging is a family affair." Indeed, families are the environment of ordinary domestic life from birth to death. Kinship, in its variations, shapes that environment by defining the significant people one should be able to count on and shaping the residential environment by conditioning those with whom one is coresident. Bilateral descent can leave an elder in extreme old age at risk of out-surviving their relatives. The care work of kinship is shouldered by a truncated core of descendants. Unilineal descent with the emphasis on a corporate group affords some protection from the risks of survivorship. In performing the work of kinship and care, families face a host of other environmental issues. With limited technology and high mobility, families under stress face difficult decisions about the care of members with limited mobility. Families in urban industrialized societies differ in many ways and face challenges not faced in the smaller domestic scaled cultures that have existed ever since humans became human. The size and function of families change along with the meanings of kinship and care. Yet, care and support remains the work of kinship. However, with the creation of a service market, care work is not exclusively a family affair.

REFERENCES

Barker, J. C. (2002). Neighbors, friends and other nonkin caregivers of community-living dependent elders. *Journal of gerontology: Social sciences, 57b*, 158-167.

Bella, R., Madsen, R. Sullivan, W., Swidler, A., & Tipton, S. (1985). *Habits of the heart: Individualism and commitment in American life.* Berkley: University of California Press.

Bengtson, V., Rosenthal, C., & Burton, L. (1990). Families in aging: Diversity and heterogeneity. In R. Binstock & L. K. George (Eds.), *The handbook of aging and the social sciences* (3rd edition, pp. 263-287). New York: Academic Press.

Bengtson, V., Rosenthal, C., & Burton, L. (1996). Paradoxes of families and aging. In R. Binstock & L. K. George (Eds.), *The handbook of aging and the social sciences* (4th edition, pp. 254-283). New York: Academic Press.

Blieszner, R., & Bedford, V. H. (Eds.). (1996). *Aging and the family: Theory and research.* Westport, CT: Prager.

Climo, J. (1992). *Distant parents.* New Brunswick, NJ: Rutgers University Press.

Ember, C. R., &. Ember, M. (2001). *Cross-cultural research methods.* Walnut Creek, CA: AltaMira.

Foley, R. A. (1992). Evolutionary ecology of fossil hominids. In E. A. Smith & B. Winterhalder (Eds.), *Evolutionary ecology and human behavior* (pp. 131-164). New York: Aldine De Gruyder.

Fry, C. L. (1995). Kinship and individuation: Cross-cultural perspectives on intergenerational relations. In V. L. Bengtson, K. W. Schaie, & L. M. Burton (Eds.), *Adult intergenerational relations: Effects of social change* (pp. 126-156). New York: Springer.

Fry, C. L. (2003). The life course as a cultural construct. In R. A. Settersten, Jr., (Ed.), *Invitation to the life course: toward new understandings of later life* (pp. 269-294), Amityville, NY: Baywood.

Glascock, A. P. (1982). Decrepitude and death-hastening: The nature of old age in third-world societies. In J. Sokolovsky (Ed.), *Aging and the aged in third world societies* (pp. 43-66). Williamsburg, VA: College of William and Mary.

Glascock, A. P., & Feinman, S. (1980). A holocultural analysis of old age. *Comparative social research, 3*, 311-333.

Glascock, A. P., & Feinman, S. (1981). Social asset or social burden: Treatment of the aged in non-industrial societies. In C. L. Fry (Ed.), *Dimensions, aging, culture and health* (pp. 13-32). South Hadley, MA: Bergin & Garvey.

Glascock, A. P., & Wagner R. A. (1986). *Death and dying in the life cycle.* New Haven, CT: Human Relations Area Files.

Gratton, B., & Haber, C. (1993). Rethinking industrialization: Old age and the family economy. In T. Cole, W. A. Achenbaum, P. L. Jakobi, & R. Kastenbaum (Eds.), *Voices and visions of aging* (pp. 134-159). New York: Springer.

Guemple, L. (1969). Human resource management: The delemma of the aging Eskimo. *Sociological Symposium, 2*, 59-74.

Katz, S. (1996). *Disciplining old age: The formation of gerontological knowledge.* Charlottsville: University Press of Virginia.

Kertzer, D. I., & Schaie, K. W. (Eds.) (1989). *Age structuring in comparative perspective.* Hillsdale, NJ: Lawrence Erlbaum Associates.

Lovejoy, C. O. (1988). The evolution of human walking. *Scientific American, 259*, 82-89.

Maxwell, E., & Maxwell R. (1980). Contempt for the elderly: A cross-cultural analysis. *Curent Anthropology, 24*, 569-570.

Microcase (1994). *Microcase analysis system; Version 3.* Bellevue, WA: Microcase Corporation.

Morgan, L. H. (1871). *Systems of consanguinity and affinity of the human family.* Washington: Smithsonian Institution.

Murdock, G. P. (1981). *Atlas of world cultures.* New Haven, CT: Yale University Press.

Murdock, G. P. (2000). *Outline of cultural materials.* New Haven, CT: Yale University Press.

Parkin, R. (1997). *Kinship: An introduction to the basic concepts.* Oxford, UK: Blackwell Publishers.

Settersten, R. A., Jr. (1999). *Lives in time and place: The problems and promises of developmental science.* Amityville, NY: Baywood.

Settersten, R. A., Jr. (Ed.). (2003). *Invitation to the life course: Toward new understandings of later life.* Amityville, NY: Baywood.

Silverman, P., & Maxwell, R. J. (1987). The significance of information and power in the comparative study of the aged. In J. Sokolovsky (Ed.), *Growing old in different societies: Cross-cultural perspectives* (pp. 43-55). Acton, MA: Copley.

Simmons, L. W. (1945). *The role of the aged in primitive society.* New Haven: Yale University Press.

Strathern, M. (1992). *After nature: English kinship in the late twentieth century.* New York: Cambridge University Press.

Troll, L. E. (Ed.). (1986). *Family issues in current gerontology.* New York: Springer.

CHAPTER 13

Environmental Gerontology Research and Practice: The Challenge of Application

PAUL G. WINDLEY
DEPARTMENT OF ARCHITECTURE
UNIVERSITY OF IDAHO

GERALD D. WEISMAN
SCHOOL OF ARCHITECTURE AND URBAN PLANNING
UNIVERSITY OF WISCONSIN—MILWAUKEE

From its inception, issues of application have been central to environmental gerontology (Wahl & Weisman, in press). However, linking research and practice remains a fundamental challenge for environmental gerontology as well as for the larger domain of environment-behavior studies (Sommer, 1997). For example, within environmental gerontology, multiple studies report that older persons overwhelmingly wish to *age in place* in their own homes and neighborhoods (cf. Lawton, 1975; Lawton & Hoover, 1981; Regnier & Pynoos, 1987; Tilson, 1990; AARP, 1996). Yet, our society continues to build low-density, auto-oriented suburban communities that will make the accommodation of aging in place increasingly difficult (Calthorpe, 1993). Similarly, although multiple studies report that older Americans view traditional "medical model" nursing homes as a residence of last resort, too many such facilities continue to be built (Koncelik, 1976; Schwarz, 1997). We know that home safety is a major concern for older persons, yet the many easy modifications that would improve safety are implemented far too infrequently (cf., Gitlin, 2000; Pynoos, Cohen, Davis, & Bernhardt, 1987).

If research in environmental gerontology is not being effectively applied, it is not because we do not know how to do so. For example, Weisman (1983) reviewed literature from diverse fields—organizational behavior, policy science, clinical psychology—highlighting both the dimensions of the problem of research utilization and the proposed strategies for its resolution. The problem is rooted in the institutionalized separation of research and practice with some variant of *action research* commonly proposed as the means of resolution. Sommer (1997) argued that the investigation of research utilization has mushroomed in the past two decades.

Parmalee and Lawton (1990) asserted that the environment and aging field stagnated in the 1980s due to the lack of theoretical development and new environmental innovation. They claimed that the field was at a crossroads, and its future direction would depend on how it integrated theory and practice. We argue that only modest progress has been made in theoretical development since that time (Scheidt & Windley, 1998), and even less progress has been achieved in research application. This chapter therefore addresses the problem of application in environmental gerontology from multiple perspectives. We begin by developing a continuum describing the range of possible strategies for linking research and practice. These strategies are synthesized from the relevant literature in environmental gerontology (Windley & Weisman, 1977; Weisman, Chaudhury, & Diaz Moore, 2001), the broader literature focused on environment-behavior studies (Seidel, 1985; Schneekloth, 1987), and research utilization in the social sciences more generally (Fishman, 1999; Polkinghorn, 1992). In the course of developing this continuum, note is taken of the quite different ways—ranging from instrumental to conceptual—in which research utilization has been defined (Weiss & Bucuvalas, 1980), as well as different models for the conduct of research itself (cf., Sommer, 1997). With this continuum in hand, we illustrate and evaluate diverse efforts to employ each of these strategies for the application of environmental gerontology research at four environmental scales: (a) regional, community, and neighborhood; (b) site and landscape; (c) building; and (d) interior design. We conclude the chapter by calling for alternative research paradigms that use what we have learned from past successful research applications, and we suggest how we might reconceptualize the roles of researchers and practitioners, and the relationship between the two.

STRATEGIES FOR LINKING RESEARCH AND PRACTICE

The linking of research and practice has been the focus of substantial attention in environmental gerontology (Windley & Weisman, 1977; Weisman, Diaz Moore, & Chaudhury, 2001) and has gained substantially more interest in the related field of environment-behavior studies, as referenced previously. By way of example, Seidel (1985) proposes three strategies for more effective research utilization: *communication*—making information available and readable, *linkage*—via implementation transfer specialists and committees, and *collaboration*—between researcher and user. Schneekloth (1987) presents three partially overlapping categories: *information transfer*—via guidelines and codes, *education*—of both professionals and users, and *action research/reflective practice*. In Schneekloth's schema, some methods, such as programming, postoccupancy evaluation, and design as inquiry, may fall into the first or the third of her categories, "depending on the process of engagement" (p. 309).

Table 13.1 builds on these previous efforts, but rather than conceptualizing each as a discreet strategy, it places them as points along a continuum. Although six specific strategies are positioned along this continuum, with each given a relatively unique identity for illustration purposes, it should be recognized that in reality the strategies substantially overlap, with one often blending into the next. Furthermore, we see these six strategies as falling along a continuum from those that are *passive and generic*, without any project-specific focus, to those that are *active* and highly *project specific*. The passive stance, without any project-specific focus, is contrasted with the other end of the continuum, where multiple actors are engaged in "action research" projects of the kind that will be described in subsequent sections.

STRATEGIES FOR RESEARCH APPLICATION

Trickle Down

Represented in the first column of Table 13.1, *trickle down* is in many ways not a formal strategy at all. To the extent that it is referenced in the research utilization literature, it is only an example of our current problematic situation where far too many researchers in environmental gerontology fail to consider if and how their studies will be disseminated to practitioners. Nevertheless, we include it because it likely remains the dominant, if far from the most desirable, mechanism for research application. We maintain it is not adequate to simply assume that research will eventually make its

TABLE 13.1   A Continuum of Research Application Strategies

Trickle Down	Communication/ Dissemination	Education	Planning/ Design Guidance	Research Application/ Applied Research	Action Research/ Reflective Practice
Passive and Generic					Active and Project-Specific

way to practitioners, much as some economists assume that wealth will "trickle down" from the most to the least affluent members of our society. Reflecting the traditions of logical positivism, particularly in the natural sciences, far too many researchers still view issues of application to be outside their purview. They see their role as limited to the generation of knowledge, with others picking up and utilizing this knowledge as they see fit (Weisman, 1983). It is likewise now widely recognized that the structure and reward systems within the research community work against an interest and engagement in issues of application where too often decisions regarding publication and promotion assume that efforts at application are at a "lower" level than "pure" research (Boyer, 1990).

However, the trickle-down model should not be dismissed out of hand. In at least selected realms, it has had a substantial impact. For example, the phenomenon of *naturally occurring retirement communities* (NORCs; Hunt & Ross, 1990), to be covered in a later section, has clearly been the beneficiary of trickle down, having been widely reviewed in popular press outlets such as *The Wall Street Journal, U.S. News & World Report, Business Week,* and *Modern Maturity.* Similarly, as reconstructed by Archea and Margulis (1979), research on the morbidity and mortality impacts of relocation of the institutionalized elderly has had an even more circuitous trickle-down path, eventually moving from the academic realm to that of the federal and state government.

Communication/Dissemination

With recognition of the limitations of the trickle-down approach and a commitment to addressing real problems, concerns about effective research utilization emerged early in the development of environmental gerontology (e.g., Windley & Weisman, 1977). The initial concern was to enhance communication and dissemination. Proposals focused on making research information more available and engaging—employing more visual material, less jargon, and fewer statistics—to attract more design practitioners. Within this communication/dissemination approach, Sommer (1997) reported success in communicating research findings in a nontechnical fashion in various trade publications. Trade magazines and even the popular press have also proven to be effective conduits for trickle-down dissemination. Within the domain of aging, the annual "Design" issue of *Nursing Homes Long Term Care Management* and the *biannual Facility Review,* published by the Design for Aging Center of the American Institute of Architects, have served as conduits for dissemination.

More recently, Web sites have emerged as an important mechanism for the communication of research-based information to care practitioners. Three examples are the sites of the National Resource Center on Supportive

Housing and Home Modification (www.homemods.org), the Center for Universal Design (www.design.ncsu.edu/cud/), and the Institute for the Future of Aging Services of the American Association of Homes and Services for the Aged (www.futureofaging.org). We will return to these sites in our consideration of interior environments and product design.

Education

The line between communication/dissemination and education strategies is often difficult to discern, especially as we move into an era of *distance learning*. Web sites, as noted, can serve an education as well as a dissemination function. In terms of more traditional notions of education, Sommer (1997) employs the example of the agricultural extension service developed in the 1920s. Some states employ housing extension specialists who often serve as important conduits for research information regarding housing for older persons. Their organization, the American Association of Housing Educators, publishes the journal *Housing & Society*. The Helen Bader Foundation and the National Office of the Alzheimer's Association have supported the National Alzheimer's Design Assistance Project. This project provides more traditional, *hands-on* educational experiences to health care, social service, and design professionals engaged in the creation of new, cutting-edge facilities for dementia care (Weisman, in press).

Planning/Design Guidance

Early efforts at more effective communication and dissemination quickly moved beyond relatively superficial issues of graphics and jargon to a more active and engaged strategy for synthesis and conveyance of research findings. The result has been a series of planning or design guidebooks characterized as *pattern books*. The origins of this approach are perhaps most clearly seen in the work of architectural theorist Christopher Alexander and colleagues (1977) who pioneered the concept of *pattern language*. Rather than simply proposing a prototype design for what was then an emerging place type, Alexander and colleagues generated guidelines or patterns, each of which dealt with a discrete facet of the total environment. Figure 13.1 provides an illustration of a pattern emerging from the work of Diaz Moore, Geboy, and Weisman (2002) on dementia day care centers. Pattern language proposes empirically supportable design hypotheses using if-then statements accompanied by a graphic illustration. The premise of this approach is that research data do not "speak for themselves." Rather it is necessary to extend research conclusions, drawing out implications based not just on the data at hand but also upon other studies and professional experience, and to link these understandings to the context of a specific place.

This pattern-book approach was quickly adapted to the field of environmental gerontology. Zeisel, Epp, and Demos (1977) produced guidelines for "low rise housing for older people," and Zeisel, Welch, Epp, and Demos (1983) published guidelines for "mid-rise elevator housing for older people." The majority of currently available guidebooks for the planning and design of buildings for older persons continue to follow this pattern-based approach (cf. Brummett, 1997; Calkins, 1988; Cohen & Weisman, 1991; Regnier, 2002; Zeisel et al., 1977). The pattern approach likely dominates in the broader field of environment-behavior studies as well; it has been suggested that patterns are a particularly apt means of

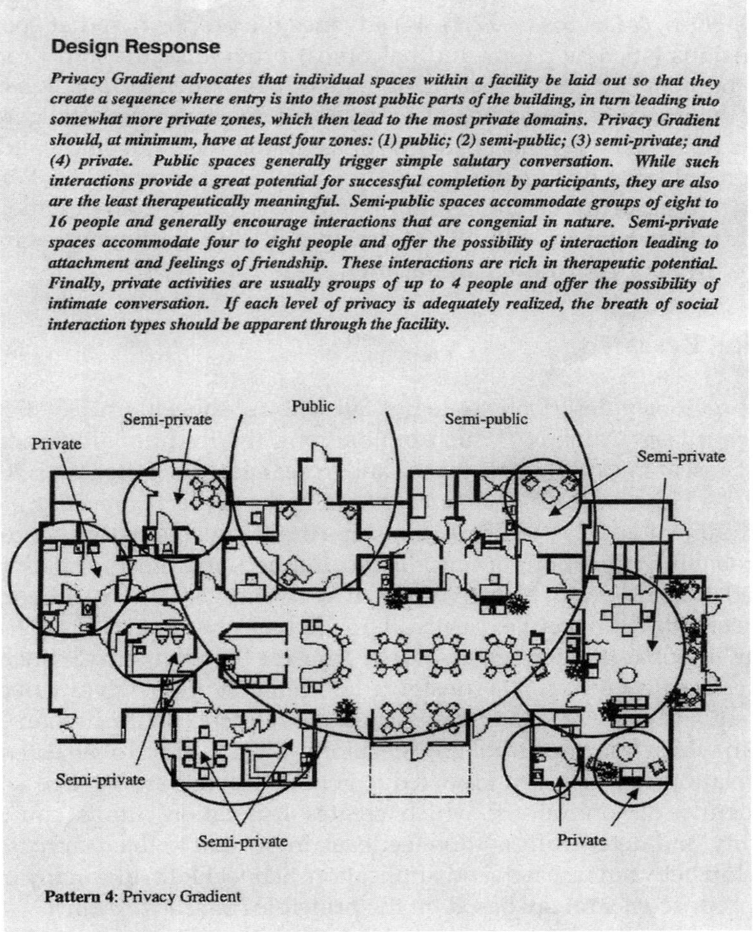
Design Response
Privacy Gradient advocates that individual spaces within a facility be laid out so that they create a sequence where entry is into the most public parts of the building, in turn leading into somewhat more private zones, which then lead to the most private domains. Privacy Gradient should, at minimum, have at least four zones: (1) public; (2) semi-public; (3) semi-private; and (4) private. Public spaces generally trigger simple salutary conversation. While such interactions provide a great potential for successful completion by participants, they are also are the least therapeutically meaningful. Semi-public spaces accommodate groups of eight to 16 people and generally encourage interactions that are congenial in nature. Semi-private spaces accommodate four to eight people and offer the possibility of interaction leading to attachment and feelings of friendship. These interactions are rich in therapeutic potential. Finally, private activities are usually groups of up to 4 people and offer the possibility of intimate conversation. If each level of privacy is adequately realized, the breath of social interaction types should be apparent through the facility.
Public
Semi-private
Semi-public
Private
Semi-private
Semi-private
Semi-private
Private
Pattern 4: Privacy Gradient

FIGURE 13.1 Example of a pattern for dementia day care centers (Diaz Moore et al., 2002).

capturing "practice knowledge" (Polkinghorn, 1992) and the systemic complexity of places (Weisman, 2001).

Research Application/Applied Research

The transition from simply communicating the products of research to a more active synthesis of research in the context of guidelines or patterns was substantial. In addition to providing a more integrated context for findings, patterns also adapted a *design-as-hypotheses* framework, describing (more or less explicitly) the expected/desired consequences of a proposed environmental configuration. By way of example, in one pattern Zeisel, Epp, & Demos (1977, p. 44) advance the proposition that "outdoor extensions (such as patios and balconies) provide secure and protected environments for casual socializing with others." Such propositions are at least theoretically amenable to testing, and some environmental gerontologists have taken up this challenge of assessing the value and validity of design guidance documents (e.g., Day, Carreon, & Stump, 2000). We characterize this sort of testing as "applied research," the goal of which is to confirm the value and validity of design guidance documents as mechanisms for effective research application.

Action Research

The previously described strategies fall within Schneekloth's (1987) *information transfer* category, which builds upon the traditional hierarchy of basic research, applied research, and research application (cf., Moore, Tuttle, & Howell, 1985). For some, the strengths of this perspective are that environment and behavior relationships are knowable within some level of probability, directions of causality are implied, and the information generated is considered objective (Groat & Wang, 2002). For others (e.g., Schneekloth), a concern exists that knowledge generation and application occur in separate spheres and time frames. Furthermore, Schneekloth argues because research is considered objective it often "gives value, and consequently power, to knowledge without reference to the human condition in which it is produced" (Schneekloth, 1987, p. 311). To the extent that the relationship between knowledge generators and knowledge users is frequently discontinuous, which creates frustration, limits contextual validity, and deters information feedback important to the reciprocal relationship between research and application, Schneekloth, like many others, has proposed a strategy based on the principles of *action research*.

The term *action research* was coined more than 50 years ago by Kurt Lewin (1946), one of the founders of social psychology, who argued that research in the social sciences should be integrated with concerns for application. Action research is collaborative knowledge building that involves clients, practitioners, consultants, and researchers whose collective aim is to produce practical knowledge useful to the everyday lives of people (Senge & Scharmer, 2001). Although slight variations occur in the procedures, action research is essentially a cyclical, multistep process composed of a circle of planning, action, and fact-finding about the result of a specific action (Lewin, 1947).

Action research emerged from Lewin's work at the Center for Group Dynamics at the Massachusetts Institute of Technology, a group that endeavored to both analyze and act on social problems. From Lewin's perspective, "research that produced nothing but books will not suffice" (1946, p. 35). At the same time, theory was not sacrificed for the sake of the practical; indeed in some cases fundamental knowledge might not have been obtainable unless it had derived from real social problems (Susman & Evered, 1978).

Weisman (1983) noted that the subsequent evolution of action research has not been a process of steadily advancing knowledge, but it is characterized by "fits and starts" yielding fragmented knowledge in different fields. An early article by Sanford (1970) suggested that a root cause for the failure of action research to "get off the ground" was the institutional separation of science and practice. Schon (1983) later described this separation as the "rigor versus relevance" dilemma where practitioners and researchers must choose between

> remaining on the high ground where they can solve relatively unimportant problems according to prevailing standards of rigor or . . . descend to the swamp of important problems and nonrigorous inquiry. (Schon, p. 3, as quoted in Friedman, 2001, p. 159)

Friedman (2001) made a strong case that this dilemma emerged from positivist science where basic research informs practice by suggesting problem-solving techniques learned through professional education. He further explained that positivist science produces theories that are too complex for practitioners to use because of requirements for precision, control, objectivity, and focusing on the means rather than the ends. Thus, "the rules that produce valid positivist explanations of social problems cannot produce the knowledge needed to do something about them" (160).

Wisner, Stea, and Kruks (1997) provided a useful update on the utilization of participatory and action research methods in environmental planning and design, as well as relatively more "remote" fields such as adult education, public health, farm systems research, and applied ethnolinguistics and anthropology. Wisner et al.'s characterization of the basic features of action research accord well with the preceding discussion of strategies for research application: "emphasis was placed upon *training* [emphasis added] social scientists to handle not just the usual forms of social research but also to translate such research into practice in the field" (p. 272). Communication was also important to Lewin's formulation, especially what is characterized as "intercultural communication between planners and clients."

Among the case studies reviewed by Wisner et al. (1997) was a participatory planning and design project for elderly housing and a community center for the Texas Farm Workers Union undertaken by students and faculty at the University of California at Los Angeles. Because many of the prospective residents spoke only Spanish, it was decided to opt for a nonverbal and highly participatory approach to communication employing extremely simply physical models and "doll house furniture." The modeling session proved to be enjoyable for the participants, and the resultant designs differed markedly from those generated by UCLA students who were not part of the participatory design exercise. Given the honor accorded the elderly within this culture, the elderly housing was located adjacent to the community center at the heart of the development. In addition, dwelling units designed by the union retirees included two or more bedrooms, reflective of the extended family structure of the society.

A high level of user involvement is also central to the emerging field of *gerotechnology* and the design of products for older persons. Mollenkopf and Fozard (2004) assert that "the consumer or end user should be involved in all phases of the development, distribution and dispersal of technologically-based products, environment and services" (p. 263).

Weisman (1983) argued that the application of action research in environmental design has been limited for the reasons cited earlier and concluded that in order to successfully translate research into design application, Lewin's action research model should be revisited. Indeed, the basic premises of action research merge translation techniques and emerging technologies employed by designers and planners (Weisman, in press). To more clearly illustrate the context and content of environmental gerontology research, we will first consider selected cells of Table 13.2. The chapter will conclude by returning to alternative models of research, application, and education.

EXAMPLES OF RESEARCH APPLICATION

Having now characterized six alternative research utilization strategies along a continuum from passive to active approaches, we can now describe selected application efforts at four scales of environmental gerontology research: (a) regional, community, and neighborhood; (b) site and landscape; (c) building; and (d) interior design. Relating scales and strategies yields the matrix displayed in Table 13.2. As described previously, research application in environmental gerontology has received far less attention than we might have hoped. This consequently limits the number of significant post-1990 examples of application we can potentially review. Thus, to flesh out our treatment of research application, we have adopted something of a "mixed model." To supplement this review, we have also included selective, often "classic," pre-1990 efforts to bridge research and practice. Our aim in presenting this mixed model of research review is to both illustrate the various application strategies and to provide a profile of significant attempts to bridge the research-application gap over the past decade. Consequently, Table 13.2 does not endeavor to include all research in environmental gerontology conducted since 1990, nor all attempts at research application. We make this selection with full awareness that what we have chosen to label "significant work" is based on our own assessment of the research application field and that others might well see it differently. However, as discussed later in the chapter, it is our judgment that the pattern of dense and sparse cells in Table 13.2 accurately illustrates the current status of significant work in application. Citations in boldface in Table 13.2 represent work to be reviewed in this chapter, and the remaining citations are recommended as further examples of research application.

Many researchers regard the late 1970s and 1980s as the *golden years* in environmental gerontology when much of the groundbreaking research that shaped the field was carried out (Wahl & Weisman, in press). As noted earlier, the field's growth in theoretical development and practice since that time has been limited (Parmalee & Lawton, 1990). Thus, some of the research reviewed throughout the sections to follow has been selected from these earlier years because we believe the conceptual frameworks and specific findings remain relevant to this day and illustrate the different application strategies in Table 13.2.

Regional, Community, and Neighborhood

As illustrated in Table 13.2 and described later, research at regional, community, and neighborhood scales has by and large trickled down to practitioners. Nevertheless, the work of Marans, Hunt, and Vakalo (1984) and Hunt and Ross (1990) is noteworthy. Marans et al. (1984) published a major Administration on Aging-funded review of retirement communities in the United States and provided a useful classification typology for these communities. This research is important in two ways. First, it builds directly on person-environment fit models, a core theoretical framework within environmental gerontology (cf. Kahana, 1982; French, Cobb, & Rogers, 1974; and Lawton & Nahemow, 1973). Second, it presents a clear and imageable typology for the analysis of retirement communities as a place type. Marans et al.

TABLE 13.2 A Continuum of Research Application Strategies for Varying Scales of the Physical Environment

Passive and Generic ————————————————→ Active and Project-Specific

Environmental Context	Trickle Down	Communication/ Dissemination	Education	Planning/ Design Guidance	Applied Research	Action Research/ Reflective Practice
Regional, Community, and Neighborhood	Marans et al. (1984), Glasgow (1990), Fuguitt et al. (1989), Beale and Johnson (1998), Carp (1986), Liang et al. (1986), Hunt and Ross (1990)	Carp (1987), Regnier (1976), Regnier & Hamburger (1978)		Calthorpe (1993)		
Site and Landscape				Carstens (1993), Regnier (2002), Cranz (1987), Cooper-Marcus et al. (1999)		
Building	Pastalan (1991), Archea & Margulis (1979)			Zeisel et al. (1977), Zeisel et al. (1983), Cohen & Weisman (1990), Regnier (2002), Day et al. (2000), Regnier and Pynoos (1987)	Kovach et al. (1997), Milke (1996), Namari et al. (1991), Silverman et al. (1995), Carp (1987)	Hartman et al. (1987), Lawton et al. (1984), Wisner et al. (1997), Coons (1991)
Interior design		Pynoos et al. (2003)	www.homemods.org, www.design. nvsu.edu/cud, www.futureof aging.org	Pynoos et al. (1987), Pynoos et al. (2003), Steinfeld (1987)	Gitlin (2000)	Mollenkopf & Fozard (2003)

(1984) noted that it is difficult to compose a single definition of a retirement community because they vary by size, density, sponsorship, levels of service, tenure arrangements, and location. Their review showed that a wide variety of retirement communities are available and that they are generally congruent with the varied needs of older residents, and that the links between these community types and the larger external environment differ (Marans et al., 1984). Larger-scale settings such as retirement new towns and subdivisions are less autonomous and obtain many needed services from the external environment, whereas more autonomous, smaller-scale settings such as continuing care retirement centers provide services internally.

An additional finding is that retirement communities are either constant or accommodating. Accommodating communities adjust their service repertoire as the needs of older residents change over time. Constant communities are initially supportive of resident needs but are nonadaptive in their supply of services as needs change (Lawton, Greenbaum, & Liebowitz, 1980). This distinction is important to practitioners in order to develop long-term design and planning strategies for retirement communities that are well integrated with the larger contexts of which they are a part. For example, Marans and colleagues noted that privately developed retirement new towns and villages pay taxes to local governments, whereas nonprofit retirement residences and continuing-care centers do not. Glasgow (1990) and Barkley and Henry (2000) reinforced Marans et al.'s (1984) findings by demonstrating that retirement-destination communities have increased per capita incomes and per-capita transfer payments, which augment dollars spent and broaden a community's tax base. Because older residents require more services and infrastructure, employment opportunities increase for younger families in the service sector within and surrounding the retirement communities. Glasgow (1990) also noted that many older residents have higher education levels and advanced skills that become resources for the larger community.

One unique category of research on retirement communities concerns NORCs, as previously discussed. NORCs are defined as "housing developments that are not planned or designed for older people but that attract a preponderance (over 50 percent) of residents at least 60 years of age" (Hunt & Ross, 1990, p. 667). NORCs can be at any scale, ranging from apartment complexes to neighborhoods, to vacation or resort areas, and are located in urban, suburban, and rural settings (Hunt, Merrill, & Gilker, 1994). Based on a series of studies in rural Wisconsin, Marshall and Hunt (1999) developed the following three-category typology of NORCs for rural areas: natural amenity, convenience, and amenity/convenience. Natural amenity NORCs attract younger, healthier, and more affluent older people from long distances who want to take advantage of an area's natural environment. Convenience NORCs are composed of individuals less educated and affluent than natural amenity residents who move relatively short distances from one rural area to another to be closer to relatives or town services. Amenity/convenience NORCs attract both amenity and support seekers. This typology provides a point of application for designers and planners who must determine the social, economic, and environmental costs and benefits of attracting older people to a specific location. However, it is not clear whether this typology applies to urban areas.

At a more regional level, Fuguitt, Brown, and Beale (1989) demonstrated that high amenity or recreation counties attract a high proportion of retirement age migrants. Thus, of the 285 recreation counties in the United States based on recreation-related employment and activity indicators, approximately 100 (35 percent) are also designated as retirement counties based on age-specific inmigration rates (Beale & Johnson, 1998). An increased understanding of the role of recreational amenities in attracting people to retirement counties would significantly aid regional and community planners. Related to this question, Longino (2004) discusses some of the motivations for elderly migration to retirement destinations.

In summary, this body of regional and community-level research aids application by generating data linked to specific environmental contexts, and in some cases it provides environmental descriptors. The various taxonomic schemes by Marans et al. (1984), Hunt et al. (1994), and Beal and Johnson (1998) describe these environmental contexts in terms of size, context, and infrastructure. These typologies also begin to identify possible place types that serve as vehicles for research application, designer and practitioner education, and points of possible intervention. Although potentially related to application, this body of research mostly exemplifies the trickle-down approach, with NORCs as an especially clear example.

Krause's (2004) chapter provides a useful and comprehensive review of broad neighborhood factors that affect the health and well-being of older people. Tracing the effects of objective neighborhood dimensions, such as noise and environmental toxins, and subjective dimensions, such as a sense of community and fear of crime, partially demonstrates the significance of neighborhoods in the lives of older people. However, it is not clear from such reviews how the physical environment of neighborhoods can be better planned to enhance the well-being of older residents. Relatively few studies have provided neighborhood data that can guide practitioners in important planning decisions. The following summarized projects are exceptions to this trend and also illustrate communication/dissemination as well as the trickle-down strategy.

Regnier (1976) reported a series of neighborhood studies in Los Angeles and San Francisco that demonstrated how older persons' cognitive representations of their neighborhood yielded a consensus map that identified delimiters and incentives to neighborhood use by older residents. Topography, traffic patterns, land use, bus routes, and district designations were physical environmental dimensions of perceived neighborhoods that shaped neighborhood use and activities. Social factors such as ethnic identity, population density, and income were found to be significant components of perceived neighborhoods as well. Regnier (1976) showed how consensus maps help planners identify areas in neighborhoods where services should be located, identify potential sites for elderly housing and neighborhood centers, preserve areas of neighborhoods that have cognitive significance to older residents, identify street routes for public transportation, and regulate traffic lights to ease pedestrian movement.

Subsequent neighborhood research in Los Angeles conducted by Regnier and Hamburger (1978) showed how consensus maps created by older residents revealed areas in the neighborhood judged to be unsafe and compared these perceptions with actual police records of street and residential crime. Although older residents accurately identified unsafe areas within the larger neighborhood, they were less aware of specific environmental features that increased the probability of victimization. Consistent with the communication/dissemination strategy, Regnier and Hamburger (1978) outlined actions community planners could take to reduce the fear of crime among older people. These included assigning police patrols to areas perceived as unsafe and educating older people to identify safe pedestrian routes and to avoid areas where victimization is likely, such as parking lots and alleys. Another solution included forming partnerships with local authorities to create a defensible neighborhood by locating bus stops at surveillance areas and patrolling parking lots.

In a similar vein, Liang, Sengstock, and Hwalek (1986) summarized a series of findings on the physical environmental correlates of crime and fear of crime among older residents in different urban neighborhoods. To reduce victimization and fear of crime through environmental design, these investigators recommended that community planners establish clear boundaries between public and private spaces, eliminate open and uncontrolled areas, remove shrubbery in strategic areas that conceal potential criminals, and develop neighborhood plans in concert with other social and regulatory agencies.

Moving beyond typologies, Carp (1986) attempted to bridge the research-application gap in her studies of neighborhood quality among older people by developing perceived environmental-quality indices and the methods to measure them. Her assumption was that if planners are to manipulate environmental attributes to support older residents, they must be able to measure these attributes. Thus, Carp developed objective environmental measurements of neighborhoods. These focused on residential type and population density; topography; the distance from the residence to public transportation and arterials; the presence of land barriers between home and public transportation; land uses and the presence of open space, vegetation, and water; and the type of residential construction, including adequate plumbing. The proximity of environmental amenities and services to the residence was the single most important predictor of neighborhood quality, resource utilization, and activity rate. Community planners were encouraged to use objective measures of neighborhood attributes as a way of linking neighborhood-planning decisions to improving the quality of life for older residents. Carp moved her neighborhood research further toward application when she developed a series of design directives and policy considerations for practitioners and policy makers (Carp, 1987).

In summary, this series of neighborhood studies encompasses both trickle-down and communication/dissemination strategies, and it provides practitioners with potential solutions for neighborhoods more accommodating to older residents.

Site and Landscape

Cranz (1987) reported findings on site development from 280 older residents of eight housing projects in New Jersey. These findings were translated into design directives and policy implications that place this study squarely in the planning/design guidance strategy. Design directives emerging from the preferences of the study sample regarding housing site design included outdoor spaces that support a variety of activities ranging from sitting in the sun to sitting unobserved in secluded but safe areas. These outdoor spaces also included benches that allow easy entry and egress and that support social interaction, areas for accessible gardening, and walkways with varying textures and gradual grades. They also offered points of interest such as fountains, mobiles, and bird feeders; open space protected from the surrounding neighborhood but is visually accessible to neighborhood activity; and nonglare surfaces properly lighted at night.

Carstens (1993) provided an excellent review of research related to site design and outdoor spaces for older people living in residential settings ranging from congregate housing to nursing homes. Her design guidelines were comprehensive and detailed, and although they cannot be reviewed in any depth in this chapter, Table 13.3 outlines her framework for organizing these guidelines and offers illustrative examples of selected recommendations. These guidelines are unique because they are based on an environment and behavior perspective with a special focus on (a) a prosthetic approach to design, (b) the need for variety and choice, (c) enhancing autonomy and independence, (d) providing personalization and control, (e) promoting environmental adaptability, (f) increasing accessibility, and (g) proposing facility management policies. This body of research is an example of planning/design guidance in our research application continuum. Cranz and Carstens' work provides clear examples of how planning design guidelines can generate research questions leading to a program of applied research.

Regnier's (2002) recent studies of assisted-living housing in northern Europe also fall within the planning/design guidance category of our continuum. Using observational and postoccupancy evaluation approaches (including interviews and surveys) to gather data on 100 assisted-living facilities, Regnier identified 12 issues that help practitioners plan more accommodating sites for assisted-living housing. Among his key concerns are that housing sites should (a) fit a community's cognitive map, which will promote community connection and place identity, (b) serve older residents in the surrounding neighborhood by providing a critical mass of services useful to all elderly in the area, (c) employ mixed land-use models to promote social diversity and economic vitality in the surrounding neighborhood, (d) capture views beyond the dwelling and site to enhance spatial orientation and facilitate resident involvement through observation of activities, and (e) create courtyards to capture views, ensure privacy, and enhance social interaction.

Also in the spirit of planning and design guidelines, Cooper-Marcus and Barnes (1999) presented a large body of research that deals with the concept of healing gardens. The basic premise of this concept is that nature has restorative powers that promote health, healing, and overall well-being. The conceptual foundations of this notion reside in stress and stress management through coping mechanisms aided by the natural environment. Researchers in this field come from a variety of disciplines, including landscape architecture, architecture, planning, the social sciences, horticulture, and medicine. Most of the research compiled by Cooper-Marcus and Barnes (1999) was conducted in medical facilities and frequently included older people as subjects. The research specifically relates to acute care hospitals, psychiatric hospitals, healing gardens for children, nursing homes including Alzheimer's facilities, and hospices. In some instances, case studies and resulting design guidelines are reported. This body of research is large and comprehensive and cannot be reviewed in depth in this chapter. However, among the most important of their recommendations are (a) plan the hospital site early in the planning process, creating a variety of outdoor spaces that take advantage of views, permit seclusion, and allow for jurisdictional control; (b) create awareness of the availability of outdoor spaces by providing directions and information; (c) enhance views to the outdoors by the appropriate placement of windows, balconies, and items that attract wildlife; (d) create easy access to outdoor spaces in close proximity to potential users and use automatic doors, floor surfaces that facilitate movement, handrails that support recovering patients, and varying grades to accommodate a person's ability; (e) plan the garden itself to be imageable with a central focus and defined edges, use familiar materials, create larger and smaller subspaces, and provide

TABLE 13.3 Organizing Framework for Carsten's (1993) Site Design Guidelines with Illustrative Recommendations

Development Type	Neighborhood Conditions	Site-Planning Elements	Amenities and Details	Special Considerations
Mid- to High-Rise Connect outdoor activity spaces to indoor activity. **Low-Rise and Mixed** Define activity spaces. **Care on Site** Separate outdoor zones for different levels of care.	**Access** Maintain 5% slope to services. **Wayfinding** Create recognizable site plan using radial or linear layouts. **Circulation Patterns** Separate access to residences from activity spaces. **Social Spaces** Provide options for privacy and meeting others.	**Site Entry** Provide adequate site distance in all directions. **Resident Parking** Avoid a mixture on one-way and two-way aisles. **Public Patios** Locate near indoor and outdoor activity. **Garden and Nature Areas** Provide some close for easy access and others far away for exploration. **Rooftop Developments** Protect from harsh winds, sun, and glare.	**Site Entry** Provide "you are here" signs. **Resident Parking** Provide wide stalls, driving alleys, and turning radii. **Public Patios** Nearby storage and easy access to bathrooms. **Garden and Nature Areas** Provide raised planters and amenities to attract wildlife. **Rooftop Developments** Provide railings and balustrades for safety and security.	**Spatial Scale** Provide small outdoor areas with defined edges to enhance legibility and social interaction. **Level of Detailing** Provide more design detail to compensate for sensory loss. **Lighting and Glare** High-density lighting at entries, drop-off areas, and parking lots for safety. **Climate Control** Moderate shade, sun, and wind to accommodate sensitivity to temperature changes. **Ramps** Ramps should not exceed 8% slope.

overhead protection; and (f) develop administrative policies that educate employees and volunteers about the therapeutic effects of gardens, use organic methods of maintenance, allow for smoking and nonsmoking areas, and keep the gardens open all the time.

Buildings

Though difficult to demonstrate in any definitive fashion, it appears likely that the majority of efforts to apply research in environmental gerontology has occurred at the building scale. This in part reflects the building scale focus of much research in the field. A search on a computerized database of psychological literature from 1989 to 2000 yielded between 71 and 104 studies per year with a clear focus on aging, the socio-physical environment, and behavioral processes (Wahl & Weisman, in press). In most years, substantially more studies focused on "institutional environments" (including assisted living and retirement communities) than on issues of residential relocation, residential decision making, or neighborhood or outdoor mobility. This focus at the architectural scale may also reflect that implementation and interventions are less complex and time-consuming than at the urban or regional scales. The action research perspective, yet to be fully implemented, is reflected in a number of projects, including a sequence of environments created for the care of the cognitively impaired.

As described previously, planning/design guidance has been a particularly active and effective strategy for research application in environmental gerontology, with the majority of this work focused at the building scale. Guidelines and pattern books generated by Welch, Parker, and Zeisel (1984); Zeisel, Epp, and Demos (1977); Zeisel, Welch, Epp, and Demos (1983); Brummett, (1997); Calkins, (1988); Cohen, Weisman, Ray, Steiner, Rand, and Toyne (1988); and Regnier (2002) have all had substantial impact. One application effort worthy of special note is Regnier and Pynoos's (1987) publication that directly engaged researchers, including many of the leading figures in environmental gerontology, in the generation of design and policy guidelines. Chapters include four multisite evaluation (i.e., applied research) studies and two planning and design case studies.

Currently, few examples of a fully implemented action research/reflective practice approach can be found in environmental gerontology. Hartman, Horowitz, and Herman (1987) reported one early, and all too rare, effort at participation by the elderly in the planning and design of housing. Low-income older persons, displaced as a consequence of urban redevelopment in San Francisco, participated in focus groups where slides and scripts were employed to illustrate key issues (e.g., building style, high- versus low-rise construction, relation of building entry to the street). Participants were then invited to express their preferences and related opinions. As previously described, Wisner et al. (1997) employed a participatory modeling strategy with elderly farm workers.

Although it includes less in the way of resident participation than Hartman et al. (1987), a three-decade history of projects for dementia care reflects much of the action research perspective. As described by Weisman (1997, in press), care providers across the United States have created a series of "model facilities" that incorporate a number of defining features from Lewin's model of action research. These model facilities, including the Weiss Institute at the Philadelphia Geriatric Center (Lawton, Fulcomer, & Kleban, 1984) and Wesley Hall in Chelsea, Michigan (Coons, 1991), have served first of all to open our society to new and different forms of accommodation (organizational as well as architectural) for the elderly and cognitively impaired. Although residents are too often, though not always, precluded from participation as a consequence of their impairments, these model projects are notable for the active, long-term involvement of staff, administration, and sometimes residents' families in the planning/design process. Consistent with Lewin's belief in training as an essential part of the action research process, these model facilities have educated large numbers of visitors and staff who have developed considerable expertise in both substantive and process issues. These people have then gone on to share this expertise by serving as consultants to other care providers or designers.

Finally, and of great importance, the majority of these model projects has been the focus of some form of summative evaluation essential to the "spiral of steps" that includes planning, action, and fact-finding fundamental to action research. Such evaluations typically build upon the "hypotheses" articulated during the generation of planning/design guidelines. As a form of "meta-evaluation," Day et al. (2000) reviewed roughly 20 years of research on environments for the cognitively impaired, finding substantial support for guidelines synthesized from the then-current research literature by Cohen and Weisman (1991). (See also Day & Calkins, 2002.) We believe that this sequence of dementia care projects provides a model for forging closer links between research and practice in environmental gerontology.

Interior Design

Two substantial and partially overlapping bodies of research are relevant at the interior scale. The first focuses on issues of accessible, "barrier-free," or "universal" design, and the second deals with the topic of home modification. Both of these bodies of research begin with the recognition that most older persons desire to "age in place" in their own homes, rather than in any form of congregate setting, and that with advancing age, the home environment may present obstacles or "barriers" to independent and adaptive functioning.

Universal design differs from virtually all other planning and design issues raised in this chapter by virtue of being mandated by the federal government, primarily through the Americans with Disabilities Act, and enforced by the U.S. Department of Justice. As described by the Center for Universal Design (www.design.ncsu.edu/cud/), seven fundamental principles must be kept in mind: (a) accommodate diverse populations without segregation or stigmatizing, (b) accommodate individual preference and choice, (c) ensure that designs are easily used by anyone, (d) communicate information in a manner perceptible by the user, (e) minimize hazards of accidental action, (f) enable designs to be operable with minimum physical effort, and (g) provide adequate space for approach and use of any environmental element.

Pynoos, Tabbarah, Angelleli, and Demiere (1998) defined home modifications as "environmental adaptations aimed at creating a more supportive environment, enhancing participation in major life activities, preventing accidents, facilitating caregiving, and minimizing the need for more costly personal care services." Pynoos et al. (1987) emphasized five complementary strategies whereby the older person can better adapt to the environment and/or adapt the environment to better meet his or her needs. These include (a) structural changes, (b) special equipment, (c) assistive devices, (d) material adjustments, and (e) behavior changes. Steinfeld (1987) effectively bridged the issues of accessibility and home modification, focusing on how to adapt housing for disabled older persons.

Research reviewed by Pynoos, Nishita, and Perelman (2003) indicated a rising prevalence in the use of home modifications, with the greatest increase in what would be characterized as quite modest (if not impermanent) modifications such as raised toilet and shower seats and grab bars. Modifications, such as ramps, meant to enhance the accessibility of dwelling units, were substantially less common. Pynoos et al. (2003) suggested that a substantial unmet need among the elderly and impaired could be met by home modification. Of the over 5 million households that have a member with a functional disability, less than a quarter (1.14 million) have the modifications they desire.

The National Resource Center on Supportive Housing and Home Modification clearly operates at the scale of the dwelling unit interior and effectively employs both communication/dissemination and education strategies. In terms of making information maximally accessible, the Center Web site includes a virtual library that provides information on topics ranging from research on ramp slopes to color contrast to NORCs. The site likewise provides a products file with information on everything from automatic door openers to accessible closet storage systems. Finally, the Center offers an Internet course for care managers on "six steps to integrating home modification in your care plan."

At an even smaller environmental scale, the field of *gerontechnology* focuses on the design of products supportive of people as they age. Mollenkopf and Fozard (2004) review a broad range of devices that independently or networked into a "smart house" can assist with mobility, communication, medical diagnosis, and treatment.

FUTURE CHALLENGES

Linking research and practice has been the focus of only limited attention in environmental gerontology. This work ranges from describing different research domains in terms of application potential (cf., Pynoos & Regnier, 1991; Regnier, 2002) to matters of linking environmental assessment and measurement to theoretical frameworks—an important precursor to application (cf., Moos, Lemke, & David, 1987; Norris-Baker, Weisman, Lawton, Sloane, & Kaup, 1999; Carp, 1994). In an attempt to stress application, several individuals have developed design, policy, and implementation guidelines for the creation of various environmental settings (cf. Chambliss, 1989; American Institute of Architects (AIA) Foundation, 1985).

Although useful at one level, many of these guidelines lack a sound conceptual basis and are insensitive to the reciprocal nature of theory and application. A few exceptions to this trend are the guidelines for nursing homes developed by Koncelik (1976), assisted living units described by Regnier (2002), and dementia environments developed by Diaz Moore, Geboy, and Weisman (2002) and Calkins (1988). However, our overall assessment is that the broad landscape of research and practice in environmental gerontology is highly fragmented in conceptual as well as methodological terms. In our review of the literature, we found no attempt to present a comprehensive picture of the range of application approaches in environmental gerontology. This is an important conceptual challenge to take because certain approaches are more suitable to research application in some environmental domains than others.

As a first step toward this goal, Table 13.2 builds on a number of previous efforts to illustrate what we view as a *continuum* of six basic approaches relating research and practice ranging from passive to active and generic to specific approaches (Schneekloth, 1987; Seidel, 1985; and Sommer, 1997). Although each approach has a relatively unique identity, the boundaries clearly overlap.

The aim of Table 13.1 is twofold: (a) to illustrate research application strategies and (b) to provide a profile of what we judge to be significant examples of research application since 1990. The pattern of dense and void cells in Table 13.2 reflects what we believe to be the current state of the art.

As represented in the table, most of the application efforts are at the scale of the building and interior environment. As noted previously, this likely reflects the intertwined traditions of research focusing on the building scale and using the individual as the unit of analysis. As we work toward more broadly based application efforts, it seems useful to consider some possible reasons for this incomplete record.

In terms of limited research application across all of environmental gerontology, the most significant factor is the epistemological differences between traditional positivism and the more recent philosophical positions. The positivist position stated clearly by Fishman (1999, p. 1) is that "the search for general theory precedes application." This institutionalized separation has yielded frustration and limitations in conceptual validity. It has also made feedback from practitioners to researchers more problematic (cf., Schneekloth, 1987).

A second contributing factor may be the focus in much of environmental gerontology on psycho-social processes. It was asserted some years ago by Lawton, Windley, and Byerts (1982) that the "most relevant approach" to the creation of theory in environmental gerontology was in terms of such processes as environmental perception and cognition, communication, or territoriality. Associated with the traditional focus of psycho-social processes has been a reliance on the individual as the primary unit of analysis. Although research at the level of the individual is readily applicable at the building scale, finding linkages to the neighborhood and community scales is often more problematic. Approaches rooted in place by contrast are gauged by Lawton et al. (1982) to be only "moderately strong." However, in the intervening years, a number of researchers in environmental gerontology and environmental psychology (Weisman et al., 2001; Wahl & Lang, 2003) have advocated a focus on place as fundamental to both theory and application. Such a place-based approach is congruent with and supportive of an action research perspective of the kind sketched out in the following section.

A Revised Action Research Paradigm

Given this array of factors mitigating against effective research application, we advocate—along with others who have grappled with this problem—for an expanded action research paradigm for environmental gerontology. Although the full development of such an expanded framework is beyond the scope of this chapter, it is possible to outline some of its defining characteristics.

First, research within an action research perspective must be problem focused. This creates an imperative for application. Often a first step in this process is what Lewin (1947) referred to as "unfreezing the situation"

(p. 330). For example, in the context of long-term care in the United States, this meant rethinking the form of nursing homes organizationally as well as architecturally. Care providers, regulators, designers, and users had to change their views of nursing homes: smaller in scale and less institutional in appearance and operation—in broad terms, more like home. To the extent that research has supported this change in perspective (e.g., Day et al., 2000), the momentum for change has been enhanced.

A second defining characteristic is that the planning, action, and fact-finding (evaluation) phases of action research be as participatory as possible. Some important questions in this regard are as follows: Is it possible to engage all relevant actors (care providers, patients, families, staff, and designers) in the formulation of the problem to be solved and in the process of studying that problem? Is it possible to take a systemic approach to the problem at hand? Can the problem be embedded in an integrative place-based conceptualization such as the Social-Physical Places Over Time (SPOT) model developed by Wahl and Lang (2004)?

> . . . [P]laces necessarily combine both a physical-spatial as well as a social-cultural dimension . . . . We should always think of places as socially constructed, socially filled-out, and socially shaped physical environments. (Wahl & Lang, 2004)

Finally, an action research perspective must involve education and training. Substantial literature has been written on reforming teaching in both the social sciences and the environmental planning/design professions to bring it into greater congruence with an action research perspective. In a recent critique of the design professions, Boyer and Mitgang (1996) called for designers and planners to dedicate themselves to "building for human needs." This mandate is the consequence of the design professions' long-standing and deeply engrained preoccupation with architecture as form-making, often at the expense of meeting human needs. We believe that refocusing the design professions' mission on human needs within an action research perspective will require comprehensive and sustained efforts over an extended period of time to educate both researchers and practitioners. We now discuss three specific initiatives that can be undertaken to fulfill this important education objective of action research.

The Design Studio

The design studio, the teaching vehicle of choice in environmental design education, should adopt real design problems involving real clients. This requires a knowledge-based approach to design. Two attempts to encourage this approach in environmental gerontology were carried out by the Gerontological Society of America's Housing and Environment Project

(1975) and the AIA/Association of Collegiate Schools of Architecture (ACSA) Council on Architectural Research's Design for Aging Curriculum Project (1995). The aim of these projects was to encourage design schools to devote a studio project each year to designing a facility for older people within an environment and behavior perspective. These projects were immediately effective in accomplishing this objective and have had some lingering influence in many participating schools of architecture. From these projects, we learned that students involved in knowledge-based design with real projects and clients are more adept at dealing with research information, developing design solutions from conceptual frameworks found within environmental gerontology, and participating in designer-client collaboration—an important component of action research.

Research Methods

Design students should learn methods of evaluating and using existing research information, as well as generating new information. This requires an understanding of different research paradigms and their corresponding methodologies and how they can be applied to various design problems and user groups. A recent book by Groat and Wang (2002) identified different systems of inquiry and research strategies specifically applicable to architects and planners. In complementary fashion, Lawton and Herzog (1989) reviewed various research methods particularly useful for gerontology. Perhaps the most useful research methods for designers are those predominately used in the action research perspective, such as case studies, large group processes (Martin, 2001), and focus groups (Morgan, 1988). Techniques such as causal modeling (Asher, 1983; Evans & Lepore, 1997) and simulation (Clipson, 1993) can make both heuristic and analytical contributions to action research. Understanding these techniques helps students develop objectives for buildings based on human needs in collaboration with participants, and it promotes the concept of design hypotheses testable through a post-occupancy evaluation.

Researcher and Practitioner Education

It is important to educate both researchers and practitioners in the tradition of action research. Action research requires a collaborative relationship between researchers and practitioners. Many universities are reluctant partners in this collaboration, as noted by Schon (1983) who argues that "institutions are committed, for the most part, to a particular epistemology, a view of knowledge that fosters selective inattention to practical competence and professional artistry" (Schon, 1983, p. viii). However, some land-grant universities are an exception to this prevailing view, where they have a mandate to transfer knowledge that helps citizens in their respective states to solve practical problems. The land-grant philosophy is consistent with Brulin's (2001) position that progress in information transfer is "rather a matter of changing forms for knowledge formation than finding the 'very right theoretical' foundation" (Brulin, 2001, p. 440).

So what can we learn from the land grant philosophy that will facilitate a collaboration between the researcher and practitioner? Some academics now stress the need to develop joint ventures between researchers and consumers if research findings are to have any practical use (cf. Gibbons, Limoges, Nowotony, Schwartzmann, Scott, & Trow, 1994; and Brulin, 2001). "Researchers have to form knowledge in interactive relationships with practitioners. Research cannot aspire to solve problems *for* the practitioners but has to work *with* the practitioners" (Brulin, 2001, p. 441). This requires that researchers must enter into a continuous dialogue with potential stakeholders if successful collaborations and mutual education are to occur. In this regard, van Beinum (1998) stated the following:

> We sometimes tend to emphasize the importance of the dialogue with regard to the beginning of a project and underplay the fact that the "dialogue" is an ongoing condition, the "glue," the foundation of any action-oriented and developmental approach, irrespective of whether the focus is on the individual organization, networks, regional development or programmatic strategies. (van Beinum, 1998, p. 13)

We propose that the model employed by the Cooperative Extension Service at land grant universities would be helpful in furthering educational objectives in action research. Researcher and practitioner education in environmental gerontology would benefit greatly from a key feature of this model—the collaborative dialogue. A review of collaborative problem-solving between researchers and practitioners in enhancing everyday competence among older persons is provided in Diehl and Willis's (2004) chapter. In addition to the collaborative dialogue between researchers and practitioners, this same dialogue should take place among researchers, practitioners, and students.

CONCLUSIONS

In this chapter, we have attempted to make the case that new ways of thinking about research application in environmental gerontology are imperative if significant improvement in the quality of the physical environment is to be achieved. Most research application in environmental gerontology to date falls within the trickle-down and communication/dissemination approaches, with only limited examples available at the more active end of the continuum. A modified action research approach was suggested as a means to more effectively bridge research and practice in environmental gerontology. This approach requires changes in the way designers, planners, and researchers are educated. Perhaps future reviews of environmental gerontology will fill more of the cells toward the active end of the continuum described in Table 13.2, and the objective Lewin (1947) envisioned for an applied social and environmental science will be realized.

REFERENCES

Alexander, C., Ishikawa, S., & Silverstein, M. (1977). *A pattern language*. New York: Oxford University Press.

American Institute of Architects Foundation. (1985). *Design for aging: An architect's guide*. Washington, DC: American Institute of Architects Press.

American Institute of Architects/Association of Collegiate Schools of Architecture Council on Architectural Research. (1995). *Design for aging curriculum*. Washington, DC: American Institute of Architects and the Association of Collegiate Schools of Architecture.

American Association of Retired Persons (AARP). (1996). *Understanding senior housing into the next century: Survey of consumer preferences, concerns, and needs*. Washington, DC: American Association of Retired Persons.

Archea, J., & Margulis, S. (1979). Environmental research inputs to policy and design programs. In T. Byerts, S. Howell, & L. Pastalan (Eds.), *The environmental context of aging* (pp. 217-228). New York: Garland STPM Press.

Asher, H. (1983). *Causal modeling*. Beverly Hills, CA: Sage Publications.

Barkley, D., Mark, S., & Henry, D. (2000). Local economic and fiscal impacts of a planned retirement community. In P. Schaeffer and S. Loveridge (Eds.), *Case studies in small town and rural economic development* (pp. 69-80). Westport, CT: Praeger Press.

Beal, C., & Johnson, K. (1998). The identification of recreational counties in nonmetropolitan areas of the USA. *Population Research and Policy Review, 17*, 37-53.

Boyer, E. (1990). *Scholarship reconsidered: Priorities of the professoriate*. Princeton, NJ: The Carnegie Foundation for the Advancement of Teaching.

Boyer, E., & Mitgang, L. (1996). *Building community: A new future for architectural education and practice*. Princeton, NJ: The Carnegie Foundation for the Advancement of Teaching.

Brulin, G. (2001). The third task of universities or how to get universities to serve their communities. In P. Reason & H. Bradbury (Eds.), *Handbook of action research: Participative inquiry and practice* (pp. 440-445). Newbury Park, CA: Sage.

Brummett, W. (1997). *The essence of home: Design solutions for assisted living*. New York: Van Nostrand Reinhold.

Calkins, M. (1988). *Design for dementia: Planning environments for the elderly and confused*. Owings Mills, MD: National Health Publishing.

Calthorpe, P. (1993). *The next American metropolis: Ecology, community, and the American dream*. New York: Princeton Architectural Press.

Carp, F. (1986). Neighborhood quality perception and measurement. In R. Newcomer, M. P. Lawton, & T. Byerts (Eds.), *Housing an aging society: Issues, alternatives, and policy* (pp. 127-140). New York: Van Nostrand Reinhold.

Carp, F. (1987). The impact of planned housing: A longitudinal study. In V. Regnier & J. Pynoos (Eds.), *Housing the aged: Design directives and policy considerations* (pp. 43-79). New York: Elsevier.

Carp, F. (1994). Assessing the environment. In M. P. Lawton & J. Teresi (Eds.), *Annual review of gerontology and geriatrics* (Vol. 14, pp. 324-352). New York: Springer.

Carstens, D. (1993). *Site planning and design for the elderly: Issues, guidelines, and alternatives.* New York: Van Nostrand Reinhold.

Chambliss, B. (1989). *Creating assisted living housing.* Denver, CO: Colorado Association of Homes and Services for the Aging.

Clipson, C. (1993). Simulation for planning and design. In R. Marans & D. Stokals (Eds.), *Environmental simulation* (pp. 42-45). New York: Plenum Press.

Cohen, U., & Weisman, G. (1991). *Holding on to home: Designing environments for people with dementia.* Baltimore, MD: Johns Hopkins University Press.

Cohen, U., Weisman, G., Ray, K., Steiner, V., Rand, J., & Toyne, R. (1988). *Environments for people with dementia: Design guide.* The Health Facilities Research Program, Washington, DC: American Institute of Architects/ Association of Collegiate Schools of Architecture Council on Architectural Research.

Coons, D. (1991). A model of residential living. In D. Coons (Ed.), *Specialized dementia care units* (pp. 36-54). Baltimore, MD: Johns Hopkins University Press.

Cooper-Marcus, C., & Barnes, M. (Eds.). (1999). *Healing gardens: Therapeutic benefits and design recommendations.* New York: John Wiley & Sons.

Cranz, G. (1987). Evaluating the physical environment. In V. Regnier & J. Pynoos (Eds.), *Housing the aged: Design directives and policy considerations* (pp. 81-104). New York: Elsevier.

Day, K., & Calkins, M. (2002). Design and dementia. In R. Bechtel & A. Churchman (Eds.), *Handbook of environmental psychology* (pp. 374-393). New York: John Wiley and Sons.

Day, K., Carreon, D., & Stump, C. (2000). The therapeutic design of environments for dementia: A review of the empirical research. *The Gerontologist, 40*(4), 397-416.

Diaz Moore, K., Geboy, L., & Weisman, G. (2002). *Designing a better day: Planning and design guidelines for adult and dementia day care.* Milwaukee, WI: Center for Architecture and Urban Planning Research, University of Wisconsin-Milwaukee.

Diehl, M., & Willis, S. (2003). Everyday competence and everyday problem solving in aging adults: The role of physical and social context. In H. W. Wahl, R. Scheidt, & P. Windley (Eds.), *Annual review of gerontology and geriatrics.* New York: Springer.

Evans, G., & Lepore, S. (1997). Moderating and mediating processes in environment-behavior research. In G. Moore & R. Marans (Eds.), *Advances in environment, behavior, and design: Toward the integration of theory, methods, research, and utilization* (Vol. 4, pp. 255-285). New York: Plenum Press.

Fishman, D. (1999). *The case for pragmatic psychology*. New York: New York University Press.

French, J., Cobb, S., & Rogers, W. (1974). A model of person-environment fit. In G. Coelho, D. Hamburg, & J. Adams (Eds.), *Coping and adaptation* (pp. 316-333). New York: Basic Books.

Friedman, V. (2001). Action science: Creating communities of inquiry in communities of practice. In P. Reason & H. Bradbury (Eds.), *Handbook of action research: Participative inquiry and practice* (pp. 159-170). Newbury Park, CA: Sage.

Fuguitt, G. V., Brown, D. L., & Beale, C. L. (1989). *Rural and small town America*. New York: Russell Sage Foundation.

Gerontological Society of America. (1975). *Housing and environment project*. A special report to the Administration on Aging, U.S. Department of Health, Education, and Welfare (HEW).

Gibbons, M., Limoges, C., Nowotony, H., Schwartsmann, S., Scott, P., & Trow, M. (1994). *The new production of knowledge: The dynamics of science and research in contemporary societies*. London: Sage Publications.

Gitlin, L. (2000). Adjusting "person-environment systems:" Helping older people live the "good life" at home. In R. Rubinstein, M. Moss, & M. Kleban (Eds.), *The many dimensions of aging: Essays in honor of M. Powell Lawton* (pp. 41-54). New York: Springer.

Glasgow, N. L. (1990). Attracting retirees as a community development option. *Journal of the Community Development Society, 21*(1), 103-114.

Groat, L., and Wang, D. (2002). *Architectural research methods*. New York: John Wiley and Sons.

Hartman, C., Horovitz, J., & Herman, R. (1987). Involving older persons in designing housing for the elderly. In V. Regnier & J. Pynoos (Eds.), *Housing the aged: Design directives and policy considerations* (pp. 153-176). New York: Elsevier.

Hunt, M., Merrill, & Gilker. (1994). Naturally occurring retirement communities in urban and rural settings. In E. Folts & D. Yeatts (1994), *Housing and the aging population: Options for the new century* (pp. 107-120). New York: Garland Publishing.

Hunt, M., & Ross, L. (1990). Naturally occurring retirement communities: A multiattribute examination of desirability factors. *The Gerontologist, 30*(5), 667-674.

Kahana, E. (1982). A congruence model of person-environment transaction. In M. P. Lawton, P. G. Windley, & T. O. Byerts (Eds.), *Aging and the environment: Theoretical approaches* (pp. 97-121). New York: Springer.

Koncelik, J. (1976). *Designing the open nursing home*. Stroudsburg, PA: Dowden, Hutchinson, & Ross.

Kovack, C., Weisman, G., Chaudhury, H., & Calkins, M. (1997). Impacts of a therapeutic environment for dementia care. *American Journal of Alzheimer's Disease, 12*, 99-116.

Krause, N. (2003). Neighborhoods, health, and well-being in late life. In H. W. Wahl, R. Scheidt, & P. Windley (Eds.), *Annual review of gerontology and geriatrics*. New York: Springer.

Lawton, M., Fulcomer, M., & Kleban, M. (1984). Architecture for the mentally impaired. *Environment and Behavior, 16*(6), 730-757.

Lawton, M., Windley, P., & Byerts, T. (1982). *Aging and environment: Theoretical approaches*. New York: Springer.

Lawton, M. P. (1975). *Planning and managing housing for the elderly*. New York: John Wiley and Sons.

Lawton, M. P., Greenbaum, M., & Liebowitz, B. (1980). The lifespan of housing environments for the aging. *The Gerontologist, 20*(1), 56-64.

Lawton, M. P., & Herzog, A. (Eds.). (1989). *Special research methods for gerontology*. New York: Baywood.

Lawton, M. P. & Hoover, S. (Eds.). (1981). *Community housing choices for older Americans*. New York: Springer.

Lawton, M. P., & Nahemow, L. (1973). Ecology and the aging process. In C. Eisdorfer & M. P. Lawton (Eds.), *Psychology of adult development and aging* (pp. 619-674). Washington, DC: American Psychological Association.

Lewin, K. (1946). Action research and minority problems. *Journal of Social Issues, 1*, 34-46.

Lewin, K. (1947). Frontiers in group dynamics, *Human Relations, 1*, 2-38. Reprinted in G. W. Levin, *Resolving social conflict and field theory in social science*. Washington, DC: American Psychological Association.

Liang, J., Sengstock, M., & Hwalek, M. (1986). Environment and criminal victimization of the aged. In R. J. Newcomer, M. P. Lawton, & T. Byerts (Eds.), *Housing an aging society: Issues, alternatives, and policy* (pp. 141-150). New York: Van Nostrand Reinhold.

Longino, C. (2003). Socio-physical environments at the macro level: The impact of population migration. In H. W. Wahl, R. Scheidt, & P. Windley (Eds.), *Annual review of gerontology and geriatrics*. New York: Springer.

Marans, R., Hunt, M., & Vakalo, K. (1984). Retirement communities. In I. Altman, M. P. Lawton, & J. Wohlwill (Eds.), *Elderly people and the environment* (pp. 57-93). New York: Plenum.

Marshall, L., & Hunt, M. (1999). Rural naturally occurring retirement communities: A community assessment procedure. *Journal of Housing for the Elderly, 13*(1/2), 19-34.

Martin, A. (2001). Large group processes as action research. In P. Reason & H. Bradbury (Eds.), *Handbook of action research: Participative inquiry and practice* (pp. 200-208). Newbury Park, CA: Sage Publications.

Milke, D. (1996). *McConnell Place North post-occupancy evaluation*. Edmonton, Alberta, Canada: Capital Care Group.

Mollenkopf, H., & Fozard, J. (2003). (Title is under possible revision for the present volume).

Moore, G., Tuttle, D., & Howell, S. (1985). *Environmental design research directions*. New York: Praeger.

Moos, R., Lemke, S., & David, T. (1987). Priorities for design and management in residential settings for the elderly. In V. Regnier & J. Pynoos (Eds.), *Housing the aged: Design directives and policy considerations* (pp. 179-206). New York: Elsevier Press.

Morgan, D. (1988). *Focus groups as qualitative research*. Beverly Hills, CA: Sage Publications.

Namazi, K., Whitehouse, P., Rechlin, L., Calkins, M., Brabender, B., & Hevener, S. (1991). Environmental modifications in a specially designed unit for the care of patients with Alzheimer's disease. *American Journal of Alzheimer's Care and Related Disorders, 6*, 3-9.

Norris-Baker, L., Weisman, G., Lawton, M. P., Sloane, P., & Kaup, M. (1999). Assessing special care units for dementia. In E. Steinfeld & G. S. Danford (Eds.), *Enabling environments: Measuring the impact of environment on disability and rehabilitation* (pp. 165-181). New York: Kluwer Academic/Plenum Publishers.

Parmalee, P., and Lawton, M. P. (1990). The design of special environments for the aged. In J. Birren & W. Schaie (Eds.), *Handbook of the psychology of aging* (pp. 464-488). San Diego, CA: Academic Press.

Pastalan, L. (Ed.). (1991). Optimizing housing for the elderly: Homes not houses. *Journal of Housing for the Elderly, 7*(1, Special Issue).

Polkinghorn, D. (1992). Post-modern epistemology of practice. In S. Kvale (Ed.), *Psychology and post modernism* (pp. 146-165). Newbury Park, CA: Sage.

Pynoos, J., Cohen, E., Davis, L., & Bernhardt, S. (1987). In V. Regnier & J. Pynoos (Eds.), *Housing the aged: Design directives and policy considerations* (pp. 91-117). New York: Elsevier Press.

Pynoos, J., Nishita, C., & Perelman, L. (2003). Advances in the home modification field: A tribute to M. Powell Lawton. In R. Scheidt & P. Windley (Eds.), Physical environments and aging: Critical contributions of M. Powell Lawton to theory and practice. *Journal of Housing for the Elderly, 17*(1-2, Special Issue), 105-116.

Pynoos, J., & Regnier, V. (1991). Improving residential environments for frail elderly: Bridging the gap between theory and application. In J. Birren, J. Lubben, J. Rowe, & D. Deitchman (Eds.), *The concept and measurement of quality of life in the frail elderly* (pp. 91-117). San Diego, CA: Academic Press.

Pynoos, J., Tabbarah, M., Angelelli, J., & Demiere, M. (1998). Improving the delivery of home modifications. *Technology and Disability, 8*, 3-14.

Regnier, V. (1976). Neighborhoods as service systems. In M. P. Lawton, R. J. Newcomer, and T. O. Byerts (Eds.), *Community planning for an aging society* (pp. 240-257). Stroudsburg, PA: Dowden, Hutchinson, & Ross.

Regnier, V. (2002). *Design for assisted living.* New York: John Wiley & Sons.

Regnier, V., & Hamburger, J. (1978). *Comparison of perceived and objective crime against the elderly in an urban neighborhood.* Paper presented at the 31st Annual Meeting of the Gerontological Society, Dallas, Texas.

Regnier, V., & Pynoos, J. (Eds.). (1987). *Housing the aged: Design directives and policy considerations.* New York: Elsevier Press.

Sanford, N. (1970). Whatever happened to action research? *Journal of Social Issues, 26*, 3-23.

Scheidt, R., & Windley, P. (Eds.). (1998). *Environment and aging theory: A focus on housing.* Westport, CT: Greenwood Press.

Schneekloth, L. (1987). Advances in practice in environment, behavior, and design. In E. Zube & G. Moore (Eds.), *Advances in environment, behavior, and design* (Vol. 1, pp. 307-334). New York: Plenum Press.

Schon, D. (1983). *The reflective practitioner. How professionals think in action.* New York: Basic Books.

Schwarz, B. (1997). Nursing home design: A misguided architectural model. *Journal of Architectural and Planning Research, 14*(4), 343-359.

Seidel, A. (1985). What is success in E&B research utilization? *Environment and Behavior, 17*(1), 47-70.

Senge, P., & Scharmer, O. (2001). Community action research: Learning as a community of practitioners, consultants, and researchers. In P. Reason & H. Bradbury (Eds.), *Handbook of action research: Participative inquiry and practice* (pp. 238-249). Newbury, CA: Sage Publications.

Silverman, M., Ricci, R., Saxton, J., Ledowitz, S., McAllister, C., & Keane, C. (1995). *Woodside Place: The first three years of a residential Alzheimer's facility.* Pittsburgh, PA: Presbyterian Senior Care.

Sommer, R. (1997). Utilization issues in environment-behavior research. In G. Moore & R. Marans (Eds.), *Advances in environment, behavior, and design: Toward the integration of theory, methods, research, and utilization* (Vol. 4, pp. 347-368). New York: Plenum Press.

Steinfeld, E. (1987). Adapting housing for older disabled people. In V. Regnier & J. Pynoos (Eds.), *Housing the aged: Design directives and policy considerations* (pp. 307-340). New York: Elsevier.

Susman, G., and Evered, R. (1978). An assessment of the scientific merits of action research. *Administrative Quarterly, 23,* 582-603.

Tilson, D. (Ed.). (1990). *Aging in place: Supporting the frail elderly in residential environments.* Glenview, IL: Scott Foresman and Company.

van Beinum, H. (1998). On the practice of action research. *Concepts and transformations, 3*(12) 1-29.

Wahl, H. W., & Lang, F. (2003). Aging in context across the adult life course: Integrating physical and social environmental research perspectives. In H. W. Wahl, R. Scheidt, & P. Windley (Eds.), *Annual review of gerontology and geriatrics.* New York: Springer.

Wahl, H. W., & Weisman, G. (in press). Environmental gerontology at the beginning of the new millennium: Major achievements and some concerns. *The Gerontologist.*

Weisman, G. (1983). Environmental programming and action research. *Environment and Behavior, 15*(3), 381-408.

Weisman, G. (1997). Environments for older persons with cognitive impairments. In G. Moore & R. Marans (Eds.), *Advances in environment, behavior, and design* (Vol. 4, 315-346). New York: Plenum.

Weisman, G. (2001). The place of people in architectural design. In A. Pressman (Ed.), *The architect's portable design handbook: A guide to best practice* (pp. 158-170). New York: McGraw-Hill.

Weisman, G. (in press). Creating places for people with dementia: An action research perspective. In K. W. Schaie, H. W. Wahl, M. Mollenkopf, and F. Oswald (Eds.), *Aging in the community: Living arrangements and mobility.* New York: Springer.

Weisman, G., Chaudhury, H., & Diaz Moore, K. (2001). Theory and practice of place: Toward an integrative model. In R. Rubinstien, M. Moss, & M. Kleban (Eds.), *The many dimensions of aging* (pp. 3-21). New York: Springer.

Weiss, C., & Bucuvalas, M. (1980). *Social science research and decision-making.* New York: Columbia University Press.

Welch, P., Parker, V., & Zeisel, J. (1984). *Independence through interdependence: Congregate living for older people.* Boston, MA: Department of Elder Affairs, Commonwealth of Massachusetts.

Windley, P., and Weisman, G. (1977). Social science and environmental design: The translation process. *Journal of Architectural Education, 31*(1), 16-19.

Wisner, B., Stea, D., & Kruks, S. (1997). Participatory and action research methods. In E. Zube & G. Moore (Eds.), *Advances in environment, behavior, and design* (Vol. 4, pp. 271-295). New York: Plenum.

Zeisel, J., Epp, G., & Demos, S. (1977). *Low-rise housing for older people.* U.S. Department of Housing and Urban Development, Office of Policy Development and Research.

Zeisel, J., Welch, P., Epp, G., & Demos, S. (1983). *Midrise elevator housing for older people: Behavioral criteria for design.* U.S. Department of Housing and Urban Development, Office of Policy Development and Research.

INDEX

Note: Boldface numbers indicate illustrations and tables.

Association of Collegiate Schools for
   Architecture (ACSA), 357
avunculocal descent, **316**

Baby Boom generation, population
   migration and, 123–124
Baltes, Margaret, 2, 10, 16, 26
Barker, Roger, 10, 42–43
barometric functions, in general
   ecological model (Lawton), 47–49
barriers to accessibility, 97
basic level of (BaCo) competence, 133
Basic Skills Assessment Test, 145
Beales or Rural-Urban Continuum
   code categories, in urban vs. rural
   populations, 281
behavior setting, 74
beta press, 40, 51
   ecological theory of aging (ETA), 67
Big Five personality factors, 148–149
bilateral descent kinship, in family
   caregiving, 317, **316**, 318–321, **320**,
   322–325, 326–327, 329
bilocal descent, **316**
bodily changes, illness (*See also* health
   status), self, ecology and aging in,
   72–73
bottom-up approach, general
   ecological model (Lawton) and, 43
building design for elderly and
   gerontology research, 351–352
built environment, in self, ecology and
   aging, 74–75
Burmedi, David, 195

California, population migration and,
   110–128
Canadian Model of Occupational
   Performance (CMOP), accessibility
   and, 91, 102
caregiving (*See* kinship and supportive
   environments of aging)
Carstensen, Laura, 15
census data, population migration
   and, 111
Center for Group Dynamics, 341
challenge zone, general ecological
   model (Lawton) and, 36, 67–68

change (*See also* adaptation; relocation)
   general ecological model (Lawton)
   and, 50–52, 54
   interior living environments and,
   168, 176, 185
   residential satisfaction and, 198–199
   technology and, acceptance of,
   262–264
classes of environment, general
   ecological model (Lawton) and,
   40–44
classic approaches aging theories,
   12–14
cognitive abilities (mental health)
   collaborative cognition and, 150–152
   competence and problem solving,
   146–148
   environmental complexity and,
   147–148
   Everyday Cognition Battery (ECB)
   in, 152
   interior living environments and,
   172–173
   person–environment fit and, 147
   Seattle Longitudinal Study and,
   146–147
   technology and, 261–262
   urban vs. rural populations, 294–295
collaboration, in research and practice
   of environmental gerontology, 336
collaborative cognition, 150–152
comfort zone, general ecological model
   (Lawton) and, 36, 67–68
communication
   information and communication
   technology (ICT) and, 251,
   253–254, 259, 261, 264
   research and practice in
   environmental gerontology
   and, 335
   Telematics for the Integration of
   Disabled and Older People in
   Europe (TIDE) program and, 253
community (*See* neighborhood
   satisfaction)
community application of gerontology
   research, 343–348